Congenital Vascular Malformations

Young-Wook Kim • Byung-Boong Lee
Wayne F. Yakes • Young-Soo Do
Editors

Congenital Vascular Malformations

A Comprehensive Review of Current Management

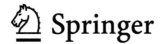

Editors
Young-Wook Kim
Division of Vascular Surgery
Department of Surgery
Samsung Medical Center
Seoul
South Korea

Byung-Boong Lee
Professor of Surgery and Director
Center for the Lymphedema and
  Vascular Malformations
George Washington University
Washington, DC
USA

Adjunct Professor of Surgery
Uniformed Services
University of the Health Sciences
Bethesda, MD
USA

Wayne F. Yakes
Swedish Medical Center
Vascular malformation Center
Englewood
Colorado
USA

Young-Soo Do
Department of Radiology
Samsung Medical Center
Seoul
South Korea

ISBN 978-3-662-46708-4   ISBN 978-3-662-46709-1   (eBook)
DOI 10.1007/978-3-662-46709-1

Library of Congress Control Number: 2017945379

Printed on acid-free paper

This Springer imprint is published by Springer Nature
The registered company is Springer-Verlag GmbH Germany
The registered company address is: Heidelberger Platz 3, 14197 Berlin, Germany

Foreword

It is with genuine pleasure that I write this Foreword for a book whose material has been painstakingly studied, treated, and collected during several decades by a multidisciplinary cadre of dedicated physicians deeply interested in a discipline that has not been the favorite among our colleagues in the medical field.

As I have written elsewhere[1], "our three vascular systems, arterial, venous and lymphatic, form a complex seamless network of miles of intricate vessels with specific vital physiologic functions. They intertwine, twist and cross in different directions continuously moving large volumes of blood and lymph. These systems are critically important for our normal life. By the miracle of nature, they are automatically separated from each other at birth. However, due to still obscure genetic derangement, distorted errors of nature result in vascular anomalies. After birth, these systems may maintain their fetal characteristics and produce either diffuse or circumscribed clusters of vessels where arteries and veins are still connected mixing arterial with venous blood (arteriovenous shunts) or mixed venous and lymphatic vessels as occurs in cases of malformations of veno-lymphatic predominance such as in the syndrome of Klippel-Trenaunay."

Since their initial description, congenital vascular malformations have been a difficult and complicated sector of the vascular system. They have always been a classification, diagnostic, and therapeutic challenge, and therein lies the reason for their mysterious and captivating attraction to a group of masochistic physicians who love the challenge of a bizarre, malformed limb or a disfiguring craniofacial malformation. It is not necessary for me to delve deeply into the reasons that have rekindled the interest in the field of vascular anomalies to recognize that the diagnosis and management of this large group of diseases has had a monumental impulse with the radiological, endovascular, and genetic revolutions.

In the year 1996, I received an invitation from Professor B.B. Lee, a coeditor of this book and at that time chairman of the Department of Surgery at Samsung Medical Center in Seoul South Korea, to visit his Department. During the week that I spent with Dr. Lee's team, I made daily rounds seeing patients with an array of vascular malformations and observing some

---

[1] Villavicencio JL. Classification of peripheral arteriovenous and venous malformations. A review. In: Stanley J, Veith JF, Wakefield TW editors. Therapy in vascular and endovascular surgery 5th ed. Elsevier Saunders, Philadelphia; 2014. p 829–30.

challenging cases being thoroughly investigated and treated using ethanol and other therapeutic modalities. I was witnessing the birth of an outstanding multidisciplinary group of physicians interested in tackling the challenging group of anomalies of the vascular system. Throughout the years, this group has become one of the leading centers in the world for the study, investigation, and management of congenital vascular malformations. I had the opportunity to verify my previous statement during a second visit in 2004. I met then Professor Young-Wook Kim and most of the coauthors of this book. Dr. Lee had surrounded himself by a group of several prestigious investigators such as the late Dr. John Bergan, Corinne Becker, Dirk Loose, Wayne Yakes, and Raul Mattassi, just to mention a few. Through visits to Seoul and conferences with his team, these experts contributed to cement the basis for the creation of a first-class center for the study and care of patients with congenital vascular malformations. This book is the proud child of those efforts. It is rewarding indeed to notice the renovated interest that this subject has had in recent years with its inclusion in excellent international symposiums dedicated to congenital vascular anomalies in the most important congresses of the world.

The authors of this book ought to be commended for their effort. I am sure that this book will find a warm welcome among many of our puzzled colleagues facing a child with a monstrous vascular malformation and will guide and assist them in finding the best possible tactic to assist their patient. Behind its pages, as a solid shield, lays the experience and expertise of the collaborators who are compassionate experts who have experienced the great satisfaction of seeing again the smile of an afflicted patient.

Washington DC, USA   J. Leonel Villavicencio, MD, FACS

Preface

It has been a long way since we dared to challenge the enigma of modern medicine, especially in congenital vascular malformations (CVMs). Indeed, it took over 20 years for us to master these ever-confusing vascular birth defects, starting from scratch like a blind man feeling an elephant.

Taking the advantage of unconditional support by the newly founded institute Samsung Medical Center, we were able to organize a dream team including so many world experts of multispecialty we invited from the four corners of the world as critical consultants and became a world leading group within a decade.

Finally, based on extraordinary experiences we accumulated through the last two decades with nearly 3000 patients, we were able to organize *Handbook of Congenital Vascular Malformation* with so many collaborators to share this hard-earned dividend with the rest of our colleagues who were not as fortunate as we were.

Indeed, CVMs are still the most confusing type of vascular disorder showing thousands of different faces due to their nature as vascular embryonal developmental anomalies. These anomalies as the outcome of developmental arrest from various stages of embryogenesis affect all three circulation systems so that they present an extreme variety of clinical manifestations in arteries, veins, lymphatics, and/or cutaneous/capillary vasculature throughout the body in various combinations.

Therefore, the CVM patients would present not only the primary lesion, either as an independent or mixed/combined condition, but also the secondary complications and morbidity caused by the primary lesion.

CVM is often found scattered throughout the body in varying extent and severity with varying symptoms and signs and become clinically detectable in various ages throughout life. Therefore, these CVM patients with extreme age distribution from infant to old age with garden-variety complaints would wind up seeking for help from a vast array of clinicians/specialties such as vascular surgery, orthopedic surgery, and plastic surgery, as well as pediatrics and other specialties. Hence, CVMs remain an enigma, difficult to define including the specialty dealing with this unique disease process.

In the past, before modern contemporary concept was established, even for those who became interested in CVMs, it was virtually impossible to comprehend all of the different forms of malformations. Definition and classification of the CVMs then were based only on singular if not sporadic anecdotal experiences at best so that the nature of these unique developmental defects was scantly understood and studied/documented purely based on the clinical findings alone.

It must have been as if observing a subject through a small buttonhole without realizing the whole subject. But through the last three decades in particular, the old concept of the CVMs established on name-based eponyms has been successfully replaced with contemporary concept with new definition and classification based on current advanced diagnostic and therapeutic technology.

Through these trials and tribulations, the current understanding of CVM has grown by leaps and bounds for the last two decades and continues to accelerate at a blinding rate. Mandated research in this unique field has grown exponentially to include understanding of the development of fetal vascular systems using animal research protocols as well as understanding of CVM pathogenesis at molecular or submolecular levels through human embryology research.

Nevertheless, therapeutic modalities of CVM have been far from being satisfactory. The surgical/excisional treatment with chance of cure is extremely limited by significantly high recurrence rates due to their nature. The outcome of deep-seated infiltrating lesion in particular is still far from satisfactory despite the variety of endovascular sclerotherapies or embolotherapies.

Some of the leading sclerosing agents, for example, have such restrictions and limitations with many serious side effects including systemic toxicity and extravasation causing further perivascular tissue damage.

In light of current difficulties in clinical practices associated with CVM, we invited world-renowned CVM specialists throughout the international community for each carefully selected topic/issue to share their experiences and elucidate the current state of understanding in CVM classification, pathogenesis, clinical features, diagnostic approaches, treatment of the lesions, and management of their complications.

Indeed, all our collaborator colleagues gave such generous donation of their time and knowledge unconditionally with no proper compensation; we are eternally grateful.

To conclude, we also would like to acknowledge and offer our heart-filled gratitude to those researchers and medical practitioners who have paved the way for continued enrichment of knowledge and understanding of the CVM. Furthermore, even with the shortcomings that we acknowledge associated with the treatment and understanding of this disease process, for those who entrust themselves to us for treatment, we would like to offer sincere gratitude to them as well.

Lastly, it is with our utmost desire that this book becomes a valuable source of understanding of this relatively uncommon vascular disorder, congenital vascular malformations, to those students as well as clinical practitioners who may have an interest in CVM.

Seoul, South Korea   Young-Wook Kim
Bethesda, MD, USA   Byung-Boong Lee
Seoul, South Korea   Young-Su Do
Englewood, CO, USA   Wayne Yakes

Contents

Part I Introduction

**1 Congenital Vascular Malformations:
An Historical Account**............................... 3
J. Leonel Villavicencio

**2 Embryological Background of Congenital Vascular
Malformations**.. 7
Hiroo Suami and Byung-Boong Lee

**Part II Pathogenesis of Congenital Vascular
Malformation (CVM)**

3 Angiogenesis and Vascular Malformations 17
Patricia E. Burrows

4 Genetic Aspects of Vascular Malformations................. 23
Francine Blei

**5 Epidemiologic Aspect of Congenital Vascular
Malformation**.. 31
Young-Wook Kim and Byung-Boong Lee

**6 Provoking Factors for Aggravation of Congenital
Vascular Malformation**................................ 35
Francine Blei

Part III Classification and Definition/Nomenclature

7 General Overview..................................... 41
Byung-Boong Lee, James Laredo, and Richard Neville

8 ISSVA Classification of Vascular Anomalies 47
Francine Blei

9 Hamburg Classification: Vascular Malformation 51
Dirk A. Loose and Raul E. Mattassi

10   **Angiographic Classification: Arteriovenous
     Malformation and Venous Malformation**.................. 55
     Kwang Bo Park and Young Soo Do

11   **New Arteriographic Classification of AVM
     Based on the Yakes Classification System**.................. 63
     Wayne F. Yakes, Robert L. Vogelzang, Krasnodar Ivancev,
     and Alexis M. Yakes

**Part IV   Contemporary Diagnosis of CVM: Clinical Features
            and Evaluation**

12   **General Overview**...................................... 73
     James Laredo and Byung-Boong Lee

13   **Differential Diagnosis from Hemangioma**................. 77
     Francine Blei

14   **Venous Malformation of the Head and Neck
     and Extremities**.. 83
     Patricia E. Burrows

15   **Venous Malformation: Truncular Form**................... 91
     Young-Wook Kim and Raul Mattassi

16   **Hemolymphatic Malformation: Mixed Form Congenital
     Vascular Malformation**.................................. 97
     James Laredo and Byung-Boong Lee

17   **Arteriovenous Malformations (AVMs): Clinical Features
     and Evaluation**.. 105
     Young Soo Do, Young-Wook Kim, Byung-Boong Lee,
     and Wayne F. Yakes

18   **Lymphatic Malformation (LM) (Extratruncular):
     Lymphangioma**.. 113
     Jovan N. Markovic and Cynthia K. Shortell

19   **Truncular Lymphatic Malformation (LM):
     Primary Lymphedema**.................................... 121
     Ningfei Liu

20   **Clinical Features and Evaluation of Superficial
     & Deep Capillary Malformation (CM)**.................... 129
     Peter Berlien

Part V   Contemporary Diagnosis of CVM: Imaging Modalities

21   **Contemporary Diagnosis: Imaging Modalities – Overview**.... 141
     Jovan N. Markovic and Cynthia K. Shortell

22   **Contemporary Diagnosis: MRI and MRA**.................. 147
     Jovan N. Markovic and Cynthia K. Shortell

23 **Ultrasonography in the Diagnosis of Congenital
    Vascular Malformation**................................ 155
    Massimo Vaghi

24 **CT and CT Angiogram in the Diagnosis of Congenital
    Vascular Malformations**............................... 161
    Massimo Vaghi and Andrea Ianniello

25 **Radionuclide Scintigraphy for Congenital
    Vascular Malformations**............................... 165
    Joon Young Choi

26 **Indocyanine Green (ICG) Lymphography**.................. 173
    Takumi Yamamoto

27 **Microscopic Lymphangiography**........................ 179
    Claudio Allegra, Michelangelo Bartolo,
    and Anita Carlizza

28 **MR Lymphangiography**................................ 185
    Ningfei Liu

Part VI   Contemporary Management of CVM

29 **Management of Congenital Vascular
    Malformation: Overview** 195
    Young-Wook Kim, Young Soo Do, and Byung-Boong Lee

30 **Endovascular Treatment of Vascular Malformation:
    An Overview** 197
    Wayne F. Yakes, Alexis M. Yakes, Robert L. Vogelzang,
    and Krasnodar Ivancev

31 **Endovascular Treatment of Venous Malformation
    in the Head and Neck, Trunk, and Extremities** 211
    Patricia E. Burrows

32 **Endovascular Treatment of AVMs: Head and Neck** 223
    Wayne F. Yakes, Krasnodar Ivancev, Robert L. Vogelzang,
    and Alexis M. Yakes

33 **Endovascular Treatment of AVM: Trunk and Extremity** 233
    Young Soo Do and Kwang Bo Park

34 **Management of Lymphatic Malformations** 241
    Kurosh Parsi

35 **Complications of Endovascular Treatment
    of Peripheral Congenital Vascular Malformations** 257
    Kurosh Parsi and Young Soo Do

36 **Surgical Treatment of Low-Flow CVM** 269
    Raul Mattassi

37 **Surgical Treatment for High-Flow CVM** 275
    Dirk A. Loose

38 Combined Surgical and Endovascular Approaches 283
    Byung-Boong Lee, James Laredo, and Richard Neville

39 Management of Deep Vein Aplasia, Hypoplasia,
    and Lateral Marginal Vein 291
    Raul Mattassi

40 Surgical Treatments for Lymphedema 297
    Dong-Ik Kim and Je Hoon Park

41 Complex Decongestive Therapy of Primary
    Lymphedema 307
    Ji Hye Hwang

42 Laser Therapy of Superficial and Deep Capillary
    Malformation (CM): Principles of Laser Technology 315
    Peter Berlien

43 Conservative/Medical Treatment of CVM 323
    Iris Baumgartner and Byung-Boong Lee

Part VII Special Issue in the CVM Management

44 Multidisciplinary Team Approach for Patients
    with Congenital Vascular Malformation (CVM):
    Experience at Samsung Medical Center 331
    Young-Wook Kim, Young Soo Do, Dong Ik Kim,
    and Byung-Boong Lee

45 Congenital Vascular Bone Syndrome:
    Limb Length Discrepancy 335
    Young-Wook Kim and Raul Mattassi

46 Biological Approaches to the Aggressive CVM Lesion
    (Antiangiogenic Therapy) 343
    Patricia E. Burrows

47 Pelvic Arteriovenous Malformation (AVM) 349
    Young-Wook Kim, Young Soo Do, Dong-Ik Kim,
    and Byung-Boong Lee

48 Treatment Strategy on Chylolymphatic/
    Lymphatic Reflux 355
    Cristóbal Miguel Papendieck and Miguel Angel Amore

49 Treatment Strategy on Neonatal and Infant CVMs 363
    Cristóbal Miguel Papendicek and Miguel Angel Amore

50 Strategy in Pediatric Patients 369
    J.C. Lopez Gutierrez

Epilogue 375

Index 377

Part I

Introduction

Congenital Vascular Malformations: An Historical Account

J. Leonel Villavicencio

An Overview

Mild as well as severe vascular anomalies have been described in ancient documents by authors such as Hippocrates [1], Ambrose Pare [2], Galen [3], and others.

Some anomalies have been named after those who first described them, such as the Klippel-Trenaunay, Maffucci, Servelle, Martorell, and Parkes Weber syndromes. Others have been named after Greek or Roman mythological monstrosities. As we review the features and names of some of the congenital vascular anomalies heretofore described, we cannot avoid but to notice the striking relationship with creatures and myths of the Greek and Roman mythology. It is fascinating to review the Pantheon of Greek and Roman gods and realize that the monstrous aspect and names of some of the congenital vascular anomalies that we observe in our clinics were often inspired by mythological creatures.

The cirsoid aneurysm of the scalp, an arteriovenous malformation, resembles Medusa's head where the hair was replaced by a nest of snakes [4], and the caput medusae, a net of paraumbilical veins, is formed in patients with portal hypertension due to liver cirrhosis. The sirenomelia, a severe and often fatal congenital anomaly, received its name by its resemblance to the Sirens mythological creatures [5]. Let's review the reasons behind these names.

The Sirens were beautiful but dangerous creatures that lured the sailors with their beautiful voices to their doom, causing the ships to crash on the reefs near their island. They were the daughters of the river god Achelous while their mother may have been Terpsichore the music goddess. Although closely linked to marine environments, they were not considered sea deities. The Sirens were probably considered companions of Persephone, daughter of the goddess Demeter. The latter had given them wings in order to protect her daughter; however, after Persephone's abduction from Hades, Demeter cursed them. The Siren's song was a beautiful but sad melody eternally calling for Persephone's return.

The Argonauts encountered the Sirens but successfully evaded them; Orpheus who was on board, started playing his lyre so beautifully that his music completely drowned the Sirens' song. The tenth century Byzantine encyclopedia Suda says that from their chests up, Sirens had the form of sparrows, below, they were women, or alternatively, that they were little birds with women's faces (Fig. 1.1).

The Sirens of Greek mythology, are sometimes portrayed as fully aquatic and mermaid-like. The facts that in Spanish, French, Italian, and Portuguese the word for mermaid is respectively Sirena, Sirene, Syrena, Sereia, and that in Biology the Serenia comprises an order of fully aquatic mammals that include the manatee, adds to the confusion.

Sirenomelia, also known as mermaid syndrome, is a rare congenital malformation in

J.L. Villavicencio, MD, FACS
Distinguished Professor of Surgery,
The Norman M. Rich Department of Surgery,
Uniformed Services University of the Health
Sciences, Walter Reed National Military
Medical Center, Bethesda, MD, USA
e-mail: jvillavicencio@me.com;
j.villavicencio@usuhs.edu

© Springer-Verlag Berlin Heidelberg 2017
Y.-W. Kim et al. (eds.), *Congenital Vascular Malformations*, DOI 10.1007/978-3-662-46709-1_1

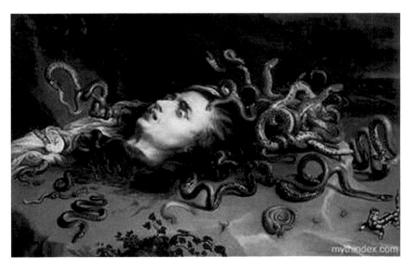

Fig. 1.1 Medusa's head severed by Perseus [4]

which the legs are fused giving them the appearance of a mermaid tail (Fig. 1.2). This condition is found in approximately one out of 100,000 live births (about as rare as conjoined twins) and is usually fatal within a day or two after birth due to complications associated with abnormal kidney and urinary bladder development and function. More than half the cases of sirenomelia result in stillbirth, and this condition is more likely to occur in identical twins than in single births or fraternal twins. It is due to a failure of the normal vascular supply from the lower aorta in utero. Maternal diabetes has been associated with "caudal regression syndrome and sirenomelia" although a few sources question this association [5–8].

> Medusa was a monster, one of the Gorgon sisters and daughter of Phorkys and Keto, the children of Gaea (Earth) and Oceanus (Ocean). She had the face of an ugly woman with snakes instead of hair; anyone who locked into her eyes was immediately turned to stone. Her sisters were Sthenno and Euryale, but Medusa was the only mortal of the three.
>
> Medusa was originally a golden-haired, fair maiden, who, as a priestess of Athena, was devoted to a life of celibacy; however, after being wooed by Poseidon and falling for him, she forgot her vows and married him. For this offense, she was punished by the goddess in a most terrible manner. Each wavy lock of the beautiful hair that had charmed her husband, was changed into a venomous snake; her once gentle love-inspiring eyes turned into blood-shot, furious orbs, which incited fear and disgust in the mind of the onlooker; whilst her former roseate hue and milk white skin assumed a loathsome greenish tinge (Fig. 1.3).
>
> Seeing herself transformed into such a repulsive creature, Medusa fled her home never to return. Wandering about, abhorred, dreaded, and shunned by the rest of the world she turned into a character worthy of her outer appearance. In her despair, she fled to Africa where, while wandering restlessly from place to place, young snakes dropped from her hair; that is how according to the ancient Greeks, Africa became a hotbed of venomous reptiles. With the curse of Athena upon her, she turned into stone whomever she gazed upon, till at last, after a life of nameless misery, deliverance came to her in the shape of death at the hands of Perseus.

As I have written on the subject before [9].

We must recognize those who preceded us trying to sort out the large variety and complexity of the congenital vascular malformations. In 1863, the German pathologist Rudolf Virchow in an effort to establish some kind of order into the maze of this pathology, called "angiomas" to all vascular malformations. He divided them into simplex, cavernosum and racemosum. This terminology was recognized in the Anglo-Saxon writings and thinking during the entire century [10].

Edmondo Malan categorized the vascular malformations according to their embryological characteristics and in 1974 published a scholarly written monograph where he classified 451 cases of vascular anomalies that he studied and treated in: predominantly venous, predominantly arterial, predominantly arterio-venous and predominantly lymphatic. Each of these categories could be localized, or diffuse" [11].

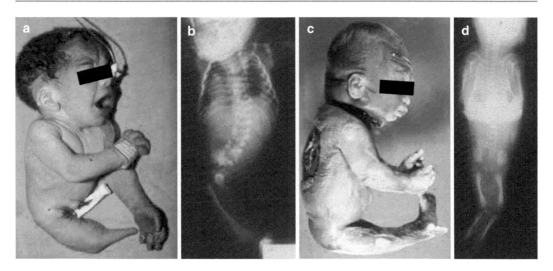

Fig. 1.2 Sirenomelia [6]. Fusion of lower extremities (**a**) Newborn child with sirenomelia (**b**) Total body film showing the fusion of the lower extremities and bone abnormalites (**c**) Lateral view of a fetus with complete fusion of both lower exremities (**d**) Total body Xray of child showing both poorly developed lower extremities fused

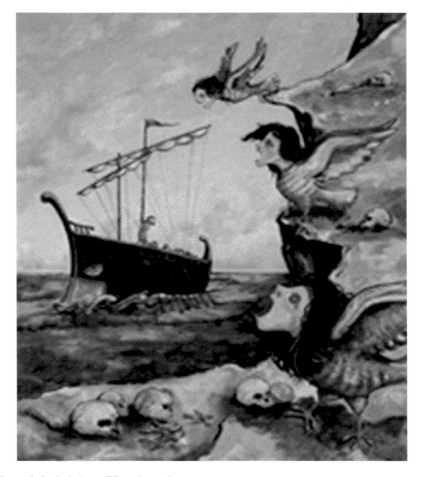

Fig. 1.3 The mythological sirens. Winged aquatic women

Efforts of classification, however, have only contributed to increase confusion among physicians who are often bewildered by the bizarre and often grotesque presentation of congenital vascular anomalies. There is in this book a section dedicated to the very important topic of classification of congenital vascular anomalies, and for that reason, we will not dwell into this subject.

Great progress has occurred during the last 50 years in the puzzling field of the congenital vascular anomalies. My trip into this challenging pathology began in 1957 in Boston. Throughout these years I have been fortunate to observe that in spite of the often repugnant aspect of some patients afflicted by these malformations, there is a group of physicians who have realized that we are here to care for those who cannot care for themselves and who in desperation turn their eyes to us hoping to find relief [9].

References

1. Adams F. The genuine works of hippocrates. XL1. On superfoetation. New York: William Wood and Co; 1844. p. 94.
2. Pare A. The works of the famous Chirurgion Ambrose Parey, Book 25 Translated by Thomas Johnson. London: Thomas Cote and R Young; 1634. p. 979.
3. Ballantyne JW. Teratogenesis. An inquiry into the causes of Monstrosities. Edinburgh: Oliver and Boyd; 1897. p. 15.
4. Medusa. Wikipedia. The free encyclopedia. Google Scholar. http:www.history.com/topics/ancienthistory/greek-mythology/videos/story-of-medusa.
5. Assimakopoulos E, Athanasiadis A, Zafrakas M, Dragoumis K, Bontis J. Caudal regresion syndrome and sirenomelia in only one twin in two diabetic pregnancies. Clin Exp Obstet Gynecol. 2004;31(2):151–3.
6. Garrido-Allepuz C, Haro E, Gonzalez D, Martinez ML, et al. A clinical and experimental overview of sirenomelia: insight into the mechanisms of congenital limb malformations. Dis Model Mech. 2011;4:289–99.
7. Duhamel B. From the mermaid to anal imperforation: the syndrome of caudal regression. Arch Dis Child. 1961;36:152–5.
8. Kallen B, Castilla EE, Lancaster PA, Mutchinick O, Knudsen LB, Martinez-Frias ML, Mastroiacovo P, Robert E. The Cyclops and the mermaid: an epidemiological study of two types of rare malformation. J Med Genet. 1992;29(1):30–5.
9. Villavicencio JL. Venous malformations: introduction; historical background. Phlebology. 2007;22(6):247.
10. Virchow R.. Angiome. In: Die krankhaften Geschwulste. Berlin August Hirschwald, vol. 3; 1863. p. 306–425.
11. Malan E. Vascular malformations (Angiodysplasias). Milan: Carlo Erba Foundation; 1974.

Embryological Background of Congenital Vascular Malformations

Hiroo Suami and Byung-Boong Lee

Introduction

The study of the embryological development of the circulatory system began in earnest during the nineteenth century. Early pioneer researchers in this field used intravascular injection of various dye solutions of India ink, silver nitrate, and Prussian blue for demonstration of minute vessels [1, 2]. The injected tissues were fixed and histological investigation was conducted. The researchers' extensive and careful observations enabled them to map the development of the vascular and lymphatic systems in both humans and other mammals.

During the development of the arterial system, construction of aortic arch goes through the most complicated process and is thus recognized as the key to most congenital vascular malformations. The aortic arch originates from symmetrical brachial arches. After tremendous alteration, involving systemic and segmental fusion and separation, the brachial arches transform into the aortic arch. Rathke's diagram is useful and provides a general idea of which components persist and which degenerate to enable transformation into the matured structure [3].

In the development of the venous system, formation of paired anterior and posterior cardinal veins is a significant event. The paired veins take on the important roles of blood drainage in this early developmental stage, but most of their parts degenerate after completion of their roles. Formation of the inferior vena cava is a complex process. Chronological diagrams by McClure and Butler demonstrate precisely how the primitive venous system transforms into the inferior vena cava [4]. Following a sequential, elaborate process, any misplaced degenerations trigger rerouting of blood drainage to the heart and cause persistence of the primary veins.

Sabin used swine embryos and Lewis used rabbit embryos to investigate the development of the lymphatic system [5, 6]. They proposed that the lymphatic system originates from several sites on the primary vein and sprouts centrifugally. In contrast, Huntington and McClure proposed that lymphatic vessels arise in the mesenchymal tissue, independently from the primary veins, growing centripetally, and then subsequently connecting to the venous system [7]. A recent study using molecular markers suggests that in fact both centripetal and centrifugal growths appear to contribute to the development of the lymphatic system [8].

H. Suami, MD, PhD (✉)
Australian Lymphoedema Education, Research and Treatment, Faculty of Medicine and Health Sciences, Macquarie University, Level 1, 75 Talavera Rd, Sydney, NSW 2109, Australia
e-mail: hiroo.suami@mq.edu.au

B.-B. Lee, MD, PhD, FACS
Professor of Surgery and Director, Center for the Lymphedema and Vascular Malformations, George Washington University, Washington, DC, USA

Adjunct Professor of Surgery, Uniformed Services, University of the Health Sciences, Bethesda, MD, USA
e-mail: bblee38@gmail.com

© Springer-Verlag Berlin Heidelberg 2017
Y.-W. Kim et al. (eds.), *Congenital Vascular Malformations*, DOI 10.1007/978-3-662-46709-1_2

Maldevelopment of the lymphatic system causes dysfunction of interstitial fluid drainage, namely, heredity or primary lymphedema.

Development of the Blood Vascular System

The blood vascular system develops in two distinct, consecutive phases: (1) vasculogenesis, the de novo differentiation of blood vessels from mesoderm-derived precursor cells, and (2) angiogenesis, the remodeling of these vessels to form arteries and veins [9].

Vasculogenesis first occurs in the yolk sac. Structures called blood islands form as hemangioblasts differentiate into endothelial and red blood cells. The endothelial cells migrate from the blood islands and form a random vascular network called the capillary plexus. Meanwhile, the dorsal aorta forms inside the embryo; eventually, it connects the heart to the capillary plexus of the yolk sac thus completing the circulation loop.

In human embryos, angiogenesis begins at day 21 of embryogenesis, when the heart begins to beat and blood starts circulating in the capillary plexus. Biomechanical and hemodynamic input induces active vascular remodeling. The capillary plexus is remodeled into a functional structure that includes large-caliber vessels for low-resistance rapid flow and small-caliber capillaries for diffusional flow. This remodeling occurs by the regression, sprouting, splitting, or fusion of preexisting vessels. Endothelial cells in the capillary plexus start differentiating into cells with arterial and venous identities.

Biomechanical factors and fluid dynamics have long been recognized as important regulators of angiogenesis. Thoma, a pioneer angiogenesis research, observed that within embryos, increases in local blood flow cause vessel diameters to enlarge, whereas decreases in local blood flow cause vessel diameters to shrink [10]. Chapman studied the angiogenesis of chicken embryos in which he removed the hearts and observed that the initial vessel patterns laid down during vasculogenesis remained undisturbed. He hypothesized that subsequent angiogenesis occurred by mechanical forces [11]. Murray

proposed that vessel caliber is proportional to the amount of shear stress at the vessel wall [12].

Development of the Arterial System

After the heart starts circulating blood through the primitive vascular network, two aortas form at the dorsal region. Fusion starts in the middle section and then extends cranially and caudally; thus the single dorsal aorta develops (Fig. 2.1) [13, 14]. The dorsal aorta connects to the vitelline arteries in the mid portion and to the umbilical arteries in the caudal portion. In the cranial portion of the embryo, five pairs of aortic arches form sequentially at both sides. They originate from the aortic sac and connect to the ipsilateral dorsal aorta.

The layout of the primitive aortic arches is transformed to the adult aortic arch from week 6–8 of development. The first asnd second aortic arches exist only for a short period of time and then regress (Fig. 2.2a). The vertebral arteries form on the lateral side of the dorsal arteries and the intersegmental arteries connect between them horizontally. After the first and second aortic arches disappear, the segment of the dorsal aorta between the third

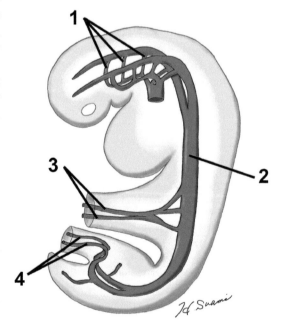

Fig. 2.1 Embryonic arteries at the fourth week of gestation (*1* aortic arches, *2* dorsal aorta, *3* vitelline arteries, and *4* umbilical arteries)

and fourth aortic arches regresses on both sides (Fig. 2.2b). The sixth pair of aortic arches forms from the aortic sac, and they give branches to the lung (Fig. 2.2c). A segment of only the right dorsal artery involutes between the bifurcation and the right seventh intersegmental artery. The pair of seventh intersegmental arteries elongates laterally; however other pairs of intersegmental arteries regress because of maturation of the vertebral arteries. The intermammary arteries derive from the seventh intersegmental arteries and extend cau-

dally. The next involution occurs at the segment of the right sixth aortic arch between the right dorsal artery and pulmonary branch (Fig. 2.2d). The same segment of the left sixth aortic arch persists as the ductus arteriosus until the time of birth. The pulmonary trunk is separated from the aortic sac and with the sixth aortic arches. The seventh intersegmental arteries move cranially and elongate to limb buds to start supplying blood to the upper limbs.

In summary, the first and second aortic arches regress completely. The third aortic arches form a

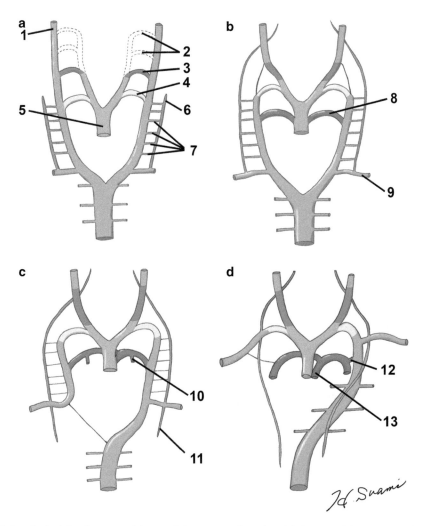

Fig. 2.2 Embryological development of the arterial system from the sixth to eighth week of gestation. (**a**) The first and second aortic arches exist only for a short period of time (*1* dorsal aorta, *2* the first and second aortic arches, *3* the third aortic arch, *4* the fourth aortic arch, *5* aortic sac, *6* vertebral artery, and *7* intersegmental arteries). (**b**) The sixth aortic arch forms from the aortic sac (*8* the sixth

aortic arch and *9* the seventh intersegmental artery). (**c**) A segment of the right dorsal artery involutes between the bifurcation and the right seventh intersegmental artery (*10* pulmonary artery and *11* internal mammary artery). (**d**) A segment of the right sixth aortic arch involutes between the right dorsal artery and pulmonary brunch (*12* ductus arteriosus and *13* pulmonary trunk)

part of the carotid arteries. The fourth aortic arches form a part of the aortic arch and a part of the right subclavicular artery. The sixth aortic arches form the pulmonary arteries and the ductus arteriosus. The seventh intersegmental arteries form the subclavicular arteries.

Anomalous Development of the Aortic Arch

Due to the complex nature of the evolution and involution that occurs during the development of the major arteries, and the fact that multiple processes must occur correctly, anomalous conditions of the aortic arch can occur. For example, a patent ductus arteriosus is one of the most common abnormalities, occurring in around 8 out of 10,000 births [14]. Coarctation of the aorta is another one of the more commonly occurring at around 3.2 out of 10,000 births [14]. This abnormality is classified into two types: pre-ductal and post-ductal corresponding to the anatomic position of the lesion with the ductal arteriosus.

Abnormal involution and persistence of primitive arteries cause several other malformations. "Abnormal origin of the right subclavicular artery" occurs when the right fourth aortic arch and a part of the right dorsal artery cranial to the seventh intersegmental artery involute and the right dorsal artery caudal to the seventh intersegmental artery persists. "Double aortic arch" occurs when all parts of the right dorsal artery persist. "Interrupted aortic arch" occurs when both fourth aortic arches involute and the right dorsal artery caudal to the seventh intersegmental artery persists. Thus, knowledge of abnormal involution and persistence during the early stages of embryological development helps our understanding of the pathogenesis of congenital arterial malformations.

Development of the Venous System

The primitive vascular structure in capillary and reticular plexuses in the early embryonic stage soon develops distinguishable arteries and veins.

The part of the body distal to the developing heart drains through paired anterior cardinal veins, whereas the caudal portion of the body drains through paired posterior cardinal veins (Fig. 2.3) [15].

In the fifth week, paired anterior cardinal veins and posterior cardinal veins form, and they are the first embryonic veins to drain the cerebral and caudal portion of the body, respectively. Soon, subcardinal veins sprout from the posterior cardinal veins (Fig. 2.4a) [4]. The following alterations occur over the fifth to seventh week. Paired supracardinal veins form from the posterior cardinal veins. The sub- and supracardinal veins anastomose on both sides to form the "subsupracardinal anastomoses" (Fig. 2.4b). The posterior cardinal veins regress because now subcardinal and supracardinal veins supersede them (Fig. 2.4c). Longitudinal segments of left subcardinal vein cranial to the subcardinal anastomosis also regress. Paired anterior cardinal veins form a new anastomosis to let the blood drain from the left anterior cardinal vein into the right anterior cardi-

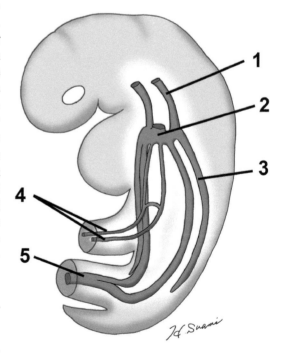

Fig. 2.3 Embryonic veins at the fourth week of gestation (*1* anterior cardinal vein, *2* sinus venosus, *3* posterior cardinal vein, *4* vitelline veins, and *5* umbilical vein)

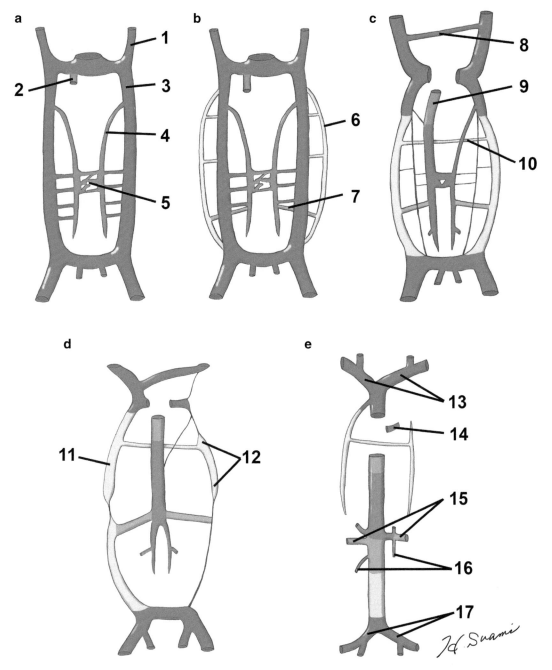

Fig. 2.4 Embryological development of the venous system from the fifth to seventh week of gestation. (**a**) The subcardinal veins form from the posterior cardinal veins (*1* anterior cardinal vein, *2* right vitelline vein, *3* posterior cardinal vein, *4* subcardinal vein, and *5* subcardinal anastomosis). (**b**) Paired supracardinal veins form from the posterior cardinal veins (*6* supracardinal vein and *7* subsupracardinal anastomosis). (**c**) The posterior cardinal veins regress. New anastomoses form between the anterior cardinal veins and between the posterior cardinal veins (*8* anastomosis between the anterior cardinal veins, *9* hepatic vein, and *10* anastomosis between the posterior cardinal veins). (**d**) Cranial part of the supracardinal veins remains as azygos, hemiazygos, and accessory hemiazygos veins (*11* azygos vein and *12* hemiazygos and accessory hemiazygos veins). (**e**) A right-sided inferior vena cava forms (*13* brachiocephalic veins, *14* coronary sinus, *15* renal veins, *16* spermatic or ovarian veins, and *17* common iliac veins)

nal vein via the newly formed "brachiocephalic vein." A new anastomosis forms between supracardinal veins. The right supracardinal vein remains as the "azygos vein" together with the cranial part of the right posterior cardinal veins forms the "arch of azygos vein," while the left supracardinal vein becomes the "hemiazygos vein" and also the "accessory azygos vein" (Fig. 2.4d). Most of the veins on the left side regress, resulting in a right-sided "inferior vena cava" (IVC), to meet the new conditions to be faced upon birth (Fig. 2.4e). The portion of the left anterior cardinal vein caudal to the brachicephalic anastomosis regresses, and it transforms into the "oblique vein" of the left atrium (vein of Marshall) on the back of the left atrium and the "coronary sinus." The right anterior cardinal vein forms the superior vena cava (SVC) [16].

Anomalous Development of the Superior and Inferior Vena Cava

Due to the complex evolutional process to form the SVC, from various segments of three different embryonic/cardinal veins, there is a high risk of defective development of the SVC. In addition, there are various conditions of the stenosis or dilatation and/or aneurysm formation, either with or without internal defect. "Double superior vena cava" is the outcome of the persistence of the left caudal anterior cardinal vein [17]. It is due to the failed degeneration and/or involution of the left anterior cardinal vein proximal to brachiocephalic anastomosis. Left SVC is the outcome that results from persistence of the entire left cardinal vein. In the absence of the right proximal superior vena cava, the blood from the right upper body drains to the "left SVC" via right brachiocephalic vein.

There is a high risk of developmental anomalies arising as a result of errors of the IVC developmental process. "Absence of the suprarenal inferior vena cava" (IVC) may arise as a result of the complexity of fusion process of multiple blocks of three different cardinal veins, which needs to occur to meet the new conditions following birth [18]. It occurs when the right subcardinal

vein fails to make a connection with the liver. The IVC drains into the arch of the azygos and the hepatic veins drain independently to the right atrium. "Double inferior vena cava" occurs when iliac anastomosis of the postcardinal vein regresses or shrinks and the left subcardinal vein, caudal to anastomosis of the subcardinal veins, persists to maintain drainage from the left iliac veins [19].

Development of the Lymphatic System

Development of the human lymphatic system begins in the sixth or seventh week of embryogenesis following development of the primitive vascular system. First, paired jugular lymph sacs, which originate from the anterior cardinal veins, develop near the junction of the subclavicular and internal jugular veins [5, 6]; lymphatic capillaries and vessels sprout centrifugally toward the head and neck, upper extremities, and upper torso. Each jugular sac maintains connection to the subclavicular vein. Secondary to this, the retroperitoneal lymph sac derives from the mesonephric veins and lies in the root of the mesentery. The sac forms visceral lymphatic vessels including the thoracic duct. The retroperitoneal sac joins the cisterna chili and they drain into the thoracic duct. Initially, two thoracic ducts form connecting the jugular sacs and the cisterna chili. Anastomoses form between them. The single thoracic duct develops from the cranial left thoracic duct, the anastomosis, and the right distal thoracic duct. Lastly, paired posterior lymph sacs develop near the junctions of the primitive iliac veins and posterior cardinal veins. The lymphatic vessels from these sacs spread toward the lower torso and lower extremities (Fig. 2.5).

Anomalous Development of the Lymphatic System

Lymphatic malformations often manifest clinically as congenital or heredity lymphedema resulting from insufficient development of the lymphatic system during the late stages of embryological development. Lymphatic congenital defects present in various forms, including hypoplastic, hyperplastic, or aplastic lesions of the lymphatic vessels and/or lymph nodes. Such lesions are associated with malfunctions of the lymphatic system.

Truncular lymphatic malformations do not always result in an evident morphological defect of the lymphatic system, however. For example, patients with "Milroy-Meige syndrome," or inherited primary lymphedema, which occurs right after birth, do not have any apparent structural defects of the lymphatic system but rather have functional impairment at the capillary lymphatic or initial lymphatic level [20]. In addition, patients with "lymphedema-distichiasis syndrome" have impairment of the endoluminal valves, which causes lymphatic reflux. The syndrome is associated with other clinical symptoms including cardiac malformations, cleft palate, ptosis, double eyelashes, and yellow nails.

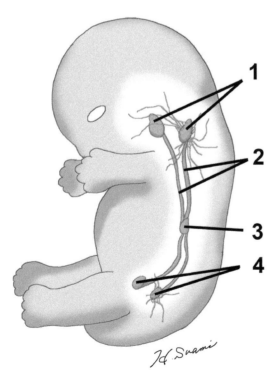

Fig. 2.5 Embryonic lymphatics at the seventh week of gestation (*1* jugular lymph sacs, *2* thoracic ducts, *3* retroperitoneal lymph sac, and *4* posterior lymph sacs)

Summary

Embryological development of the vascular system is an intricate sequential process involving evolution, involution, generation, and degeneration. Anomalous involution often triggers formation of abnormal circulation that then requires and promotes persistence of the primitive vascular structure. Congenital vascular malformations demonstrate a wide variety of clinical manifestations in terms of not only their pathological presentation but also their response to therapy. Understanding the embryological background of these lesions, which also relates to their clinical prognoses, is fundamental to comprehending dynamic circulatory alterations following treatment.

References

1. Gladstone RJ. Development of the inferior vena cava in the light of recent research, with especial reference to certain abnormalities, and current description of the ascending lumber and azygos veins. J Anat. 1929;64:70–93.
2. Barry A. The aortic arch derivatives in the human adult. Anat Rec. 1951;111:221–38.
3. Rathke H. Bemerkungen über die Entstehung der bei manchen Vögeln und den Krokodilen vorkommenden unpaarigen gemeinschaftlichen Carotis. Archiv Anat Physiol. 1858;315-322
4. McClure CFW, Butler EG. The development of the vena cava inferior in man. Am J Anat. 1925;35:331–83.
5. Sabin FR. On the origin of the lymphatic system from the veins and the development of the lymph hearts and thoracic duct in the pig. Am J Anat. 1902;1:367–91.
6. Lewis F. The development of the lymphatic system in rabbits. Am J Anat. 1905;5:95–111.
7. Huntington GS, McClure CFW. The anatomy and development of the jugular lymph sac in the domestic cat (Felis demestica). Am J Anat. 1910;10:177–312.
8. Butler MG, Isogai S, Weinstein BM. Lymphatic development. Birth Defects Research (Part C). 2009;87:221–31.
9. Flamme I, Frolich T, Risau W. Molecular mechanisms of vasculogenesis and embryonic angiogenesis. J Cell Physiol. 1997;173:206–10.
10. Thoma R. Untersuchungen uber die histogenese und histomechnikdes gefasssystems. Stuttgart: Ferdinand Enke; 1893.
11. Chapman WB. The effect of the heart-beat upon the development of the vascular system in the chick. Am J Anat. 1918;23:175–203.

12. Murray PDF. The development in vivo of the blood of the early chick embryo. R Soc Med (London Ser B). 1932;3:497–521.

13. Moore KL, TVN P, editors. The developing human: clinical oriented embryology. 8th ed. Philadelphia: Saunders; 2008.

14. Sadler TW. Langman's medical embryology. 12th ed. Philadelphia: Lippincott Williams & Wilkins, a Wolters Kluwer business; 2012.

15. Collins P. Embryology and development. In: PL W, LH B, MM B, et al., editors. Gray's anatomoy: the anatomical basis of medicine and surgery. 38th ed. Edinburgh: Churchill Livingston; 1995. p. 327.

16. FitzGerald DP. The study of developmental abnormalities as an aid to that of human embryology, based on observations on a persistent left superior vena cava. Dublin J Med Sci. 1909;127:14–8.

17. Beattie J. The importance of anormalies of the superior vena cava in man. Canad Med Assoc J. 1931;25:281–4.

18. Gil RJ, Perez AM, Arias JB, Pascual FB, Romeo ES. Agenesis of the inferior vena cava associated with lower extremities and pelvic venous thrombosis. J Vasc Surg. 2006;44:1114–6.

19. Hashmi ZA, Smaroff GG. Dual inferior vena cava: two inferior vena cava filters. Ann Thorac Surg. 2007;84:661–3.

20. BB L. Lymphatic malformations. In: LL T, CL N, BB L, et al., editors. Lymphedema: diagnosis and treatment. London: Springer-Verlag; 2008. p. 31–42.

Part II

Pathogenesis of Congenital Vascular Malformation (CVM)

Angiogenesis and Vascular Malformations

3

Patricia E. Burrows

In the process of vasculogenesis, blood and lymphatic channels form in the embryo from clusters of angioblasts that differentiate into endothelium and other mesenchymal cells that form the vessel wall [smooth muscle cells, fibroblasts] and surrounding mesenchyme. Early vascular channels form the primary vascular plexus and vascular remodeling leads to development of arteries, veins, and capillaries. Subsequently, new blood vessels form from sprouting, intussusceptive vascular growth, and splitting of vessels from preexisting channels. Specification is believed to be related to expression of Efrin B2 in arterial and EphB2 in venous endothelium. Lymphatic channels form from veins. Defects in any of the proteins involved in the regulation of vasculogenesis and angiogenesis can result in abnormal channels that can subsequently expand and cause symptoms. After birth, abnormal regulation of angiogenesis can lead to increased cell proliferation or reduced apoptosis, thrombosis, and other changes that contribute to the clinical manifestations of a vascular malformation. Congenital vascular malformations, in general, enlarge in proportion to the growth of the affected child, but it is well known that they may expand episodically, espe-cially during periods of accelerated somatic growth and increased hormonal stimulation. The recent finding that endothelial cells in vascular malformations have increased receptors to human growth hormone and somatostatin compared with those in normal tissue explains the increased growth and symptomatology of vascular malformations that is seen during growth spurts as well as at puberty and during pregnancy [1, 2]. In addition, animal models have confirmed the responsiveness of vascular malformations to angiogenic growth factors [3].

Venous Malformations

Familial mucocutaneous venous malformations and 50 % of sporadic VM are caused by mutations in the tyrosine kinase receptor TIE2. Experiments show that in human endothelial cells, mutant tie2 and its ligands, angiopoietins 1 and 2, cause increased activation of AKT signaling and reduced production of platelet-derived growth factor-B, which is important in mural cell recruitment. These molecular changes, both in the lab setting and in humans, cause VMs characterized by a defective endothelial cell monolayer, deficient smooth muscle in the vessel wall, and defects in thrombospondin function, while abnormalities result in formation of enlarged, disfigured, and fragile venous channels, as well as intralesional thrombosis and clotting protein consumption [4]. The cause and effect of TIE2

P.E. Burrows, MD
Medical College of Wisconsin, Interventional
Radiologist, Children's Hospital of Wisconsin,
9000 West Wisconsin Ave., MS 721, Milwaukee,
WI 53226, USA
e-mail: pburrows@chw.org

© Springer-Verlag Berlin Heidelberg 2017
Y.-W. Kim et al. (eds.), *Congenital Vascular Malformations*, DOI 10.1007/978-3-662-46709-1_3

mutation in the etiology of VM is supported by the observation that treatment of patients with sirolimus, which suppresses AKT, appears to control the growth and improve the consumption coagulopathy of extensive VM [5]. Rapid recurrence of symptomatic VM after partial resection is common, presumably due to stimulation of venous angiogenesis. In a similar fashion, even after effective endovascular ablation of malformed venous channels, similarly abnormal channels, presumably collaterals, can develop in the adjacent soft tissue. Intralesional thrombi created by sclerotherapy can be recanalized by circulating endothelial progenitor cells, leading to new abnormal channels. This is the reason that sclerotherapy should be repeated until the vessel is occluded permanently by fibrosis.

Abnormal angiogenesis can also occur in veins without TIE2 mutation. Angiogenesis in a partly thrombosed vein can lead to development of a focal vascular mass termed Masson's tumor.

Arteriovenous shunts can develop in the walls of partly occluded veins after venous thrombosis, or after incomplete endovascular ablation (Fig. 3.1). In fact, dural sinus thrombosis is believed to be the trigger for development of acquired dural AVMs in adults.

Arteriovenous Malformations [AVMs]

AVMs are also caused by abnormal regulation of blood vessel development. More than 860 genes are known to be upregulated or downregulated in cerebral AVMs [6]. The study of familial forms of AVM has revealed a number of causative genetic mutations, including ENDOGLIN (ENG), ACTIVIN RECEPTOR-LIKE KINASE 1 [ALK1], and SMAD4 in patients with hereditary hemorrhagic telangiectasia [HHT], RASA1 in patients with capillary malformation-arteriovenous

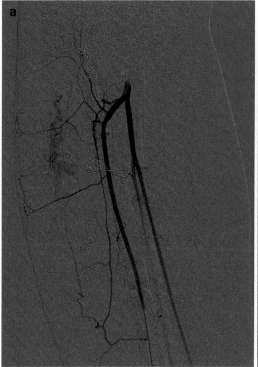
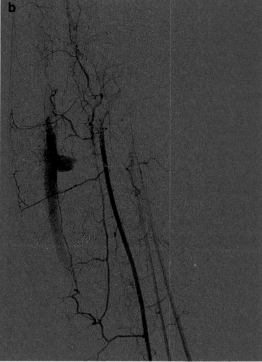
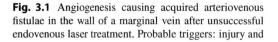

Fig. 3.1 Angiogenesis causing acquired arteriovenous fistulae in the wall of a marginal vein after unsuccessful endovenous laser treatment. Probable triggers: injury and hypoxia. (**a**, **b**) Sequential images from a right anterior tibial angiogram showing tiny arteriovenous shunts into the distal segment of the partly occluded vein

malformation [CM-AVM], and PTEN in patients with AVM associated with Cowden syndrome and Bannayan-Riley-Ruvalcaba syndrome. A number of animal models have been developed, mainly by creating mutations in endoglin (eng), activin receptor-like kinase 1 [Alk1], RASA1, and notch pathways [7–9]. In the lab setting, angiogenesis in normal and abnormal endothelial cell models can be stimulated by vascular endothelial growth factors (VEGF). In the Alk1 mouse model, AVMs establish from newly formed arteries and veins, rather than from remodeling of a preexistent capillary network. Creation of a wound or stimulation with VEGF is needed to create the AVM in ALK1-deficient adult mice. In this model, VEGF blockade can prevent the formation of AVM and arrest the progression of AVM development [10]. Clinically, most AVMs evolve over time, and it has been known for many years that quiescent lesions can become more active [increased shunting, swelling, pain] during periods of active somatic growth and as a result of conditions that are known to upregulate vascular growth factors, such as surgery, embolization, trauma, inflammation, puberty, and pregnancy (Figs. 3.2 and 3.3). Histochemistry of resected AVM tissue has revealed increased numbers of endothelial cell receptors for human growth factor and somatostatin, as well as upregulation of MMP9, inflammatory markers, and VEGF [11]. Recently, it has been found that suppression of VEGF pharmacologically [bevacizumab and thalidomide] can result in decreased arteriovenous shunting and improved symptomatology in some patients with HHT [12]. Doxycycline appears to decrease cerebral MMP-nine activity and angiogenesis induced by VEGF. Endothelial cells from resected AVMs respond to doxycycline and minocycline in cell culture, but clinical response in patients with symptomatic AVMs has not been well documented. One child with sporadic AVM had an excellent, dose-dependent, sustained response to treatment with marimastat, a preclinical broad-spectrum MMP inhibitor. Other patients with AVMs have been treated with angiogenesis inhibitors anecdotally, but, aside from a small trial of minocycline in patients with cerebral AVMs, there have not been any prospective clinical trials.

While it has been widely believed that AVMs are congenital, there is increasing evidence that AVMs can be acquired [13]. Triggers for postnatal development of AVM include venous thrombosis [deep vein thrombosis in the lower extremities and dural sinus thrombosis resulting in dural AVM], ischemia [e.g., cerebral infarct], and trauma [e.g., chronic posttraumatic AV fistula, uterine AVMs]. While the mechanisms leading to acquired AVM have not been studied in detail, the presence of increased numbers of endothelial progenitor cells in thrombosed blood vessels as well as higher grade AVMs suggests a role for these cells, likely in response to upregulation of vascular growth factors [11, 14].

Summary

Vasculogenesis, normal and aberrant angiogenesis, and pathological angiogenesis stimulated by extrinsic factors are all involved in development and progression of vascular malformations. Antiangiogenic drug treatment appears to be effective in controlling the development and progression of AVM in animal models as well as in patients with HHT, who have mutations in ALK1 and ENG. Further study of patients with sporadic AVM and patients with VM will hopefully lead to effective pharmacotherapy in the future.

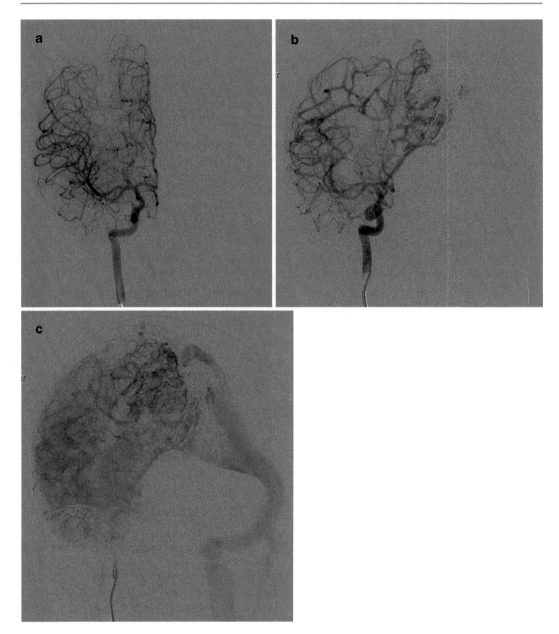

Fig. 3.2 Stimulated angiogenesis in an 11-year-old girl with dural AVM, most likely triggered by somatic growth, embolization, and onset of puberty. (**a**) *Right* internal carotid angiogram, frontal projection in 2008, showing no arteriovenous shunting. (**b, c**) *Right* internal carotid arteriogram, frontal oblique projection, shows multiple new arteriovenous fistulae between pial branches of the anterior and middle cerebral arteries and the superior sagittal sinus. In the interval, the patient had undergone additional embolization of the dural AVM and started her menstrual cycles

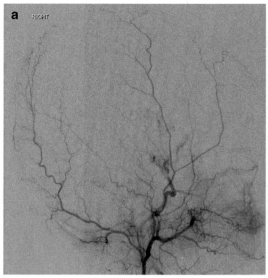
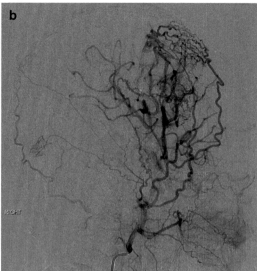

Fig. 3.3 Angiogenesis in a one-year-old girl with severe stenosis of the right internal carotid artery treated by synangiosis surgery. Probable stimuli: ischemia, hypoxia, surgical trauma, and somatic growth. (**a**) *Right* external carotid arteriogram, lateral projection prior to surgery shows normal size and distribution of the external carotid artery branches. (**b**) *Right* external carotid angiogram 1 year after synangiosis shows increased size and tortuosity of the superficial temporal artery with extensive anastomoses with the right middle cerebral artery branches

References

1. Kulungowski AM, Hassanein AH, Nose V, Fishman SJ, Mulliken JB, Upton J, et al. Expression of androgen, estrogen, progesterone, and growth hormone receptors in vascular malformations. Plast Reconstr Surg. 2012;129(6):919e–24e.
2. Maclellan RA, Vivero MP, Purcell P, Kozakewich HP, DiVasta AD, Mulliken JB, et al. Expression of follicle-stimulating hormone receptor in vascular anomalies. Plast Reconstr Surg. 2014;133(3):344e–51e.
3. Choi EJ, Kim YH, Choe SW, Tak YG, Garrido-Martin EM, Chang M, et al. Enhanced responses to angiogenic cues underlie the pathogenesis of hereditary hemorrhagic telangiectasia 2. PLoS One. 2013;8(5):e63138.
4. Soblet J, Limaye N, Uebelhoer M, Boon LM, Vikkula M. Variable somatic TIE2 mutations in half of sporadic venous malformations. Mol Syndromol. 2013;4(4):179–83.
5. Boscolo E, Limaye N, Huang L, Kang KT, Soblet J, Uebelhoer M, et al. Rapamycin improves TIE2-mutated venous malformation in murine model and human subjects. J Clin Invest. 2015;125(9):3491–504.
6. Rangel-Castilla L, Russin JJ, Martinez-Del-Campo E, Soriano-Baron H, Spetzler RF, Nakaji P. Molecular and cellular biology of cerebral arteriovenous malformations: a review of current concepts and future trends in treatment. Neurosurg Focus. 2014;37(3):E1.
7. Choi EJ, Chen W, Jun K, Arthur HM, Young WL, Su H. Novel brain arteriovenous malformation mouse models for type 1 hereditary hemorrhagic telangiectasia. PLoS One. 2014;9(2):e88511.
8. Murphy PA, Kim TN, Lu G, Bollen AW, Schaffer CB, Wang RA. Notch4 normalization reduces blood vessel size in arteriovenous malformations. Sci Transl Med. 2012;4(117):117 ra8.
9. Lubeck BA, Lapinski PE, Bauler TJ, Oliver JA, Hughes ED, Saunders TL, et al. Blood vascular abnormalities in Rasa1(R780Q) knockin mice: implications for the pathogenesis of capillary malformation-arteriovenous malformation. Am J Pathol. 2014;184(12):3163–9.
10. Han S, Huang Y, Wang Z, Li Z, Qin X, Wu A. Increased rate of positive penicillin skin tests among patients with glioma: insights into the association between allergies and glioma risk. J Neurosurg. 2014;121(5):1176–84.
11. Lu L, Bischoff J, Mulliken JB, Bielenberg DR, Fishman SJ, Greene AK. Increased endothelial progenitor cells and vasculogenic factors in higher-staged arteriovenous malformations. Plast Reconstr Surg. 2011;128(4):260e–9e.
12. Azzopardi N, Dupuis-Girod S, Ternant D, Fargeton AE, Ginon I, Faure F, et al. Dose – response relationship of bevacizumab in hereditary hemorrhagic telangiectasia. MAbs. 2015;7(3):630–7.
13. Neil JA, Li D, Stiefel MF, Hu YC. Symptomatic de novo arteriovenous malformation in an adult: case report and review of the literature. Surg Neurol Int. 2014;5:148.
14. Gao P, Chen Y, Lawton MT, Barbaro NM, Yang GY, Su H, et al. Evidence of endothelial progenitor cells in the human brain and spinal cord arteriovenous malformations. Neurosurgery. 2010;67(4):1029–35.

Genetic Aspects of Vascular Malformations

4

Francine Blei

Introduction

The past several years have been an exciting period for vascular anomalies for a number of reasons:

1. An escalation in basic research has been instrumental in illuminating the etiology and pathogenesis of vascular anomalies by identifying cellular properties and putative regulatory pathways [1, 2] and detecting new genetic findings [3–9].
2. Refined radiologic techniques permit more precise evaluation [10–13].
3. The identification of new effective treatments, some of which were derived from in vitro and in vivo laboratory discoveries [14–16].

This chapter will focus on genetic mutations which have been identified in vascular malformations. Selected references are updated reviews when possible. Reference to the updated ISSVA classification is recommended (ISSVA classification of vascular anomalies ©2014 available at "issva.org/classification") as well as the manuscript explaining this classification [17]. Refer to Table 8.1.

Mutations are either *germline* (in the case of familial vascular malformations) or *somatic*. Figure 4.1 illustrates the differences between the types of mutations in pictorial form. Germline mutations are autosomal recessive, autosomal dominant, or sex linked; however, other possibilities are de novo mutations, or mutations with variable expression and incomplete penetrance, with clinically unaffected family members carrying the mutation. Mutations are frequently but not exclusively activating or loss of function mutations.

Heritable (genomic, germline) mutations, which occur during meiosis, have been identified in affected family members with a variety of vascular malformations (Tables 4.1 and 4.2) including familial mucosal venous malformations (Tie2 activating mutation) [18], arteriovenous malformations with multifocal capillary malformations (CM-AVM, RASA1 gene) [19], glomuvenous malformations (glomulin) [20], hereditary hemorrhagic telangiectasia (HHT) (endoglin, Alk1, and others) [21], and cerebral cavernous malformations (CCMs) (KRIT1, MGC4607, PDCD10) [22], patients with PTEN hamartoma syndromes (Cowden's syndrome and Bannayan-Riley-Ruvalcaba syndrome), and patients with lymphatic malformations and vascular malformation syndromes with lymphatic malformations [23]. Additionally, several genetic mutations have been identified in familial lymphedema syndromes (VEGFR3/FLT4, VEGFD, FOXC2, *CCBE1*, SOX18, and others) [9]. For those

F. Blei, MD, MBA
Northwell Health System, Lenox Hill Hospital, New York, NY, USA
e-mail: fblei@northwell.edu

© Springer-Verlag Berlin Heidelberg 2017
Y.-W. Kim et al. (eds.), *Congenital Vascular Malformations*, DOI 10.1007/978-3-662-46709-1_4

Somatic   Germline   Mixed Somatic and Germline

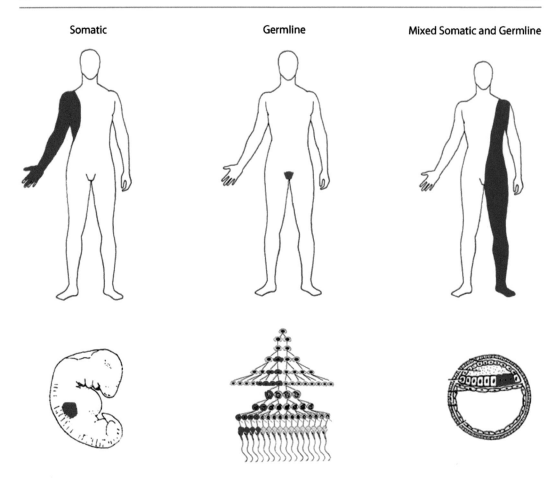

Fig. 4.1 Mosaicism and clinical genetics: This figure shows possible distributions of a mutation in adults with purely somatic, purely germline, or mixed somatic and germline patterns along the top row. The bottom figures demonstrate possible mutation patterns in the late embryo, during spermatogenesis, and in the early embryo (Copyright permission obtained. Spinner and Conlin [30])

disorders that have a defined heritable mutation, prenatal genetic testing may be possible, via amniocentesis, chorionic villus sample, or preimplantation genetic testing.

Mutations in heritable vascular anomalies syndromes are summarized in Table 4.2. The genetic basis of hereditary hemorrhagic telangiectasia was initially discovered in the late 1990s. Since then, genotype-phenotype correlations have been identified, and several causative genes have been found. However, most patients appear to have mutations in endoglin (type 1 HHT) or Alk1 (type 2 HHT) [21]. Familial venous malformations were found to be multifocal, affecting cutaneous and/or mucosal locations. A muta-tion in the angiopoietin receptor TIE2/TEK was found to be causative [3]. Patients with capillary malformation-arteriovenous malformation often present with symptoms associated with an arteriovenous malformation. Multiple small macular pink/brown cutaneous lesions (capillary malformations) of varying sizes evolve over time. A comprehensive family history may identify similarly affected asymptomatic family members, and genetic testing for the RASA1 mutation should be discussed [19]. As mentioned above, several lymphedema syndromes and familial lymphedema disorders have been characterized genetically, and at least one third of familial lymphedemas have been attributed to VEGF3

Table 4.1 Genetic mutations in overgrowth syndromes associated with vascular anomalies

Diagnosis	Clinical features	Mutation	Reference
CLOVES syndrome OMIM 612918	Congenital lipomatous overgrowth, vascular malformation, epidermal nevus, skeletal/spinal abnormalities	3q26.32 PIK3CA gene somatic mosaic activating mutations	Sapp et al. (2007), Alomari et al. (2009), Kurek et al. (2012) [32, 34, 35]
Proteus syndrome OMIM 176920	Asymmetric progressive, disproportionate overgrowth syndrome, hyperostosis, cerebriform connective tissue nevus, vascular malformation, cystic lung disease	AKT1 gene somatic mosaic activating mutations 14q32.33	Lindhurst et al. [31]
Megalencephaly-capillary malformation-polymicrogyria syndrome MCAP, M-CM OMIM 602501	Megalencephaly with brain malformation (polymicrogyria), prenatal overgrowth asymmetry, cutaneous vascular malformation, syndactyly ± polydactyly, connective tissue dysplasia	PIK3CA activating mutation 3q26.32	Mirzaa (2012), (2013) [36, 37]
Klippel-Trenaunay syndrome OMIM 149000	Capillary malformation, soft tissue overgrowth, vascular malformation	PIK3CA activating mutation 3q26.32	Luks et al. [23]
Parkes Weber syndrome OMIM 608355	Capillary malformation, arteriovenous malformation, ± soft tissue overgrowth	Somatic RASA1 5q14.3	Revencu et al. [38]
Capillary malformation-arteriovenous malformation OMIM 608354	Capillary malformation, soft tissue overgrowth, vascular malformation and arteriovenous fistula	Germline RASA1 activating mutation 5q14.3	Eerola et al. (2003), Boon (2005) [19, 39]
Sturge-Weber syndrome OMIM 185300	Facial capillary malformation (PWS), glaucoma, CNS leptomeningeal angiomatosis (encephalotrigeminal angiomatosis), bone ± soft tissue overgrowth	Somatic GNAQ 9q21	Shirley et al. [8]
PTEN hamartoma syndromes Bannayan-Riley-Ruvalcaba syndrome OMIM 153480 Cowden's syndrome OMIM 158350	Macrocephaly, vascular malformation, lipomas thyroid disorders, penile lentigines (BRRS), trichilemmomas, papillomatous	Germline PTEN 10q23.31	Eng (2001), Orloff et al. (2008), Pilarski et al. (2013), Nieuwenhuis et al. (2014), Tan et al. [40–43], [44]
Facial infiltrating lipomatosis	Unilateral facial soft tissue with skeletal overgrowth, premature dentition with macrodontia, hemimacroglossia, mucosal neuromas	Somatic PIK3CA activating mutation	Maclellan [45]
Maffucci syndrome OMIM 614569	Venous malformation, ± spindle cell hemangioma, + enchondromas	Somatic (isocitrate dehydrogenase 1 or 2), IDH1 IDH2	Amary et al. [46]
SOLAMEN	Segmental proportional overgrowth, lipomatosis, arteriovenous malformation, and epidermal nevus	PTEN 10q23.3 mosaic PTEN wild-type allelic loss	Caux et al. [47]

Table 4.2 Heritable vascular malformations

Diagnosis			Reference
Familial venous malformations OMIM 600195	Multifocal cutaneous or mucosal venous malformations	Angiopoietin receptor TIE2/TEK 9p21.2	Gallione et al. [3]
Capillary malformation-arteriovenous malformation, CM-AVM OMIM 608354	See Table 4.1	See Table 4.1	See Table 4.1
Cerebral cavernous malformations OMIM 116860	Single or multiple dilated capillaries in the brain (especially the forebrain), spinal cord, or elsewhere	Sporadic or inherited (AD, incomplete penetrance, variable expression) CCM1: 7q21–22 KRIT1 CCM2: 7p13–15 MGC4607 CCM3: 3q25.2–27 PDCD10	Cigoli et al. [25]
Hereditary hemorrhagic telangiectasia OMIM 187300, 600376, and others	Multifocal arteriovenous malformations	Genotype-phenotype correlation Most common types Type 1 Endoglin (*ENG*) 9q34.11 Type 2 Activin receptor-like kinase 1 (*ACVRL1*) 12q13.13	Review McDonald et al. [21]
Glomovenous malformations OMIM 13800	Non-mucosal venous malformation with glomus cells, may be tender, may be segmental	Autosomal dominant glomulin gene 1p22.1	[20]
PTEN hamartoma syndromes	See Table 4.1	See Table 4.1	See Table 4.1

pathway mutations [24]. Familial CNS cavernous malformations may be single or multiple and can occur in the brain or spinal cord. Several genes (on chromosome 7q and 3q) have been identified in affected families; however, the majority of mutations are associated with the KRIT1 gene (CCM1) [25].

Somatic mutations are post-zygotic mutations which occur after fertilization and only occur in the affected cells. Somatic have been identified in the affected tissue of patients with vascular malformations syndromes, as discussed below and listed in Table 4.1.

Happle [30] introduced the notion that certain genes survive by mosaic expression, since if expressed fully they would be incompatible with life. Several reviews expound upon genetic mosaicism in a multiplicity of disor-

ders [26–30]. Relevant to vascular anomalies is the left panel in Fig. 4.2, somatic mosaicism, demonstrating the mutation occurring in the developing fetus. The earlier in gestation the mutation occurs, the more extensive the involvement. This is evident with the GNAQ mutation which was identified in non-syndromic cutaneous capillary malformations (port-wine stains) and in the cutaneous capillary malformations of patients with Sturge-Weber syndrome (where the mutation presumably occurred earlier in gestation, thus affecting more cell types) [8].

PIK3CA, AKT1, and GNAQ are heretofore the most commonly identified in those syndromic vascular malformations for which somatic mutations have been identified (Table 4.1). These diagnoses include Parkes Weber syndrome,

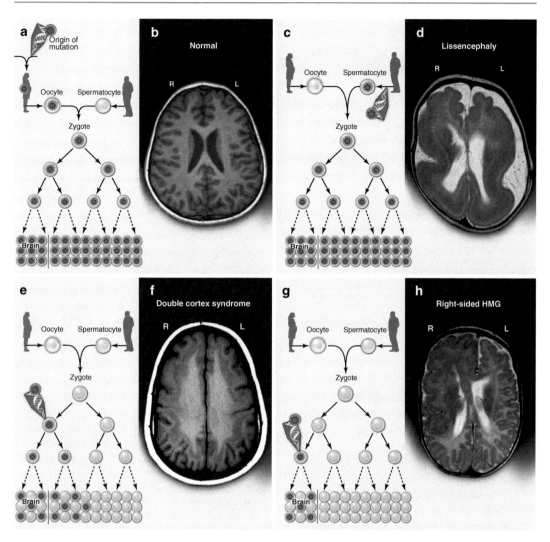

Fig. 4.2 Illustration of genomic mutations (A and C) and somatic mutations (E and G). (Poduri A, et al. Somatic mutation, genomic variation, and neurological disease. Science. 2013;341(6141). Copyright permission requested) **Image A:** Autosomal dominant inheritance – disease expression with only one mutation from one parents and affects all cells in the gamete. **Image C:** De novo mutation – all cells in gamete contain the mutation but disease expression is in a specific organ. **Image E:** Early post-zygotic mutation – somatic mutation occurring early in gestation with mosaic expression, affecting only a portion of the cells in the fetus. **Image G:** Late post-zygotic mutation – somatic mutation occurring late in gestation with mosaic expression, affecting only certain tissues in the fetus

Sturge-Weber syndrome (facial capillary malformation in trigeminal distribution, leptomeningeal angiomatosis, glaucoma, and seizures), Proteus syndrome (AKT1 gene) [31], CLOVES (congenital lipomatous overgrowth, vascular malformation, epidermal nevus, scoliosis), and Klippel-Trenaunay syndrome (PIK3CA) [32]. Entities with PIK3CA somatic mutations are collectively termed "PIK3CA-related overgrowth spectrum (PROS)" which includes diagnosis with or without vascular anomalies [33]. The PIK3-AKT pathway has been shown to be important in the etiology of these syndromes, and medications which inhibit these pathways (e.g., sirolimus) are being studied for patients with vascular anomalies (Fig. 4.3).

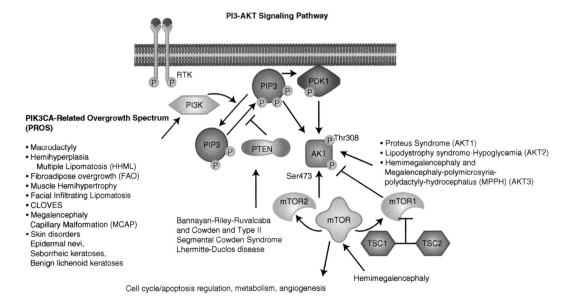

Fig. 4.3 PI3K-AKT pathway and associated clinical overgrowth disorders (Keppler-Noreuil et al. [33]. Creative Commons Attribution License)

Helpful websites to keep apprised of updated information regarding genetic mutations in vascular anomalies include the following resources:

1. OMIM (Online Mendelian Inheritance in Man) is an online catalog of human genes and genetic disorders (http://omim.org).
2. GeneTests (https://www.genetests.org/) is a website which provides genetic information including which tests can be performed for each diagnosis and where the testing is available.
3. GeneCards (http://www.genecards.org/) provides more in-depth scientific data regarding each gene. A mutation database for hereditary hemorrhagic telangiectasia is available at http://arup.utah.edu/database/hht/.
4. Vascular Anomaly and Lymphedema Mutation Database is maintained in Brussels (http://www.icp.ucl.ac.be/vikkula/VAdb/home.php?action=switch_db).

Conclusion

Much progress has been made in identifying causative genes and elaborating molecular pathways pertinent to vascular anomalies. In many cases, testing for relevant genes is not consistently covered by insurance plans. With time, one is hopeful that the clinical relevance of this genetic information will translate into routine (and reimbursable) medical tests.

Acknowledgments This author is grateful for the patients with vascular anomalies and colleagues who participate in the care of and research in this field.

References

1. Chiller KG, Frieden IJ, Arbiser JL. Molecular pathogenesis of vascular anomalies: classification into three categories based upon clinical and biochemical characteristics. Lymphat Res Biol. 2003;1(4):267–81.
2. Arbiser JL, Bonner MY, Berrios RL. Hemangiomas, angiosarcomas, and vascular malformations represent the signaling abnormalities of pathogenic angiogenesis. Curr Mol Med. 2009;9(8):929–34.
3. Gallione CJ, Pasyk KA, Boon LM, Lennon F, Johnson DW, Helmbold EA, et al. A gene for familial venous malformations maps to chromosome 9p in a second large kindred. J Med Genet. 1995;32(3):197–9.
4. Limaye N, Boon LM, Vikkula M. From germline towards somatic mutations in the pathophysiology of vascular anomalies. Hum Mol Genet. 2009;18(R1):R65–74.

5. Alders M, Hogan BM, Gjini E, Salehi F, Al-Gazali L, Hennekam EA, et al. Mutations in CCBE1 cause generalized lymph vessel dysplasia in humans. Nat Genet. 2009;41(12):1272–4.

6. Natynki M, Kangas J, Miinalainen I, Sormunen R, Pietila R, Soblet J, et al. Common and specific effects of TIE2 mutations causing venous malformations. Hum Mol Genet. 2015;24:6374–89.

7. Lo W, Marchuk DA, Ball KL, Juhasz C, Jordan LC, Ewen JB, et al. Updates and future horizons on the understanding, diagnosis, and treatment of Sturge-Weber syndrome brain involvement. Dev Med Child Neurol. 2012;54(3):214–23.

8. Shirley MD, Tang H, Gallione CJ, Baugher JD, Frelin LP, Cohen B, et al. Sturge-Weber syndrome and port-wine stains caused by somatic mutation in GNAQ. N Engl J Med. 2013;368(21):1971–9.

9. Brouillard P, Boon L, Vikkula M. Genetics of lymphatic anomalies. J Clin Invest. 2014;124(3):898–904.

10. Griauzde J, Srinivasan A. Imaging of vascular lesions of the head and neck. Radiol Clin North Am. 2015;53(1):197–213.

11. Calvo-Garcia MA, Kline-Fath BM, Adams DM, Gupta A, Koch BL, Lim FY, et al. Imaging evaluation of fetal vascular anomalies. Pediatr Radiol. 2015;45(8):1218–29.

12. Nozaki T, Matsusako M, Mimura H, Osuga K, Matsui M, Eto H, et al. Imaging of vascular tumors with an emphasis on ISSVA classification. Jpn J Radiol. 2013;31(12):775–85.

13. Rasmussen JC, Fife CE, Sevick-Muraca EM. Near-Infrared Fluorescence Lymphatic Imaging in Lymphangiomatosis. Lymphat Res Biol. 2015;13: 195–201.

14. Leaute-Labreze C, Dumas de la Roque E, Hubiche T, Boralevi F, JB T, Taieb A. Propranolol for severe hemangiomas of infancy. N Engl J Med. 2008;358(24): 2649–51.

15. Boon LM, Hammer J, Seront E, Dupont S, Hammer F, Clapuyt P, et al. Rapamycin as Novel Treatment for Refractory-to-Standard-Care Slow-Flow Vascular Malformations. Plast Reconstr Surg. 2015;136(4S Suppl):38.

16. Hammill AM, Wentzel M, Gupta A, Nelson S, Lucky A, Elluru R, et al. Sirolimus for the treatment of complicated vascular anomalies in children. Pediatr Blood Cancer. 2011;57(6):1018–24.

17. Wassef M, Blei F, Adams D, Alomari A, Baselga E, Berenstein A, et al. Vascular Anomalies Classification: Recommendations From the International Society for the Study of Vascular Anomalies. Pediatrics. 2015;136(1):e203–14.

18. Wouters V, Limaye N, Uebelhoer M, Irrthum A, Boon LM, Mulliken JB, et al. Hereditary cutaneomucosal venous malformations are caused by TIE2 mutations with widely variable hyper-phosphorylating effects. Eur J Hum Genet. 2010;18(4):414–20.

19. Eerola I, Boon LM, Mulliken JB, Burrows PE, Dompmartin A, Watanabe S, et al. Capillary malformation-arteriovenous malformation, a new clinical and genetic disorder caused by RASA1 mutations. Am J Hum Genet. 2003;73(6):1240–9.

20. Brouillard P, Boon LM, Revencu N, Berg J, Dompmartin A, Dubois J, et al. Genotypes and phenotypes of 162 families with a glomulin mutation. Mol Syndromol. 2013;4(4):157–64.

21. McDonald J, Wooderchak-Donahue W, VanSant WC, Whitehead K, Stevenson DA, Bayrak-Toydemir P. Hereditary hemorrhagic telangiectasia: genetics and molecular diagnostics in a new era. Front Genet. 2015;6:1–8.

22. Draheim KM, Fisher OS, Boggon TJ, Calderwood DA. Cerebral cavernous malformation proteins at a glance. J Cell Sci. 2014;127(Pt 4):701–7.

23. Luks VL, Kamitaki N, Vivero MP, Uller W, Rab R, Bovee JV, et al. Lymphatic and other vascular malformative/overgrowth disorders are caused by somatic mutations in PIK3CA. J Pediatr. 2015;166(4):1048–54. e1–5

24. Mendola A, Schlogel MJ, Ghalamkarpour A, Irrthum A, Nguyen HL, Fastre E, et al. Mutations in the VEGFR3 signaling pathway explain 36 % of familial lymphedema. Mol Syndromol. 2013;4(6):257–66.

25. Cigoli MS, Avemaria F, De Benedetti S, Gesu GP, Accorsi LG, Parmigiani S, et al. PDCD10 gene mutations in multiple cerebral cavernous malformations. PLoS One. 2014;9(10):e110438.

26. Biesecker LG, Spinner NB. A genomic view of mosaicism and human disease. Nat Rev Genet. 2013;14(5):307–20.

27. Erickson RP. Somatic gene mutation and human disease other than cancer: An update. Mutat Res. 2010;705(2):96–106.

28. Erickson RP. Recent advances in the study of somatic mosaicism and diseases other than cancer. Curr Opin Genet Dev. 2014;26C:73–8.

29. Frank SA. Somatic mosaicism and disease. Curr Biol. 2014;24(12):R577–81.

30. Spinner NB, Conlin LK. Mosaicism and clinical genetics. Am J Med Genet C Semin Med Genet. 2014;166C(4):397–405.

31. Lindhurst MJ, Sapp JC, Teer JK, Johnston JJ, Finn EM, Peters K, et al. A mosaic activating mutation in AKT1 associated with the Proteus syndrome. N Engl J Med. 2011;365(7):611–9.

32. Sapp JC, Turner JT, van de Kamp JM, van Dijk FS, Lowry RB, Biesecker LG. Newly delineated syndrome of congenital lipomatous overgrowth, vascular malformations, and epidermal nevi (CLOVE syndrome) in seven patients. Am J Med Genet A. 2007;143A(24):2944–58.

33. Keppler-Noreuil KM, Rios JJ, Parker VE, Semple RK, Lindhurst MJ, Sapp JC, et al. PIK3CA-related overgrowth spectrum (PROS): diagnostic and testing eligibility criteria, differential diagnosis, and evaluation. Am J Med Genet A. 2015;167A(2):287–95.

34. Alomari AI. Characterization of a distinct syndrome that associates complex truncal overgrowth, vascular, and acral anomalies: a descriptive study of 18 cases of CLOVES syndrome. Clin Dysmorphol. 2009;18(1):1–7.

35. Kurek KC, Luks VL, Ayturk UM, Alomari AI, Fishman SJ, Spencer SA, et al. Somatic mosaic activating mutations in PIK3CA cause CLOVES syndrome. Am J Hum Genet. 2012;90(6):1108–15.

36. Mirzaa GM, Conway RL, Gripp KW, Lerman-Sagie T, Siegel DH, deVries LS, et al. Megalencephaly-capillary malformation (MCAP) and megalencephaly-polydactyly-polymicrogyria-hydrocephalus (MPPH) syndromes: two closely related disorders of brain overgrowth and abnormal brain and body morphogenesis. Am J Med Genet A. 2012;158A(2):269–91.

37. Mirzaa GM, Riviere JB, Dobyns WB. Megalencephaly syndromes and activating mutations in the PI3K-AKT pathway: MPPH and MCAP. Am J Med Genet C Semin Med Genet. 2013;163C(2):122–30.

38. Revencu N, Boon LM, Mulliken JB, Enjolras O, Cordisco MR, Burrows PE, et al. Parkes Weber syndrome, vein of Galen aneurysmal malformation, and other fast-flow vascular anomalies are caused by RASA1 mutations. Hum Mutat. 2008;29(7):959–65.

39. Boon LM, Mulliken JB, Vikkula M. RASA1: variable phenotype with capillary and arteriovenous malformations. Curr Opin Genet Dev. 2005;15(3):265–9.

40. Eng C. PTEN Hamartoma Tumor Syndrome (PHTS). 2001 [Updated 2014 Jan 23]. In: GeneReviews® [Internet] [Internet]. Seattle. Available from: http://www.ncbi.nlm.nih.gov/books/NBK1488/.

41. Orloff MS, Eng C. Genetic and phenotypic heterogeneity in the PTEN hamartoma tumour syndrome. Oncogene. 2008;27(41):5387–97.

42. Pilarski R, Burt R, Kohlman W, Pho L, Shannon KM, Swisher E. Cowden syndrome and the PTEN hamartoma tumor syndrome: systematic review and revised diagnostic criteria. J Natl Cancer Inst. 2013;105(21):1607–16.

43. Nieuwenhuis MH, Kets CM, Murphy-Ryan M, Yntema HG, Evans DG, Colas C, et al. Cancer risk and genotype-phenotype correlations in PTEN hamartoma tumor syndrome. Fam Cancer. 2014;13(1):57–63.

44. Tan WH, Baris HN, Burrows PE, Robson CD, Alomari AI, Mulliken JB, et al. The spectrum of vascular anomalies in patients with PTEN mutations: implications for diagnosis and management. J Med Genet. 2007;44(9):594–602.

45. Maclellan RA, Luks VL, Vivero MP, Mulliken JB, Zurakowski D, Padwa BL, et al. PIK3CA activating mutations in facial infiltrating lipomatosis. Plast Reconstr Surg. 2014;133(1):12e–9e.

46. Amary MF, Damato S, Halai D, Eskandarpour M, Berisha F, Bonar F, et al. Ollier disease and Maffucci syndrome are caused by somatic mosaic mutations of IDH1 and IDH2. Nat Genet. 2011;43(12):1262–5.

47. Caux F, Plauchu H, Chibon F, Faivre L, Fain O, Vabres P, et al. Segmental overgrowth, lipomatosis, arteriovenous malformation and epidermal nevus (SOLAMEN) syndrome is related to mosaic PTEN nullizygosity. Eur J Hum Genet. 2007;15(7):767–73.

Epidemiologic Aspect of Congenital Vascular Malformation

Young-Wook Kim and Byung-Boong Lee

It is difficult to get exact epidemiologic data of congenital vascular malformation (CVM) due to confusing nomenclatures and definition of the CVMs in times past. Epidemiologic data available in the literatures often misguide the true incidence and prevalence of the CVMs.

Though CVM is caused by an embryonic developmental defect, it may not be clinically apparent from birth. To describe epidemiology of CVMs, we have to rely on the data of symptomatic patients with clinically apparent CVM.

Some CVM may remain quiescent throughout the remaining life. However, most of the CVM lesions grow along with age, and some of them show sudden expansion after certain events such as trauma, hormonal changes (puberty or pregnancy), or infection. We still don't know an exact mechanism to stimulate the dormant CVM lesion. Accordingly, an exact incidence of CVM cannot be estimated at the time of birth.

Y.-W. Kim (✉)
Sungkyunkwan University, School of Medicine,
Vascular Surgery, Samsung Medical Center,
Seoul, South Korea
e-mail: young52.kim@samsung.com;
ywkim52@gmail.com

B.-B. Lee, MD, PhD, FACS
Professor of Surgery and Director, Center for the
Lymphedema and Vascular Malformations, George
Washington University, Washington, DC, USA

Adjunct Professor of Surgery, Uniformed Services,
University of the Health Sciences, Bethesda, MD, USA
e-mail: bblee38@gmail.com

European Surveillance of Congenital Anomalies (EUROCAT) is a network of population-based registries (http://www.eurocat-network.eu/aboutus/whocollaboratingcentre) for the epidemiologic surveillance of congenital anomalies covering about 30 % of all births in the European Union [1].

Even in the EUROCAT data, it is difficult to estimate an exact incidence of CVM because vascular malformation is not separately listed as a congenital anomaly but may be included in the skin anomaly, limb defect, or aortic coarctation.

According to the Bogota Congenital Malformations Surveillance Program (BCMSP) between January 2005 and April 2012, congenital anomalies at birth were detected in 1.66 % (4682 out of 282,523 births). They reported that the most frequent congenital anomalies were vascular anomalies (0.03 %), followed by hypospadias (0.028 %), and anorectal malformations (0.022 %). According to the report, 84 % of vascular anomalies were blood vessel origin and 15 % were lymphatic origin. Regarding to the anatomical distribution, craniofacial lesions were the most frequently diagnosed vascular anomalies after birth, followed by vascular anomalies at the extremities, thorax, and abdomen. However, they did not differentiate CVM from the infantile hemangioma [2].

Kennedy [3] also reported the overall incidence of CVM as 1.08 % (0.83~4.5 %) based on a comprehensive review of 238 studies on the

© Springer-Verlag Berlin Heidelberg 2017
Y.-W. Kim et al. (eds.), *Congenital Vascular Malformations*, DOI 10.1007/978-3-662-46709-1_5

literatures reporting more than 20 million births. Overall incidences of CVM were obtained from hospital records, birth certificates, and also retrospective questionnaires from intensive examinations of children. However, this study highlighted the variability in reporting methods due to differences in terminology and inconsistent diagnostic criteria.

Depending upon the embryological stage when the developmental arrest has occurred, the CVMs present different clinical characteristics. CVM lesions (extratruncular form) resulting from developmental errors during an earlier stage of the vasculogenesis have "evolution potential" even after birth while CVM lesions(truncular form) derived from the later stage of the vasculogenesis do not have such property but tend to accompany with main vessel abnormalities [4, 5].

Tasnadi [6] reported overall incidence of the CVM is 1.2 % based on a study carried on 3573 three-year-old children. According to them, infiltrating or localized venous malformation (VM) and/or arteriovenous malformation (AVM) is 0.45 %, capillary malformation (CM, port wine skin lesion) is 0.42 %, lymphatic malformation (LM)/primary lymphedema is 0.14 %, and mixed from CVM showing phlebectasia, nevus, and limb length discrepancy is 0.34 %.

Among venous predominant vascular malformations, Eifert et al. [7] also reported the prevalence of deep venous anomalies (truncular VM) among the VMs using duplex ultrasonography, venography, CT, MRI, and arteriography. Among 392 patients with CVMs, 65.5 % were confirmed as truncular VM with deep venous anomalies including phlebectasia, aplasia or hypoplasia of venous trunks, aneurysms, and avalvulia of deep vein system.

Among various types of CVMs, venous malformation (VM) is reported as the most common type of CVMs, which has been reported to occur in one of 5000–10,000 childbirths [8].

If we include clinically not significant capillary malformations (CMs), CM may be much more common than the VM which occurs in 0.3 % of childbirths [9].

However, VM is certainly the most frequent type of the CVMs requiring a medical attention.

VMs are present at birth but are not always apparent at birth. They typically become more prominent as the patient grows up, and the pronounced enlargement usually occurs from infancy to puberty; thereafter, less pronounced changes occur in adulthood [10].

Majority of LM is present at birth, with the remainder presenting by 2 years of age [11].

There are two common clinical types of pure lymphatic malformation (LM): lymphedema (diffuse LM) and lymphangioma (localized, macrocystic LM). Primary lymphedema is divided into three types by age of presentation: congenital familial lymphedema (Milroy's disease), lymphedema praecox (typically presents during adolescence), and lymphedema tarda (presents after 35 years of age). Macrocystic LMs (cystic hygroma) are usually visible at birth and may be detected by prenatal ultrasound examinations. They are frequently located on the neck, axilla, retroperitoneum, or mesentery. According to a review of 305 patients with lymphangioma in our group, their anatomic distribution was most prevalent at the head and neck (46.2 %) followed by trunk surface and extremity (44.6 %) and intra-abdominal or mediastinal (9.2 %) and showed male predilection by 1.4:1 [12].

More often, LM is combined with other forms of CVM such as VM, CM, or AVM.

Lee et al. [13] made a review on the subtypes of the LM separately among 1203 CVM patients. Predominant LM lesion accounted for 32.6 % of all patients with CVM which included 271 (69 %) patients with truncular LM and 122 (31 %) patients with extratruncular LM lesions. Of 122 patients with extratruncular LM, 89 (73 %) had the macrocystic type with a predilection for the head, neck, and thorax. Of the 271 patients with truncular LM, 247 (91 %) patients showed lymphatic channel aplasia or hypoplasia and a predilection to occur in the lower extremity. LM lesion presented as combined with VM in 9 % of 1203 CVM patients.

Table 5.1 shows the demographic features and distribution of CVM lesions according to the type of CVMs.

When we reviewed our registered 2971 CVM patients at Samsung Medical Center (SMC), VM

Table 5.1 Demographic features and anatomic distribution of CVM lesions in 2971 CVM in SMC (1992–2015)

	Number of CVM patients (%)				
	VM or venous predominant	AVM	LM or lymphatic predominant	CM only	Subtotal (%)
No (%)	1576 (53 %)	502 (17 %)	861 (29 %)	32 (1 %)	2971
Age[a], mean, year	7.0	13.8	10.3	1.6	
Male/female	1: 1.2	1: 1.2	1: 1.1	1: 1.3	
Anatomic distribution					
Extremity	921(58 %)	274(55 %)	439(51 %)	14(44 %)	1648(55 %)
Lower	667(42 %)	155(31 %)	339(39 %)	11(34 %)	1172(39 %)
Upper	254(16 %)	119(24 %)	100(12 %)	3(9 %)	476(16 %)
Head and neck	416(26 %)	169(34 %)	249(29 %)	12(38 %)	846(28 %)
Trunk[b]	139(9 %)	57(11 %)	124(14 %)	1(3 %)	321(11 %)
Multiple	100 (6 %)	2(0.4 %)	49(6 %)	5(16 %)	156(5 %)
		119(24 %)	53(10 %)		3(9.4 %)
		2(0.4 %)	41(7 %)		5(16 %)

Patients with AVM involving CNS or pure arterial malformation were not included in this table

Abbreviation: *VM* venous malformation, *AVM* arteriovenous malformation, *LM* lymphatic malformation, *CM* capillary malformation

[a]Age at the initial presentation

[b]Trunk indicates chest, abdomen, and pelvis

or venous predominant CVM was the most common type of CVM (53 %). Among the VM patients, the lower extremity was the most frequently affected site (42 %), followed by head and neck (26 %), upper extremity (16 %), trunk (9 %), and multiple site involvement (6 %). Among extremity VM patients, 93 % was extratruncular and 13 % was truncular form VM (see Table 15.2).

LM and lymphatic dominant CVM comprised of 29 % of all CVM patients. It was also most prevalent in the extremities (51 %) followed by head and neck (29 %) and trunk (14 %).

AVM accounted for 17 % of CVM patients and most frequently found in the extremities (55 %) followed by head and neck (34 %) and trunk (11 %) (Table 5.1).

AVM is known as the least common type of CVMs representing approximately 10–15 % of all clinically significant CVM lesions [14]. Among them, "extratruncular" form comprises the vast majority of AVM lesions. Most of the current data regarding the incidence and prevalence of AVMs include AVM lesion affecting CNS [15, 16]. Epidemiologic data of AVM lesion affecting CNS is beyond the scope of this chapter; therefore, we excluded AVM affecting CNS from the SMC data.

Regarding the age of an initial presentation, we found that patients with AVM or LM presented at later age than patients with VM or CM. And male/female ratio was close to 1:1 in general.

AVMs are also known to occur with equal frequency in males and females. About half of the AVM lesions are recognizable at birth, and 30 % become clinically apparent during childhood. They have a predilection to the head and neck area than in other locations [17].

AVM lesions take dynamic clinical courses so that Schobinger classified AVM lesions into four stages based on the clinical features: Stage I (quiescence), Stage II (expansion), Stage III (destruction), and Stage IV (decompensation) [18].

Significant numbers of the CVMs are also known to remain mixed forms of CVM (e.g., Klippel-Trenaunay syndrome and Parkes Weber syndrome).

A substantial number of angiogenesis-related genes (i.e., *TIE2, VEGFR-3, RASA1, KRIT1, MGC4607, PDCD10,* glomulin, *FOXC2, NEMO, SOX18, ENG, ACVRLK1, MADH4, NDP, TIMP3,*

Notch3, *COL3A1*, and *PTEN*) have been identified in the pathogenesis of vascular malformations to provide a new base for further scientific epidemiological evaluation; however, more insight is required on the involved molecular mechanisms, which may lead to the development of therapeutic strategies for treating Klippel-Trenaunay syndrome (KTS) [19].

At the moment, there is no racial, demographic, or environmental risk factors for CVMs have been identified to date.

References

1. Loane M, Dolk H, Garne E, Greenlees R. Paper 3: EUROCAT data quality indicators for population-based registries of congenital anomalies. Birth Defects Res Part A Clin Mol Teratol. 2011;91(Suppl 1):S23–30. doi:10.1002/bdra.20779.
2. Correa C, Mallarino C, Pena R, Rincon LC, Gracia G, Zarante I. Congenital malformations of pediatric surgical interest: prevalence, risk factors, and prenatal diagnosis between 2005 and 2012 in the capital city of a developing country. Bogota, Colombia. J Pediatr Surg. 2014;49(7):1099–103. doi:10.1016/j.jpedsurg.2014.03.001.
3. Kennedy WP. Epidemiologic aspects of the problem of congenital malformations. In: Persaud TNV, editor. Problems of birth defects. Baltimore: Publisher University Park Press; 1977. p. 35–52.
4. Belov S. Anatomopathological classification of congenital vascular defects. Semin Vasc Surg. 1993;6(4):219–24.
5. Lee BB, Laredo J, Lee SJ, Huh SH, Joe JH, Neville R. Congenital vascular malformations: general diagnostic principles. Phlebology/Venous Forum R Soc Med. 2007;22(6):253–7.
6. Tasnadi G. Epidemiology and etiology of congenital vascular malformations. Semin Vasc Surg. 1993;6(4):200–3.
7. Eifert S, Villavicencio JL, Kao TC, Taute BM, Rich NM. Prevalence of deep venous anomalies in congenital vascular malformations of venous predominance. J Vasc Surg. 2000;31(3):462–71.
8. Vikkula M, Boon LM, Mulliken JB. Molecular genetics of vascular malformations. Matrix Biol J Int Soc Matrix Biol. 2001;20(5–6):327–35.
9. Eerola I, Boon LM, Mulliken JB, Burrows PE, Dompmartin A, Watanabe S, Vanwijck R, Vikkula M. Capillary malformation-arteriovenous malformation, a new clinical and genetic disorder caused by RASA1 mutations. Am J Hum Genet. 2003;73(6):1240–9. doi:10.1086/379793.
10. Garzon MC, Huang JT, Enjolras O, Frieden IJ. Vascular malformations: part I. J Am Acad Dermatol. 2007;56(3):353–70. quiz 371-354 doi:10.1016/j.jaad.2006.05.069.
11. Redondo P. Classification of vascular anomalies (tumours and malformations). Clinical characteristics and natural history. An Sist Sanit Navar. 2004;27(Suppl 1):9–25.
12. Whang DB, Lee SH, Lim SY, Lee SG, Seo JM. Surgical treatment of difficult cervicofacial lymphangioma in children. J Korean Assoc Pediatr Surg. 2015;21:1–7. doi:10.13029/jkaps.2015.21.2.1.
13. Lee BB, Laredo J, Seo JM, Neville R. Treatment of lymphatic malformations. In: Mattassi R, Loose DA, Vaghi M, editors. Hemangiomas and vascular malformations. Milan: Publisher Springer-Verlag Italia; 2009. p. 231–50.
14. Lee BB, Baumgartner I, Berlien HP, Bianchini G, Burrows P, Do YS, Ivancev K, Kool LS, Laredo J, Loose DA, Lopez-Gutierrez JC, Mattassi R, Parsi K, Rimon U, Rosenblatt M, Shortell C, Simkin R, Stillo F, Villavicencio L, Yakes W. Consensus document of the International Union of Angiology (IUA)-2013. Current concept on the management of arterio-venous management. Int Angiol J Int Union Angiol. 2013;32(1):9–36.
15. Jackson JE, Mansfield AO, Allison DJ. Treatment of high-flow vascular malformations by venous embolization aided by flow occlusion techniques. Cardiovasc Intervent Radiol. 1996;19(5):323–8.
16. Al-Shahi R, Warlow C. A systematic review of the frequency and prognosis of arteriovenous malformations of the brain in adults. Brain J Neurol. 2001;124(Pt 10):1900–26.
17. Kohout MP, Hansen M, Pribaz JJ, Mulliken JB. Arteriovenous malformations of the head and neck: natural history and management. Plast Reconstr Surg. 1998;102(3):643–54.
18. Schobinger R. Proceeding of ISSVA congress, Roma; 1994.
19. Delis KT, Gloviczki P, Wennberg PW, Rooke TW. Driscoll DJ (2007) Hemodynamic impairment, venous segmental disease, and clinical severity scoring in limbs with Klippel-Trenaunay syndrome. J Vasc Surg. 2006;45(3):561–7.

Francine Blei

Congenital vascular malformations, which represent developmental abnormalities of vascular or development, may affect capillaries, veins, arteries, lymphatics, or any combination of these vascular channels. Characteristically, these lesions "grow in parallel with the growth of the patient." However, there are certain scenarios in which the vascular malformation can be "aggravated," generating unwanted symptoms and potential complications. Inciting factors include time, trauma, hormonal changes (puberty, the menstrual cycle, pregnancy), infection, thromboses, and surgical intervention. Unwanted associated symptoms include thromboses, bleeding, inflammation, increased size of lesions, functional impairment, tissue hypertrophy, hypertrophic nodules, pathologic fracture, and other morbidities.

Tissue Overgrowth

Capillary malformations generally remain macular for many years; however with time, soft tissue, gingival, and skeletal overgrowth, as well as lesional thickening and nodules, can develop [1–4]. The soft tissue overgrowth occurs in the region of the capillary malformation, predominantly in the V2 distribution, and one study

suggests the onset may be delayed with early pulsed dye laser treatment [4]. The exact mechanism of the above progression is not fully understood; however, the provoking factor for capillary malformations to evolve as described is *time*, since the incidence of hypertrophy and lesional changes increases with age. Tark et al. observed histologic findings suggestive of arteriovenous malformations in resected hypertrophic nodules from adults with longstanding capillary malformations [5]. These later-stage lesions are resistant to pulsed dye laser treatment, in contrast to laser in infants, which has been shown to achieve a more favorable response [6].

Hormonal Changes: Puberty, Menstrual Cycle, and Pregnancy

Vascular malformations may remain quiescent for years, and then patients may notice a sense of fullness and intermittent pain, which may progress. Frequently this correlates with peripubertal changes. The onset of puberty is preceded biochemically by hormonal changes, which may affect a vascular malformation, manifesting as pain or discomfort. Recent evidence suggests the onset of pubertal development is occurring earlier [7–9]. The circulating hormones may trigger signs of puberty and accompanying problems in patients with vascular malformations. Kulungowski et al. reviewed hormone receptor expression in vessels of vascular malformations (arteriovenous,

F. Blei, MD, MBA
Northwell Health System, Lenox Hill Hospital,
New York, NY, USA
e-mail: francine.blei@gmail.com

lymphatic, and venous) and found increased expression of growth hormone receptor, speculating that this may be contributory to puberty-related changes in vascular malformations [10]. Patients may notice increased fullness, pain, and cyclical changes associated with the menstrual cycle. "Growth spurts" during puberty may also magnify limb length discrepancies. The use of estrogen-containing birth control pills may lead to unwanted thromboses, especially in women with a predisposing thrombophilia [11].

Pregnancy poses many challenges to patients with vascular malformations, especially lower extremity malformations. Pregnancy related complications have been studied in women with hereditary hemorrhagic telangiectasia. The rates of miscarriage and congenital anomalies were considered to be comparable to that of the general population. Wain et al. reported the results of a survey of 560 pregnancies in 226 patients with HHT [12], and De Gussem and colleagues reported the results of a retrospective study via telephone interviews of 87 women with HHT (representing 244 pregnancies) [13]. Hemothorax (2.1 %), hemoptysis (1.1 %), transient ischemic attack (possibly from a paradoxical embolus), intracranial hemorrhage, cardiac failure (in patients with hepatic AVMs), increased telangiectasias, and epistaxis were described [12–14].

Pregnancy-related complications such as intrapartum/peripartum hemorrhage and/or thrombosis, increased varicosities (e.g., vulvar), and seizures have been described in women with Klippel-Trenaunay syndrome [15–18]. Successful pregnancies in women with Klippel-Trenaunay syndrome have been reported [19, 20]; however, precautions such as prophylactic anticoagulation and high-risk surveillance are recommended [21, 22]. Anatomic variations such as May-Thurner syndrome place women at increased risk of thrombosis, especially in the setting of pregnancy, immobilization, or exposure to estrogen-containing birth control pills [11, 23, 24]. Prophylactic anticoagulation should therefore be considered in such patients.

Although the risk of intracerebral hemorrhage from intracerebral vascular malformations in pregnancy is rare, it is generally appreciated that pregnancy increases the hemorrhagic risk of AVM. In one case report, a pregnant woman with a developmental venous anomaly experienced a neurologic event, presumably due to dehydration-related thrombosis with secondary hemorrhage [25, 26].

Trauma

Trauma to a vascular malformation may cause infection, bleeding, thrombosis, fracture, or other problems. Some patients report lymphedema following sports trauma. This may be related to damage to fragile subcutaneous lymphatic vessels, e.g., in the shins.

Iatrogenic Provoking Factors: Surgery and Endovascular Therapy

Boccara et al. investigated if surgical intervention may provoke clinical aggravation of lymphatic malformations (LM) in pediatric patients. This retrospective review of 26 cases revealed that postoperative delayed wound healing, lymphatic oozing, and functional impairment were frequent [27]. Additionally, Trenor and Chaudry warn that rib biopsy can induce chronic pleural effusion in patients with complicated lymphatic anomalies [28]. Patients with vascular anomalies associated with profound thrombocytopenia (e.g., Kasabach-Merritt phenomenon in Kaposiform Hemangioendothelioma) are at risk of bleeding; thus, biopsy of these lesions and surgical intervention overall should be performed with caution.

Careful planning and staged interventional procedures by experienced interventional radiologists can abrogate serious treatment-related complications. In one series of 116 evaluable patients with venous malformations who underwent sclerotherapy with alcohol and/or sodium tetradecyl sulfate, the complications included peripheral nerve injury, deep vein thrombosis, muscle contracture, infection, skin necrosis, and others, most of which ultimately resolved [29]. Pulmonary embolism, hemoglobinuria, renal complications and coagulopathy, contour deformities, and hyperpigmentation (following bleomycin sclerotherapy) have also been reported as possible sequelae from sclerotherapy [30–34]. Foam sclerotherapy is noted to have a lower complication rate, and alcohol the highest [33, 35, 36].

Delayed wound healing, wound dehiscence, and recurrence were the most common sequelae of surgical intervention for vascular anomalies of the vermilion in a series of 38 patients [37].

In summary, there are many potential "provoking factors" which can aggravate congenital vascular malformations. It is essential to be aware of these issues and to mitigate complications when feasible.

Bibliography

1. Geronemus RG, Ashinoff R. The medical necessity of evaluation and treatment of port-wine stains. J Dermatol Surg Oncol. 1991;17(1):76–9.
2. Greene AK, Taber SF, Ball KL, Padwa BL, Mulliken JB. Sturge-Weber syndrome: soft-tissue and skeletal overgrowth. J Craniofac Surg. 2009;20(Suppl 1): 617–21.
3. van Drooge AM, de Rie M, van der Veen W, Wolkerstorfer A. Port-wine stain progression: is prevention by pulsed dye laser therapy possible? Eur J Dermatol. 2013;23(2):282–3.
4. Lee JW, Chung HY, Cerrati EW, March TM, Waner M. The natural history of soft tissue hypertrophy, bony hypertrophy, and nodule formation in patients with untreated head and neck capillary malformations. Dermatol Surg. 2015;41(11):1241–5.
5. Tark KC, Lew DH, Lee DW. The fate of long-standing port-wine stain and its surgical management. Plast Reconstr Surg. 2011;127(2):784–91.
6. Brightman LA, Geronemus RG, Reddy KK. Laser treatment of port-wine stains. Clin Cosmet Investig Dermatol. 2015;8:27–33.
7. Herman-Giddens ME. Recent data on pubertal milestones in United States children: the secular trend toward earlier development. Int J Androl. 2006;29(1): 241–6. ; discussion 86-90
8. Herman-Giddens ME, Steffes J, Harris D, Slora E, Hussey M, Dowshen SA, et al. Secondary sexual characteristics in boys: data from the Pediatric Research in Office Settings Network. Pediatrics. 2012;130(5):e1058–68.
9. Kaplowitz P. Update on precocious puberty: girls are showing signs of puberty earlier, but most do not require treatment. Adv Pediatr. 2011;58(1):243–58.
10. Kulungowski AM, Hassanein AH, Nose V, Fishman SJ, Mulliken JB, Upton J, et al. Expression of androgen,

11. estrogen, progesterone, and growth hormone receptors in vascular malformations. Plast Reconstr Surg. 2012;129(6):919e–24e.
11. Hughes RL, Collins KA, Sullivan KE. A case of fatal iliac vein rupture associated with May-Thurner syndrome. Am J Forensic Med Pathol. 2013;34(3):222–4.
12. Wain K, Swanson K, Watson W, Jeavons E, Weaver A, Lindor N. Hereditary hemorrhagic telangiectasia and risks for adverse pregnancy outcomes. Am J Med Genet A. 2012;158A(8):2009–14.
13. de Gussem EM, Lausman AY, Beder AJ, Edwards CP, Blanker MH, Terbrugge KG, et al. Outcomes of pregnancy in women with hereditary hemorrhagic telangiectasia. Obstet Gynecol. 2014;123(3):514–20.
14. Berthelot E, Savale L, Guyot A, Rahmoune FC, Bouchachi A, Assayag P. Acute high output heart failure revealing hereditary hemorrhagic telangiectasia in a pregnant woman. Presse Med. 2015;44(3):362–5.
15. Yara N, Masamoto H, Iraha Y, Wakayama A, Chinen Y, Nitta H, et al. Diffuse venous malformation of the uterus in a pregnant woman with Klippel-Trenaunay syndrome diagnosed by DCE-MRI. Case Rep Obstet Gynecol. 2016;2016:4328450.
16. Gonzalez-Mesa E, Blasco M, Anderica J, Herrera J. Klippel-Trenaunay syndrome complicating pregnancy. BMJ Case Rep. 2012;2012
17. Gungor Gundogan T, Jacquemyn Y. Klippel-trenaunay syndrome and pregnancy. Obstet Gynecol Int. 2010; 2010:706850.
18. Koch A, Aissi G, Gaudineau A, Sananes N, Murtada R, Favre R, et al. Klippel-Trenaunay syndrome and pregnancy: difficult choice of delivery from a case and a review of the literature. J Gynecol Obstet Biol Reprod (Paris). 2014;43(7):483–7.
19. Kemfang JD, Dobgima WP, Motzebo RM, Ngassam A, Fokou M, Kasia JM. Successful management of pregnancy in an African woman with Klippel Trenaunay syndrome. Pan Afr Med J. 2013;16:99.
20. Atis A, Ozdemir G, Tuncer G, Cetincelik U, Goker N, Ozsoy S. Management of a Klippel-Trenaunay syndrome in pregnant women with mega-cisterna magna and splenic and vulvar varices at birth: a case report. J Obstet Gynaecol Res. 2012;38(11):1331–4.
21. Martin JR, Pels SG, Paidas M, Seli E. Assisted reproduction in a patient with Klippel-Trenaunay syndrome: management of thrombophilia and consumptive coagulopathy. J Assist Reprod Genet. 2011;28(3):217–9.
22. Rebarber A, Roman AS, Roshan D, Blei F. Obstetric management of Klippel-Trenaunay syndrome. Obstet Gynecol. 2004;104(5 Pt 2):1205–8.
23. DeStephano CC, Werner EF, Holly BP, Lessne ML. Diagnosis and management of iliac vein thrombosis in pregnancy resulting from May-Thurner syndrome. J Perinatol. 2014;34(7):566–8.
24. Wax JR, Pinette MG, Rausch D, Cartin A. May-Thurner syndrome complicating pregnancy: a report of four cases. J Reprod Med. 2014;59(5–6):333–6.
25. Lv X, Li Y. The clinical characteristics and treatment of cerebral AVM in pregnancy. Neuroradiol J. 2015; 28(4):385–8.

26. Seki M, Shibata M, Itoh Y, Suzuki N. Intracerebral hemorrhage due to venous thrombosis of developmental venous anomaly during pregnancy. J Stroke Cerebrovasc Dis. 2015;24(7):e185–7.

27. Boccara O, Chrétien-Marquet B, Pannier S, Guéro S, Khen-Dunlop N, Hadj-Rabia S, et al. Is surgery a triggering factor for clinical worsening of lymphatic malformations? 21st Workshop, International Society for the Study of Vascular Anomalies (ISSVA); April 26–29, 2016. Argentina: Buenos Aires; 2016.

28. Trenor 3rd CC, Chaudry G. Complex lymphatic anomalies. Semin Pediatr Surg. 2014;23(4): 186–90.

29. Ali S, Weiss CR, Sinha A, Eng J, Mitchell SE. The treatment of venous malformations with percutaneous sclerotherapy at a single academic medical center. Phlebology. 2016;31(9):603–9.

30. Burrows PE. Endovascular treatment of slow-flow vascular malformations. Tech Vasc Interv Radiol. 2013;16(1):12–21.

31. Qiu Y, Chen H, Lin X, Hu X, Jin Y, Ma G. Outcomes and complications of sclerotherapy for venous malformations. Vasc Endovascular Surg. 2013;47(6): 454–61.

32. van der Vleuten CJ, Kater A, Wijnen MH, Schultze Kool LJ, Rovers MM. Effectiveness of sclerotherapy, surgery, and laser therapy in patients with venous malformations: a systematic review. Cardiovasc Intervent Radiol. 2014;37(4):977–89.

33. Aronniemi J, Castrén E, Lappalainen K, Vuola P, Salminen P, Pitkäranta A, Pekkola J. Sclerotherapy complications of peripheral venous malformations. Phlebology. 2015. [Epub ahead of print]

34. Mohan AT, Adams S, Adams K, Hudson DA. Intralesional bleomycin injection in management of low flow vascular malformations in children. J Plast Surg Hand Surg. 2015;49(2):116–20.

35. Rabe E, Pannier F. Sclerotherapy in venous malformation. Phlebology. 2013;28(Suppl 1):188–91.

36. Horbach SE, Lokhorst MM, Saeed P, de Gouyon Matignon de Pontouraude CM, Rothova A, van der Horst CM. Sclerotherapy for low-flow vascular malformations of the head and neck: a systematic review of sclerosing agents. J Plast Reconstr Aesthet Surg. 2016;69(3):295–304.

37. Park SM, Bae YC, Lee JW, Kim HS, Lee IS. Outcomes of surgical treatment of vascular anomalies on the vermilion. Arch Plast Surg. 2016;43(1):19–25.

Part III

Classification and Definition/Nomenclature

Byung-Boong Lee, James Laredo,
and Richard Neville

Congenital vascular malformations (CVMs) represent a group of "birth defects" involving the circulation – arterial, venous, lymphatic, and capillary – systems as a result of defective development that has occurred during embryogenesis (vasculogenesis/angiogenesis) [1, 2]. Hence, the CVM may present at different locations anywhere throughout the body in different conditions, shapes, extents, and severities as independent lesion (e.g., venous malformation) or as a mixed lesion with two or three different types of CVMs (e.g., hemolymphatic malformation) with different characteristics and behaviors [1–4].

B.-B. Lee, MD, PhD, FACS (✉)
Professor of Surgery and Director, Center for the Lymphedema and Vascular Malformations, George Washington University, Washington, DC, USA

Adjunct Professor of Surgery, Uniformed Services, University of the Health Sciences, Bethesda, MD, USA
e-mail: bblee38@gmail.com

J. Laredo, MD
Division of Vascular Surgery, Department of Surgery, George Washington University Medical Center, Washington, DC, USA

R. Neville, MD
Department of Surgery, Division of Vascular Surgery, George Washington University Medical Center, Washington, DC, USA

The CVM remains an enigma among the vascular disorders as a most difficult and confusing diagnostic and therapeutic clinical entity with a wide range of clinical presentations. It has a notorious reputation for extreme variety and degree of severity and location, as well as unpredictable clinical course and erratic response to treatment with high recurrence due to its embryonic characteristics.

To add more confusion, most CVMs were initially described based on the clinical findings alone and named after the clinicians who described them (e.g., Klippel-Trenaunay syndrome). These name-based eponyms (e.g., Servelle-Martorell syndrome; Sturge-Weber-Krabbe syndrome) failed to define the critical characteristics among the CVMs and provide proper anatomical and pathophysiological information on such complicated CVMs [5–8].

The old classification did not take into account the etiology, anatomy, and pathophysiology and often led to misguided and mistaken terminology (e.g., cavernous/capillary hemangioma versus infantile/neonatal hemangioma) [9, 10]. A new classification system was required to provide accurate anatomic, embryologic, and pathophysiologic information of the CVMs to allow appropriate diagnosis and treatment [11–14].

A consensus workshop held in Hamburg in 1988 was the beginning of a new, more logical classification system to replace the old name-based eponyms and meet the needs of physicians for contemporary management of the CVMs [2–4, 15, 16].

© Springer-Verlag Berlin Heidelberg 2017
Y.-W. Kim et al. (eds.), *Congenital Vascular Malformations*, DOI 10.1007/978-3-662-46709-1_7

Two new classifications were developed following the Hamburg Consensus. Both allowed precise evaluation, diagnosis, and therapeutic implementation: Hamburg classification [17–20] and ISSVA[1] classification [21–24].

Hamburg Classification [17–20]

Malan and Puglionisi proposed a new classification to distinguish the different venous, arterial, and other associated malformations [11–14], which served as the basis of the Hamburg classification and ISSVA classification. They identified two different types of lesions based on involvement of the main vessel trunks. Lesions with a direct communication with the main vessel trunks were known as "truncular" forms, and lesions occurring peripherally as separate defects were known as "arteriovenous angiomas."

Further, Belov et al. reintroduced an old embryologic term "extratruncular" borrowed from the old embryology school [25] to describe lesions consisting of vascular tissue clusters that were derived from the "early stage" of embryogenesis [17–20]. He further insisted that the use of the often misleading old term of "angioma" (c.f. hemangioma) be discontinued.

They also borrowed the term "truncular" [26] to describe lesions that directly involved the "named" vessels and were a result of defective development occurring during the "later" stage of vascular trunk formation [1–4].

The Hamburg classification, which was formulated as a new system based on the consensus through the Hamburg workshop, accommodated a new interpretation of the CVM lesions as an outcome of the developmental arrest of the vascular system during two different stages of angiogenesis. This new definition based on embryological characteristics of the CVMs later became known as the "modified" Hamburg classification [2–4, 24–27].

The Hamburg classification distinguished the morphological differences between CVM lesions

involving the main vessel trunks and lesions, previously called "angioma," remaining peripherally with no direct involvement of the vessel trunk [28–31].

Extratruncular lesions are vascular defects arising from the "earlier" stages of embryogenesis where the primitive vascular structures are still in the reticular plexiform stage and consist of an "undifferentiated capillary network" [8, 9, 32–35]. These defects present as a cluster of amorphous vascular tissue. *Truncular* lesions are the result of defective development that occurs during the "later" stages of embryogenesis where they are remnants of preexisting vascular structures [30, 31, 36, 37].

According to this embryologic concept, the worsening of CVM lesions would depend on the type of the (endothelial) cells present as the remnants of the primitive capillary network. These cells maintain the ability to grow and proliferate and may exhibit unpredictable biological behavior. [2].

Recent data on genetic mutations involving vascular malformation pathogenesis has brought additional confusion on the relationship between vessel embryology and genetic mutations affecting vessel development [2–4]. The process of vasculogenesis and the classification of vascular defects based on morphology and anatomical and pathological characteristics will remain the same regardless of the genetic mutation involved.

ISSVA Classification [21–24]

Mulliken et al. also introduced another classification system based on the Hamburg consensus. While the Hamburg classification is limited to vascular malformations, this system classifies all types of vascular anomalies – both tumors and vascular malformations [21–24]. In addition, a new classification of the CVMs was made based on the flow characteristics: fast-flow and slow-flow lesions. This new classification was subsequently adopted by ISSVA (International Society for the Study of Vascular Anomalies) officially as the ISSVA classification (1996) [2–4, 34, 35, 38, 39].

---

[1]ISSVA: International Society for the Study of Vascular Anomalies.

By ISSVA classification the term "hemangioma" was correctly defined for the first time as it had been frequently misused to describe CVMs (e.g., "cavernous/capillary" hemangioma) over many decades. The hemangioma is defined as a "vascular tumor" of benign nature that originates from endothelial cells. The term hemangioma should represent the "infantile/neonatal" hemangioma and "congenital" hemangioma as classified through ISSVA classification. [9, 10].

Vascular malformation and hemangiomas are two entirely different vascular disorders with distinct anatomical, histological and pathophysiological characteristics, and clinical behavior. Both are classified as "vascular anomalies" in ISSVA classification [21–24, 34, 35, 38, 39].

CVM is the result of defective embryologic development, an inborn vascular defect that is generally recognizable at birth and continues to grow at a rate that is proportional to the growth rate of the body regardless of its type and will never regress.

On the other hand, a "hemangioma" is a vascular tumor that originates from the endothelial cells and usually appears in the early neonatal period. Hemangioma has a distinctive growth cycle characterized by a proliferation phase of early rapid growth followed by an involutional phase of slow regression [34, 35, 38, 39]. Hence, a hemangioma has "self-limited" growth followed by subsequent involution that usually occurs before the age of 5–10 years in the majority of cases. CVMs exhibit "self-perpetuating" growth as embryologic tissue remnants.

ISSVA classification further classified the CVMs based on the flow status: fast and slow flow. The arteriovenous malformation (AVM) was further subclassified to "AV Fistula and AV malformation," both of which represent [21] AVMs that are derived from two different stages of embryogenesis as appropriately classified by the Hamburg classification.

ISSVA classification ignored the critical difference between truncular and extratruncular forms and failed to recognize one of two morphologically and functionally different groups of CVMs properly: "truncular" CVM lesion which was defined by Woolard (1922) based on the

embryological concept with the two stages of embryogenesis [26].

Based on the subclassification of the AVM by ISSVA classification into "AV fistula (AVF) and AV malformation (AVM)," many clinicians interpret erroneously there are two different AVMs, fistulous and non-fistulous, and mistakenly identify the AVM group defined by ISSVA classification as a "non-fistulous" lesion. [4, 16, 40].

The "AVF" lesion defined by ISSVA classification is equivalent to the "truncular" AVM lesion with no nidus (e.g., ductus Botalli, pulmonary AVM) defined by the Hamburg classification. The "AVM" defined by ISSVA classification is equivalent to the "extratruncular" AVM lesion with nidus defined by the Hamburg classification [16, 40].

In addition, the ISSVA classification still uses all of the preexisting name-based classifications and syndromes which were strongly advocated to be abandoned by many experts in order to reduce confusion (e.g., Hamburg consensus workshop of 1988). This remains a major controversy and possible weakness of this excellent classification system [2, 16].

The complexity of the ISSVA classification and continued use of numerous name-based syndromes as a part of a new CVM classification has limited its utility in clinical practice and implementation in the management of CVMs, although its major advantage remains in differentiating vascular tumors/hemangiomas from CVMs [2].

The current classification systems are far from the perfect, and further modification will be necessary as our knowledge of the etiology, anatomy, embryology, histopathophysiology, hemodynamics, and genetics of the CVMs continues to grow [2].

References

1. Lee BB, Laredo J, Lee TS, Huh S, Neville R. Terminology and classification of congenital vascular malformations. Phlebology. 2007;22(6):249–52.
2. Lee BB, Baumgartner I, Berlien P, Bianchini G, Burrows P, Gloviczki P, Huang Y, Laredo J, Loose DA, Markovic J, Mattassi R, Parsi K, Rabe E, Rosenblatt M, Shortell C, Stillo F, Vaghi M, Villavicencio L,

Zamboni P. Diagnosis and treatment of venous malformations consensus document of the International Union of Phlebology (IUP): updated 2013. Int Angiol. 2015;34(2):97–149.

3. Lee BB, Antignani PL, Baraldini V, Baumgartner I, Berlien P, Blei F, Carrafiello GP, Grantzow R, Ianniello A, Laredo J, Loose D, Lopez Gutierrez JC, Markovic J, Mattassi R, Parsi K, Rabe E, Roztocil K, Shortell C, Vaghi M. ISVI-IUA consensus document – diagnostic guidelines on vascular anomalies: vascular malformations and hemangiomas. Int Angiol. 2015;34(4):333–74.

4. Lee BB, Baumgartner I, Berlien HP, Bianchini G, Burrows P, Do YS, Ivancev K, Kool LS, Laredo J, Loose DA, Lopez-Gutierrez JC, Mattassi R, Parsi K, Rimon U, Rosenblatt M, Shortell C, Simkin R, Stillo F, Villavicencio L, Yakes W. Consensus Document of the International Union of Angiology (IUA)-2013. Current concept on the management of arterio-venous management. Int Angiol. 2013;32(1): 9–36.

5. Lee BB, Laredo J, Lee SJ, Huh SH, Joe JH, Neville R. Congenital vascular malformations: general diagnostic principles. Phlebology. 2007;22(6):253–7.

6. Lee BB. Changing concept on vascular malformation: no longer Enigma. Ann Vasc Dis. 2008;1(1):11–9.

7. Lee BB, Kim HH, Mattassi R, Yakes W, Loose D, Tasnadi G. A new approach to the congenital vascular malformation with a new concept: how the pioneer Prof. Stefan Belov enlightened us through the Seoul consensus. Int J Angiol. 2003;12:248–51.

8. Lee BB. Critical issues on the management of congenital vascular malformation. Ann Vasc Surg. 2004;18(3):380–92.

9. Lee BB. Venous malformation and haemangioma: differential diagnosis, diagnosis, natural history and consequences. Phlebology. 2013;28(Suppl 1):176–87.

10. Lee BB, Laredo J. Hemangioma and venous/vascular malformation are different as an apple and orange! Editorial. Acta Phlebol. 2012;13:1–3.

11. Malan E, Puglionisi A. Congenital angiodysplasias of the extremities, note II: arterial, arterial and venous, and hemolymphatic dysplasias. J Cardiovasc Surg (Torino). 1965;6:255–345.

12. Malan E. History and nosography. In: Malan E, editor. Vascular malformations (Angiodysplasias). Milan: Carlo Erba Foundation; 1974. p. 15–9.

13. Villavicencio JL. Congenital Vascular malformations: historical background. Special Issue: Phlebology. 2007;22:247–8.

14. Malan E, Puglionisi A. Congenital angiodysplasia of the extremities. J Card Surg. 1964;5:87–130.

15. Lee BB, Laredo J. Classification of congenital vascular malformations: the last challenge for congenital vascular malformations. Phlebology. 2012;27(6): 267–9.

16. Lee BB. New classification of congenital vascular malformations (CVMs). Rev Vasc Med. 2015;3(3): 1–5.

17. Belov S. Classification of congenital vascular defects. Int Angiol. 1990;9:141–6.

18. Belov S. Classification, terminology, and nosology of congenital vascular defects. In: Belov S, Loose DA, Weber J, editors. Vascular malformations. Reinbek: Einhorn-Presse; 1989. p. 25–30.

19. Belov S. Anatomopathological classification of congenital vascular defects. Semin Vasc Surg. 1993;6:219–24.

20. Van Der Stricht J. Classification of vascular malformations. In: ST B, DA L, Weber J, editors. Vascular malformations. Reinbek: Einhorn-Presse Verlag GmbH; 1989. p. 23.

21. Enjolras O, Wassef M, Chapot R. Introduction: ISSVA classification. In: Color atlas of vascular tumors and vascular malformations. New York: Cambridge University Press; 2007. p. 1–11.

22. Mulliken JB, Glowacki J. Hemangiomas and vascular malformations in infants and children: a classification based on endothelial characteristics. Plast Reconstr Surg. 1982;69:412–22.

23. Mulliken JB, Zetter BR, Folkman J. In vivo characteristics of endothelium from hemangiomas and vascular malformations. Surgery. 1982;92:348–53.

24. Mulliken JB. Classification of vascular birthmarks. In: Mulliken JB, Young AE, editors. Vascular birthmarks: hemangiomas and malformations. Philadelphia: WB Saunders; 1988. p. 24–37.

25. Sabin FR. Origin and development of the primitive vessels of the chick and of the pig. Cont Embriol Carnegie Inst. 1917;6–7:61–7.

26. Woolard HH. The development of the principal arterial stems in the forelimb of the pig. Contrib Embryol. 1922;14:139–54.

27. Bastide G, Lefebvre D. Anatomy and organogenesis and vascular malformations. In: Belov S, Loose DA, Weber J, editors. Vascular Malformations. Reinbek: Einhorn-Presse Verlag GmbH; 1989. p. 20–2.

28. Lee BB, Laredo J. Venous malformation: treatment needs a bird's eye view. Phlebology. 2013;28:62–3.

29. Lee BB, Bergan J, Gloviczki P, Laredo J, Loose DA, Mattassi R, Parsi K, Villavicencio JL, Zamboni P. Diagnosis and treatment of venous malformations – Consensus Document of the International Union of Phlebology (IUP)-2009. Int Angiol. 2009;28(6): 434–51.

30. Leu HJ. Pathoanatomy of congenital vascular malformations. In: Belov S, Loose DA, Weber J, editors. Vascular malformations, vol. 16. Reinbek: Einhorn-Presse Verlag; 1989. p. 37–46.

31. Lewis FT. Development of the veins in the limbs of rabbit embryos. Am J Anat. 1906;5:113–20.

32. Lee BB, Laredo J, Kim YW, Neville R. Congenital vascular malformations: general treatment principles. Phlebology. 2007;22(6):258–63.

33. Lee BB. Advanced management of congenital vascular malformation (CVM). Int Angiol. 2002;21(3): 209–13.

34. Mulliken JB. Cutaneous vascular anomalies. Semin Vasc Surg. 1993;6:204–18.

35. Boon LM, Enjolras O, Mulliken JB. Congenital hemangioma: evidence of accelerated involution. J Pediatr. 1996;128:329–35.
36. Lee BB. Venous embryology: the key to understanding anomalous venous conditions. Phlebolymphology. 2012;19(4):170–81.
37. Lee BB, Laredo J, Neville R. Embryological background of truncular venous malformation in the extracranial venous pathways as the cause of chronic cerebrospinal venous insufficiency. Int Angiol. 2010;29(2):95–108.
38. Enjolras O, Riche MC, Merland JJ, Escandej P. Management of alarming hemangiomas in infancy: a review of 25 cases. Pediatrics. 1990;85:491–8.
39. Mulliken JB. Treatment of hemangiomas. In: Mulliken JB, Young AE, editors. Vascular birthmarks, hemangiomas and malformations. Philadelphia: WB Saunders; 1988. p. 88–90.
40. Lee BB, Lardeo J, Neville R. Arterio-venous malformation: how much do we know? Phlebology. 2009;24:193–200.

Francine Blei

Introduction

Observations of human vascular anatomy initially described the normal vascular trees and anastomoses. The cardiovascular system materializes early in embryologic development, and much research has been focused on understanding the interplay among the various cell types and physiologic functions of the vasculature. Descriptive analyses of normal vascular development dominated early medical texts, with appreciation of the "closed circulation" model by William Harvey in the seventh century. Along with the recognition of diseases and human physiology was a growing interest in the vasculature [2–4]. Early appreciation of the cellular components of the vasculature became apparent in the nineteenth century, with anatomists, embryologists, and physiologists pioneering the notion of germ layers and, later, the cellular basis of disease. Virchow is credited as the first to describe a vascular lesion as an "angioma," a term which has been used indiscriminately to describe vascular lesions [2]. William His is attributed as the first to describe the "endothelium" (1865), and researchers focused on evolution of normal vascular differentiation [5]. Early

in the twentieth century, Sabin theorized that the hemangioblast was the source of both endothelial and hematopoietic cells and also suggested that the primitive lymphatic system was derived from the venous system, a theory which has been substantiated with more sophisticated investigations [6–8]. Early theories of arterial and venous lymphatic vascular development were later augmented by observations of vascular dysplasias. Malan and Puglionisi, in the mid-twentieth century, described angiodysplasias of the extremities [9, 10], and in 1982 Mulliken and Glowacki published their seminal paper separating vascular anomalies (based on clinical and cellular features) into vascular malformations and hemangiomas [1].

A small assemblage of interested specialists created a working group to understand vascular anomalies. This eventually led to the establishment of the International Society for the Study of Vascular Anomalies (ISSVA; www.issva.org), currently with >200 members, comprised of clinicians and researchers in multiple medical disciplines from many continents. With biennial workshops, the membership established a classification based on the original Mulliken schema which was updated to expand the initial separation into proliferative vascular lesions and vascular malformations. This classification was informally updated in 2007 by Wassef and Enjolras, who added additional diagnoses (e.g., congenital hemangiomas, kaposiform hemangioendothelioma, and others) and replaced eponymous diagnoses with names of

F. Blei, MD, MBA
Northwell Health System, Lenox Hill Hospital,
NY, New York, USA
e-mail: fblei@northwell.edu

© Springer-Verlag Berlin Heidelberg 2017
Y.-W. Kim et al. (eds.), *Congenital Vascular Malformations*, DOI 10.1007/978-3-662-46709-1_8

the involved vessels (e.g., Klippel-Trenaunay syndrome → capillary, venous, and/or lymphatic malformation ± hypertrophy) [11].

Since that time, the classification became outdated, as additional information became recognized – such as additional diagnoses, the significance of anatomic configuration (e.g., segmental distribution), and genetic mutations in some patients with vascular anomalies.

Acknowledging the need to further update the classification of vascular anomalies, a revised classification was established, which integrates the knowledge which has been acquired in this discipline. The updated ISSVA Classification of Vascular Anomalies ©2014 International Society for the Study of Vascular Anomalies is available at "issva.org/classification." A detailed explanation of the classification was also published, which provides a more comprehensive description of each diagnostic category and the history of the classification schemes [12].

The ISSVA Classification of Vascular Anomalies ©2014 is organized as a series of 20 interrelated slides, and the information will be updated as necessary. The initial slide (Table 8.1) highlights the fundamental separation of vascular anomalies into two overall categories, vascular tumors and vascular malformations. Subsequent slides expound upon each diagnostic category, with further explanations in Appendix slides. For those lesions with an associated genetic mutation, a hyperlink can be accessed by clicking on the turquoise letter *G*, which links to a subsequent slide in the Appendix, listing the genes associated with the entity. Likewise, for those diagnoses which are expounded upon, by clicking on the *underlined turquoise text*, one is taken to the relevant slides later in the deck. Table 8.2 lists the content of each slide in the updated classification. Tables 8.3 and 8.4 provide examples of the inclusion of the specific elements which have been added to the vascular tumors section, distinguishing benign, locally aggressive, and malignant entities and including morphologic pattern, type, and association with other structural and/or developmental anomalies.

Readers are referred to a detailed description of this classification published by ISSVA members in 2014 [12]. With this framework available, it is anticipated that the medical community can communicate with a uniform terminology and ameliorate the state of misinformation and confusion that has historically dominated "vascular anomalies," a field which is gradually being integrated into medical training curricula.

Acknowledgments The author is grateful for the patients with vascular anomalies, their families, and colleagues who participate in the care of and research in this field.

Table 8.1 ISSVA classification of vascular anomalies, 2014 (Copyright licensed under Creative Commons)

| | Vascular anomalies | | | |
| | Vascular malformations | | | |
Vascular tumors	Simple	Combined	Of major named vessels	Associated with other anomalies
Benign Locally aggressive or borderline Malignant	Capillary malformations Lymphatic malformations Venous malformations Arteriovenous malformations Arteriovenous fistula	Capillary-venous, capillary-lymphatic, lymphatic venous, capillary-lymphatic-venous, capillary-arteriovenous, capillary-lymphatic-arteriovenous	(Aka "channel-type" or "truncal" vascular malformations) Further characterized by involvement of artery, lymphatic, or vein and by anomaly of origin, course, number, length, diameter, etc.	For example, Klippel-Trenaunay Sturge-Weber Mafucci CLOVES Proteus Bannayan-Riley-Ruvalcaba Others

issva.org/classification for the interactive comprehensive classification

Table 8.2 Topics for each slide in the 2014 ISSVA Classification

Slide 1	Vascular anomalies	Vascular tumors and vascular malformations
Slide 2	Vascular tumors	Benign, locally aggressive or borderline, malignant
Slide 3	Simple vascular malformations I	Capillary malformations
Slide 4	Simple vascular malformations II	Lymphatic malformations
Slide 5	Simple vascular malformations IIb	Primary lymphedema
Slide 6	Simple vascular malformations III	Venous malformations
Slide 7	Simple vascular malformations IV	Arteriovenous malformations and arteriovenous fistulae
Slide 8	Combined vascular malformations	≥2 vascular malformations in one lesion
Slide 9	Anomalies of major named vessels	"Channel-type," "truncal" vascular malformations
Slide 10	Vascular malformations associated with other anomalies	
Slide 11	Provisionally unclassified vascular anomalies	
Slide 12	Appendix 1	Abbreviations used
Slide 13	Appendix 2a	Causal genes of vascular anomalies – capillary malformations
Slide 14	Appendix 2b	Causal genes of vascular anomalies – lymphatic malformations
Slide 15	Appendix 2c	Causal genes of vascular anomalies – venous malformations
Slide 16	Appendix 2d	Causal genes of vascular anomalies – arteriovenous malformations and arteriovenous fistulae
Slide 17	Appendix 2e	Causal genes of vascular anomalies associated with other anomalies
Slide 18	Appendix 2f	Causal genes of provisionally unclassified vascular anomalies
Slide 19	Appendix 3	Infantile hemangiomas – different patterns, types, and associations with other lesions
Slide 20	Appendix 4	Vascular anomalies possibly associated with platelet count/coagulation disorders

Table 8.3 ISSVA classification of vascular tumors, 2014 (Copyright licensed under creative commons)

Benign vascular tumors	
Infantile hemangioma/hemangioma of infancy	
Congenital hemangioma	
Rapidly involuting	(RICH)[a]
Non-involuting	(NICH)
Partially involuting	(PICH)
Tufted angioma[a, b]	
Spindle-cell hemangioma	
Epithelioid hemangioma	
Pyogenic granuloma (aka lobular capillary hemangioma)	
Others	
Locally aggressive or borderline vascular tumors	
Kaposiform hemangioendothelioma[a, b]	
Retiform hemangioendothelioma	
Papillary intralymphatic angioendothelioma (PILA), Dabska tumor	
Composite hemangioendothelioma	
Kaposi sarcoma	
Others	
Malignant vascular tumors	
Angiosarcoma	
Epithelioid hemangioendothelioma	
Others	

See www.issva.org/ – for interactive comprehensive classification

N.B. reactive proliferative vascular lesions are listed with benign tumors

[a]Some lesions may be associated with thrombocytopenia and/or consumptive coagulopathy; see details

[b]Many experts believe that these are part of a spectrum rather than distinct entities

Table 8.4 Appendix 3 infantile hemangioma ISSVA 2014 classification

Pattern
Focal
Multifocal
Segmental
Indeterminate
Type
Superficial
Deep
Mixed (superficial + deep)
Reticular/abortive/minimal growth
Others
Association with other lesions
PHACE syndrome
Posterior fossa malformations, hemangioma, arterial anomalies, cardiovascular anomalies, eye anomalies, sternal clefting, and/or supraumbilical raphe
LUMBAR (SACRAL/PELVIS) syndrome
Lower body hemangioma, urogenital anomalies, ulceration, myelopathy, bony deformities, anorectal malformations, arterial anomalies, and renal anomalies

See www.issva.org/ – for interactive comprehensive classification

References

1. Mulliken JB, Glowacki J. Hemangiomas and vascular malformations in infants and children: a classification based on endothelial characteristics. Plast Reconstr Surg. 1982;69(3):412–22.
2. Virchow R. Angioma in die Krankhaften Geschwülste, vol. 3. Berlin: Hirshwald; 1863. p. 306–425.
3. Wegener G. Ueber Lynmphangiome. Arch Klin Chir. 1877;20:641–707.
4. His W. The anatomical nomenclature. Nomina Anatomica. Leipzig: Veit; 1895.
5. Laubichler M, Aird W, Maienschein J. The endothelium in history. In: Aird W, editor. Endothelial biomedicine. Cambridge: Cambridge University Press; 2007. p. 5–19.
6. Eichmann A, Yuan L, Moyon D, Lenoble F, Pardanaud L, Breant C. Vascular development: from precursor cells to branched arterial and venous networks. Int J Dev Biol. 2005;49(2–3):259–67.
7. Oliver G, Detmar M. The rediscovery of the lymphatic system: old and new insights into the development and biological function of the lymphatic vasculature. Genes Dev. 2002;16(7):773–83.
8. Yang Y, Oliver G. Development of the mammalian lymphatic vasculature. J Clin Invest. 2014;124(3):888–97.
9. Malan E, Puglionisi A. Congenital angiodysplasias of the extremities. I. Generalities and classification; venous dysplasias. J Cardiovasc Surg (Torino). 1964;5:87–130.
10. Malan E, Puglionisi A. Congenital angiodysplasias of the extremities. II. Arterial, arterial and venous, and haemolymphatic dysplasias. J Cardiovasc Surg (Torino). 1965;6(4):255–345.
11. Enjolras O, Wassef M, Chapot R. Color atlas of vascular tumors and vascular malformations. Cambridge, UK: Cambridge University Press; 2007.
12. Wassef M, Blei F, Adams D, Alomari A, Baselga E, Berenstein A, et al. Vascular anomalies classification: recommendations from the International Society for the Study of Vascular Anomalies. Pediatrics. 2015;136(1):e203–14.

Hamburg Classification: Vascular Malformation

Dirk A. Loose and Raul E. Mattassi

Vascular malformations occur in such an enormous variety of forms and types that they have been a symbol of confusion among various vascular disorders through decades. Unfortunately even until today in many places, the differentiation of hemangiomas and vascular malformations is not precisely known or is not accurately used in daily clinical practice. A fundamental statement was the clear differentiation of vascular tumors and vascular malformations within the topic of vascular anomalies [1]. A concept of rational treatment of these different findings can only be gained on the basis of a classification referring to clear anatomic and pathological features [2].

That is why in 1988 following an initiative of Prof. Dr. St. Belov, a consensus conference was performed in Hamburg, Germany (Fig. 9.1) under his leadership and guidance convening international scientists of different specialties. The only topic was to create a classification of congenital vascular malformations, which should be simple, clearly arranged, comprehensible, and implementable in clinical practice. The sessions unanimously resolved that the vascular tumors have to be discussed absolutely apart from the extensive group of the congenital vascular malformations. Following the proposals of Malan [3], those "vascular malformations were differentiated into a number of anatomo-clinical pictures, each with a precise definition of the vascular abnormality, of its evolution and of the therapeutic possibilities." In addition, Malan introduced the concept of the "predominant type of the involved vessel" because he noticed that in vascular malformations, very rarely only one type of vessel alone is affected, but in most cases polyangiopathies have to be dealt with.

In order to define the vascular malformations which were formed extratruncular out of the primitive vascular network during the reticular stage of its embryonal development, the term extratruncular form was installed into the classification. Within this term the limited form is included as well as the infiltrating form which is specific for vascular malformations. In contrast, the vascular malformations which derive from a disturbance in the late phase of the vessel development affect the main vessels and such are called the truncular forms. Malan [3] and Belov [4, 5] are convinced of the idea that the truncular and the extratruncular forms are the result of a defect in the embryonic phase of development of the vessels. The latest results in molecular and genetic research and development demonstrate that this concept may be right [6].

The Hamburg classification [5] was adopted by this working group in 1988 (Table 9.1), and the conclusion in 1993 [4] was published as follows: "(1) the proposed classification of congenital vascular defects based on anatomic and pathological features has proved to be useful in

D.A. Loose (✉) • R.E. Mattassi
Bereich Angiologie und Gefäßchirurgie,
Facharztklinik Hamburg und Klinik Fleetinsel,
Hamburg, Germany
e-mail: info@prof-loose.de

© Springer-Verlag Berlin Heidelberg 2017
Y.-W. Kim et al. (eds.), *Congenital Vascular Malformations*, DOI 10.1007/978-3-662-46709-1_9

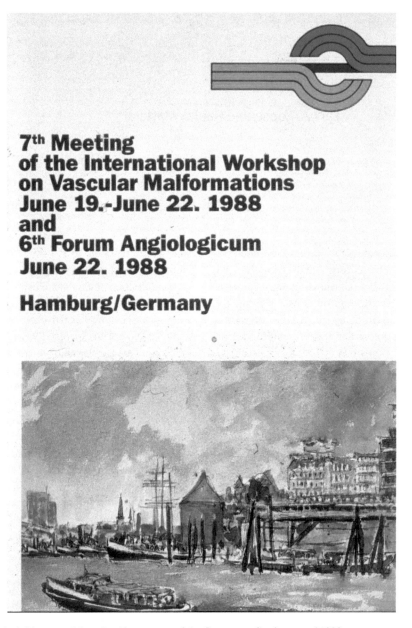

Fig. 9.1 Original title page of the scientific program of the Consensus Conference of 1988

clinical practice. It is valid for vascular defects in all locations (central, visceral, and peripheral), includes all types and anatomic forms of vascular malformations, yet is quite simplified. (2) A uniform and universal classification system is necessary for clear communication between the many different specialists dealing with congenital vascular defects. (3) It offers a clear and precise descriptive system to serve as the basis for diagnosis of congenital vascular defects. (4) A unified classification system offers the possibility of uniform analysis and comparative reporting between scientific investigators working in this field around the world" (see Table 9.1).

This conclusion, published by Belov [4], became true, and every specialist dedicated to congenital vascular malformations accepted this Hamburg classification and worked with it efficiently. However, soon the capillary/microvascular form was added, and in 2007 a modified Hamburg

Table 9.1 Classification of congenital vascular defects according to their species and anatomic form ("Hamburg Classification 1988")

	Anatomical forms	
Species	Truncular	Extratruncular
Predominantly arterial defects	Aplasia or obstruction dilatation	Infiltrating limited
Predominantly venous defects	Aplasia or obstruction dilatation	Infiltrating limited
Predominantly lymphatic defects	Aplasia or obstruction dilatation	Infiltrating limited
Predominantly AV shunting defects	Deep AV fistulae superficial AV fistulae	Infiltrating -limited
Combined vascular defects	Arterial and venous, (without AV-shunt) hemolymphatic (with or without AV-shunt)	Infiltrating hemolymphatic limited hemolymphatic

Table 9.2 Hamburg classification of congenital vascular malformations (CVMs) according to their species and embryology

A. Hamburg classification[a] of CVMs – Species
Arterial malformation
Venous malformation
Arterio-Venous malformation
Lymphatic malformation
Capillary malformation
Combined vascular malformation
B. Hamburg classification of CVMs[b, c]: forms – Embryological subtypes
Extratruncular forms
Infiltrating, diffuse
Limited, localized
Truncular forms
Obstruction or stenosis
Aplasia; hypoplasia; hyperplasia
Stenosis; membrane obturation; congenital spur
Dilatation
Localized (aneurysm)
Diffuse (ectasia)

[a]Original classification was based on the consensus on the CVM through the international workshop held in Hamburg, Germany, 1988, and subsequently modified based on the predominant lesion
[b]Represents the developmental arrest at the different stages of embryonic life: Earlier stage – Extratruncular form; Later stage – Truncular form
[c]Both forms may exist together; may be combined with other various malformations (e.g., capillary, arterial, AV shunting, venous, hemolymphatic and/or lymphatic); and/or may exist with hemangioma

classification was proposed and worldwide accepted and recommended [7] (Table 9.2).

Further modifications of the Hamburg classification were proposed by the ISSVA (International Society for the Study of Vascular Anomalies) in 1996 and in 2014. While the 1996 modification was elegant in its simplicity, but did not adequately and sufficiently reflect the current understanding of vascular malformations [8], several details were missing. That is why in 2014 another updated and expanded modification was published basing on the original Hamburg classification [9] (Table 9.3).

Table 9.3 ISSVA classification of 2014

Overview table	
Vascular tumors	*Simple vascular malformations (extratruncal)*
Benign v.t.	Capillary m. (CM)
Locally aggressive or borderline v.t.	Lymphatic m. (LM) primary lymphedema
Malignant v.t.	Venous m. (VM)
	Arteriovenous m. (AVM) AV fistulas (AVF)
	Combined vascular malformations (extratruncular)
	Truncular vascular malformations of major named vessels
	Lymphatics
	Veins
	Arteries

Again capillary (i.e., microvascular), lymphatic, venous and arteriovenous malformations, and arteriovenous fistulas are differentiated. Malformations of the main named vessels are specified again as truncal, and combined extratruncular forms are also considered. In addition, subgroups like "vascular malformations associated with other anomalies" or "provisionally unclassified vascular anomalies" are mentioned. As an appendix the causal genes of vascular anomalies as they are known today are also completely included [10, 11].

References

1. Mulliken JB, Glowacki J. Hemangiomas and vascular malformations in infants and children: a classification based on endothelial characteristics. Plast Reconstr Surg. 1982;69:412–22.
2. Malan E, Puglionisi A. Congenital angiodysplasias of the extremities. Note I: generalities and classification; venous dysplasias. J Cardiovasc Surg (Torino). 1964; 5:87–130.
3. Malan E. Vascular malformations (Angiodysplasias). Milan: Carlo Erba Foundation; 1974.
4. Belov S. Anatomopathological classification of congenital vascular defects. Semin Vasc Surg. 1993; 6(4):219–24.
5. Belov St. Classification, terminology and nosology of congenital vascular defects. In: Belov St, Loose DA, Weber J, editors. Vascular malformations. Einhorn-Presse Verlag Reinbek; 1989. p. 25–8.
6. Limaye N, Vikkula M. Molecular and genetic aspects of hemangiomas and vascular malformations. In: Mattassi R, Loose DA, Vaghi M, editors. Hemangiomas and vascular malformations: an atlas of diagnosis and treatment. 2nd ed. Milano: Springer; 2015. p. 21–38.
7. Lee BB, Bergan J, Gloviczki P, Laredo J, Loose DA, Mattassi R, Parsi K, Villavicencio JL, Zamboni P. Diagnosis and treatment of venous malformations. Consensus document of the International Union of Phlebology (IUP)-2009. Int Angiol. 28(6):434–51.
8. Enjolras O, Mulliken JB. Vascular tumors and vascular malformations (new issues). Adv Dermatol. 1997;13:375–423.
9. Michel Wassef, Francine Blei, Denise Adams, Ahmad Alomari, Eulalia Baselga, Alejandro Berenstein, Patricia Burrows, Ilona J. Frieden, Maria C. Garzon, Juan-Carlos Lopez-Gutierrez, David J.E. Lord, Sally Mitchel, Julie Powell, Julie Prendiville, Miikka Vikkula ISSVA Board and Scientific Committee. Vascular anomalies classification: recommendations from the International Society for the Study of Vascular Anomalies. Pediatrics. 2015. doi:10.1542/peds.2014–3673. Originally published online June 8 2015.
10. Mattassi R, Loose DA. Classification of vascular malformations. In: Mattassi R, Loose DA, Vaghi M, editors. Hemangiomas and vascular malformations. 2nd ed. Italia: Springer; 2015. p. 181–6.
11. Green AK. Vascular anomalies. Classification, diagnosis and management. Quality Medical Publishing Inc., St.Louis, 2013 9-18

Angiographic Classification: Arteriovenous Malformation and Venous Malformation

10

Kwang Bo Park and Young Soo Do

Introduction

Angiography is the gold standard of confirmative diagnosis as well as therapeutic tools in arteriovenous malformation (AVM). Typically, artery angiography in AVM shows feeding artery, nidus, and early draining veins. These malformed vascular structures can be imaged through the full-shot arteriography, but it is hard to separate individual vascular component only with a single overall angiographic image. Angiographic findings of AVM are totally different in every single patient, and the malformed vasculature is very complex to figure out the detailed vascular connection at a glance. Not infrequently, untrained physician cannot discriminate even between the artery and vein on angiography because the vessels are numerous, tortuous, and overlapped with each other. Therefore, systematized angiographic classification for the AVM seldom appears in the medical literatures. Complex vascular connection in AVM can be imaged better with selective arteriography, and sometimes direct puncture arteriography is helpful for understanding detailed vascular connection and hemodynamic status of AVM components vessel. Without

understanding vascular anatomy and its hemodynamic interaction of the malformed vessels in the AVM, adequate treatment plan is difficult to make. As for the endovascular treatment, some type of AVM responds to treatment dramatically, but some AVM is hard to relieve even with repetitive procedures. Therefore, types and patterns of different AVMs have been required to be classified systematically to correlate with the treatment response.

For the intracranial AVM, several attempts were made to suggest systematized classification since 1977. Among them, Spetzler and Martin grading system [1] graded AVM with point scale considering the size of AVM nidus, cortical location, and the deep venous drainage. However, the number and connection pattern of feeding artery was not included in the classification system. Feeding artery in AVM can be single or multiple, and they usually show extremely tortuous appearance due to the increased arterial flow volume heading to arteriovenous shunt. Shi-Chen scale divided the size of AVM, the location and depth, arterial blood supply, and venous drainage into grades 1–4, and then the final grade was determined from each of four patterns of grades [2]. However, unlike the intracranial AVM, the importance of location factor is not so great in torso and extremity AVM. Furthermore, although the feeding artery, nidus, and draining vein can be seen on angiography, anatomical lesion location requires additional cross-sectional image data such as magnetic resonance imaging or

K.B. Park, MD (✉) • Y.S. Do, MD (✉)
Department of Radiology, Samsung Medical Center,
Sungkyunkwan University School of Medicine,
Jongno-gu, South Korea
e-mail: kbjh.park@samsung.com; ys.do@samsung.com

computed tomography. Therefore, simplified angiographic classification of intracranial AVM proposed by Houdart et al. on 1993 considered to be an adequate model for application in peripheral AVM [3]. In this simplified classification system, AVM was divided into three different types, and the number and size of the feeding artery and vein as well as the vascular connection between the feeding artery and vein were the main consideration for the angiographic description and classification.

Based on these concept, Cho et al. proposed modified angiographic classification for the AVMs in the torso and extremity on 2006 [4]. Diagram in the Fig. 10.1 describes the vascular anatomical connection between feeding artery and draining veins. Type I was defined as an arteriovenous fistulae that consist with not more than three different feeding arteries shunt to a single draining vein which was a single direct arteriovenous fistula. Type II refers to arteriolovenous fistulae that consist with multiple arterioles shunt to

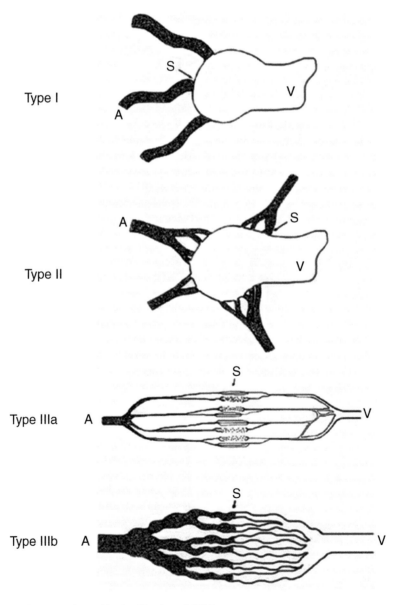

Fig. 10.1 Diagram for the angiographic classification of AVM

a single draining vein. Arterial components in type II AVM show a plexiform appearance on angiography. Ordinarily, both feeding arteries and draining vein are hypertrophied and tortuous, but the degree of vascular tortuosity does not influence on the angiographic classification in type II. Type III AVMs have multiple feeding arteries and multiple draining veins and subdivided into type IIIa which is arteriolovenulous

fistulae with non-hypertrophied feeding artery and draining vein. Type IIIb is arteriolovenulous fistulae with hypertrophied feeding arteries and draining veins. Figure 10.2 shows typical angiographic appearance of AVM corresponding to each subtype of AVM. Response to embolization therapy is relatively good in types I and II. Both type I and II AVMs have dominant outflow vein, and the rate of cure in embolization was reported

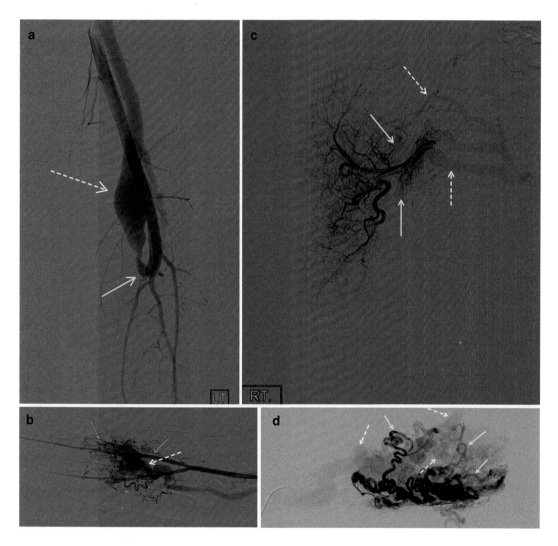

Fig. 10.2 Four subtypes of AVMs according to the angiographic classification. (**a**) Type I AVM with arteriovenous fistulae. Single feeding artery from tibioperoneal trunk (*arrow*) connected to single draining vein (*dotted arrow*). (**b**) Type II AVM with single early draining vein in the right forearm. Multiple feeding arteries (*red arrows*) are connected to single early draining vein (*white dotted*

arrow). (**c**) Type IIIa AVM in the right buttock. Non-hypertrophied arterial feeders (*arrows*) are connected to multiple non-hypertrophied draining veins (*dotted arrows*). (**d**) Type IIIb AVM in the left upper arm. Multiple hypertrophied feeding arteries (*yellow arrows*) are connected to multiple hypertrophied draining veins (*white dotted arrows*)

up to 68 % [5]. On the other hand, types IIIa and IIIb show less therapeutic response to embolization. Although the modified angiographic classification system provided clear category between each type of AVM, not all the AVM falls into these four specific types completely. Twenty-four to thirty-two percent of patients are classified into complex AVM that shows more than two different types of AVM are combined [6]. Therefore, perfect angiographic classification is almost impossible to establish to stratify these complex vascular lesions clearly into individual patterns. One study showed that lesion extent is also related with treatment response [6]. Even with type IIIb AVM, localized lesion can show good result with repetitive treatment. However, extensive AVMs involving whole extremity are hard to show satisfactory result. Because recent angiographic classification system for AVM lacks the consideration of lesion extent, further research and treatment experience is required for revising the modified angiographic classification into more reliable and well correlated with therapeutic results.

Venous Malformation: Angiographic Classification

Venous malformations occupy the largest population in the congenital vascular anomaly and are responsible for more than 50 % of patient referrals to vascular anomaly centers [7, 8]. VMs are composed of abnormal veins that show variable luminal diameter and wall thickness, and they usually lack of venous valve [7]. Certain VMs consist with fine small diameter dysplastic veins but large proportion of VM consists with markedly ectatic and serpentine venous channels. Dysplastic veins are connected with each other in an irregular and disorganized pattern, and VMs have normal venous connection with superficial or deep venous system.

Although full-shot arteriography in AVM is easy to get an overall image for the vascular malformation, VM is hard to be imaged in a single injection phlebography through transvenous approach. Also, the routine ascending or descending phlebography cannot show the whole VM in a single image because the venous flow is coming out from the VM frequently. Therefore, direct puncture phlebography is useful to understand the dysplastic venous connection of the VM in detail, but even with direct puncture phlebography, whole VM cannot be filled with contrast media because the venous drainage of VM component that is apart from the needle insertion point passes through the different venous connection. Furthermore, direct puncture venography is an invasive procedure so that the exact phlebographic classification can be obtained with simultaneous sclerotherapy in many cases. Direct puncture phlebographic findings in VM are very complex in most of the patients; however, careful analysis of direct puncture phlebography provides detailed information for the patterns of normal venous connection and the appearances of dysplastic vein. Phlebographic evaluation sometimes requires manual compression or dispersion of contrast media to the rest of nonopacified VM component and nonopacified normal venous connection. Unless adequate phlebographic evaluation is done, VM cannot be characterized thoroughly. Former biological and clinical classification system like Hamburg classification or ISSVA classification did not reflect venous anatomical and hemodynamic factors [9].

Phlebographic classification for the VM has few data. In 1991, Dubois et al. suggested classification for the VM according to the type of venous drainage as type I was an excluded, well-circumscribed VM without visible draining veins; type II was venous lakes drained into a normal venous system; and type III was VM having ectatic abnormal draining veins [10]. In 2001, Dubois et al. described direct phlebographic findings into three simplified categories: cavitary, spongy, and dysmorphic veins [11]. However, this simple description is insufficient for stratifying the complex malformed venous structures in torso and extremity VMs. In 2003, Dr. Puig proposed modified phlebographic classification system [12]. Puig also considered the pattern of venous drainage and normal venous connection as a clue to stratify four different types of VMs. Figure 10.3 shows typical

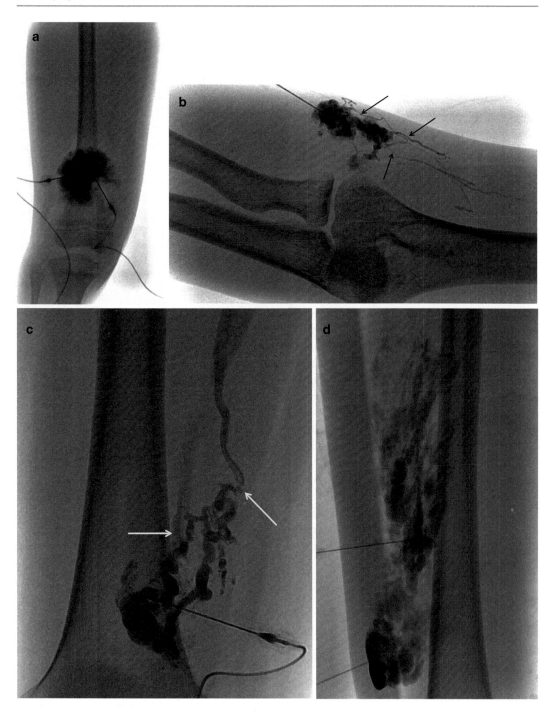

Fig. 10.3 Phlebographic classification of venous malformations. (**a**) Type I isolated VM without peripheral venous drainage. (**b**) Type II VM in the right elbow that drains into normal superficial veins (*arrows*). (**c**) Type III VM that drains into dysplastic veins (*arrows*). (**d**) Type IV VM with diffuse venous dysplasia. Complex, irregular, and ectatic veins are spread in the left thigh

phlebographic appearance of four types of VMs. Type I was defined as an isolated malformation without peripheral venous drainage (Fig. 10.3a). Type II was venous malformation that drains into normal veins (Fig. 10.3b). Type III was venous malformation that drains into dysplastic veins (Fig. 10.3c). Type IV was venous malformation that represents a venous dysplasia (Fig. 10.3d). Incidences of each type of VMs were reported as 30 % for type I, 37 % for type II, 21 % for type III, and 12 % for type IV [12]. However, these incidences can be varied from center to center because the data were derived from small population (43 patients) phlebographic study. The importance of Puig classification was that it emphasized venous anatomical factors including normal venous communication with dysplastic veins. Understanding the vascular anatomy of VM and the hemodynamic connection between dysplastic veins and normal venous channel is helpful to establish the treatment scheme. Puig classification (reference) is well correlated with percutaneous sclerotherapy results. Types I and II show good therapeutic response to sclerotherapy because the sclerosing agent can be confined within VM for sufficient time and sclerosant washout into normal venous system can be minimized. Type I and II VMs showed higher cure rate with lower number of treatment sessions [10]. However, sclerosing agent is hard to stay enough in type III and IV VMs that lead to less therapeutic response. Furthermore, type III and IV VMs have risks for embolic material spillage into the normal venous system that gives rise to systemic complication. Therefore, rate of exclusion from sclerotherapy is higher (up to half of patients) in type III and IV VMs [12]. This phlebographic classification system can be applied to simple VMs on ISSVA classification 2014 [9, 13], not for the combined types. Combined VMs are often more complex in phlebographic findings, and some of the lesions are difficult to get direct puncture venography because the dysplastic veins are too small. Current phlebographic classification lacks in consideration of lesion extent, location, and multiplicity. In a simple manner, phlebographically localized VMs are easy to treat, and the therapeutic response is better because the lesion extent is restricted, and sclerosing effect can

be maximized. However, diffuse VMs are less likely to show good therapeutic response because the lesion extent is too broad. Diffuse VMs require too many number of treatment sessions to achieve satisfactory result or even impossible to treat with either sclerotherapy or surgery. The number of treatment sessions and the invasiveness of treatment are also related with the life quality of individual patient. There is a limitation that the phlebographic classification consider only the dysplastic vein, but some VMs have large proportion of solid or fibrous connective tissue stroma as a lesion component. The ratio of vascular component and solid component also affects the result of sclerotherapy [14]. Certain types of VM are hard to get direct puncture phlebography because of the abundant stroma with relative paucity of dysplastic venous channel. Therefore, further research, discussion, and agreement would be required to make improved, reliable, and outcome-related phlebographic classification system for VMs.

References

1. Spetzler RF, Martin NA. A proposed grading system for arteriovenous malformations. J Neurosurg. 1986;65(4):476–83.
2. Shi YQ, Chen XC. A proposed scheme for grading intracranial arteriovenous malformations. J Neurosurg. 1986;65(4):484–9.
3. Houdart E, Gobin YP, Casasco A, Aymard A, Herbreteau D, Merland JJ. A proposed angiographic classification of intracranial arteriovenous fistulae and malformations. Neuroradiology. 1993;35:381–5.
4. Cho SK, Do YS, Shin SW, et al. Arteriovenous malformations of the body and extremities: analysis of therapeutic outcomes and approaches according to a modified angiographic classification. J Endovasc Ther. 2006;13:527–38.
5. Cho SK, Do YS, Kim DI, et al. Peripheral arteriovenous malformations with a dominant outflow vein: results of ethanol embolization. Korean J Radiol. 2008;9:258–67.
6. Park KB, Do YS, Kim DI, et al. Predictive factors for response of peripheral arteriovenous malformations to embolization therapy: analysis of clinical data and imaging findings. J Vasc Interv Radiol. 2012;23:1478–86.
7. Legiehn GM, Heran MKS. Venous malformations: classification, development, diagnosis, and interventional radiologic management. Radiol Clin North Am. 2008;46:545–97.

8. Vikkula M, Boon LM, Mulliken JB. Molecular basis of vascular anomalies. Trends Cardiovasc Med. 1998;8:218–92.

9. Lee BB, Baumgartner I, Berlien P, et al. Diagnosis and treatment of venous malformations consensus document of the international union of phlebology (IUP): updated 2013. Int Angiol. 2013;32:1–53.

10. Dubois JM, Sebag GH, Prost YD, Teillac D, Chretien B, Brunelle FO. Soft-tissue venous malformations in children: percutaneous sclerotherapy with ethibloc. Radiology. 1991;180:195–8.

11. Dubois JM, Soulez G, Oliva VL, Berthiaume MJ, Lapierre C, Therasse E. Soft-tissue venous malformations in adult patients: imaging and therapeutic issues. Radiographics. 2001;21:1519–31.

12. Puig S, Aref H, Chigot V, Bonin B, Brunelle F. Classification of venous malformations in children and implications for sclerotherapy. Pediatr Radiol. 2003;33:99–103.

13. Wassef M, Blei F, Adams D, Alomari A, Baselga E, Berenstein A, et al. Vascular anomalies classification: recommendations from the international society for the study of vascular anomalies. Pediatrics. 2015;136(1):e203–14.

14. Park HS, Do YS, Park KB, Kim KH, Woo SY, Jung SH, et al. Clinical outcome and predictors of treatment response in foam sodium tetradecyl sulfate sclerotherapy of venous malformations. Eur Radiol. 2016;26(5):1301–10.

New Arteriographic Classification of AVM Based on the Yakes Classification System

11

Wayne F. Yakes, Robert L. Vogelzang, Krasnodar Ivancev, and Alexis M. Yakes

The world's literature certainly verifies the extreme challenges in the diagnosis and treatment of AVMs. The purpose of this chapter is to present a new Yakes AVM Classification System that has proven therapeutic implications to effectively treat complex AVMs in any anatomical area [1, 2]. By employing the Yakes AVM Classification System, a physician is now able to accurately classify AVMs and determine specific endovascular treatment strategies to consistently treat AVMs, and patients can enjoy long-term excellent outcomes. Defining the angioarchitecture of the high-flow AVM determines accurately the endovascular management strategy to best permanently ablate the AVM requiring treatment. Further, employing this new Yakes AVM Classification System will lower complication rates in treating these complex congenital vascular pathologies.

The Houdart Classification of Intracranial Arteriovenous Fistulae and Malformations of high-flow lesions [3] and the Do Classification of AVMs of the peripheral arterial circulation [4] are strikingly similar despite their anatomic locational differences (CNS vs. peripheral vasculatures). Both authors also suggest similar therapeutic approaches based on their similar arteriographic classification.

The Houdart Type a and Type b and Do Types I and II proffer retrograde approaches to occlude the vein aneurysm outflow as being a potential for curative treatment of these AVM types. Yakes et al. illustrated the retrograde vein occlusion techniques for high-flow malformations in 1990 [5]. Later, Jackson et al. published the success of the retrograde vein approach in 1996 [6]. The Do Group in Seoul, South Korea (also the publisher of the Do AVM Classification and editor of this text), published the retrograde vein approach in 2008 [7].

The Yakes AVM Classification System has some similarities to both classification systems and some stark differences. The Yakes classification system is as follows: Type I is a direct arteriovenous fistula, a direct artery to vein connection, typified by pulmonary AVF and renal AVF, for example. This angioarchitecture type is not specifically described in the Houdart or Do classification systems. Type II (AVM characterized usually by multiple inflow arteries into a

W.F. Yakes, MD (✉) • A.M. Yakes, BM
The Yakes Vascular Malformation Center,
Englewood, CO 80113, USA
e-mail: Wayne.yakes@vascularmalformationcenter.com

R.L. Vogelzang, MD
Northwestern Medical Center, Chicago, IL, USA

K. Ivancev, MD, PhD
Division of Vascular Surgery,
University of Hamburg Medical Center,
Hamburg, Germany

© Springer-Verlag Berlin Heidelberg 2017
Y.-W. Kim et al. (eds.), *Congenital Vascular Malformations*, DOI 10.1007/978-3-662-46709-1_11

63

"nidus" pattern with direct artery-arteriolar to vein-venular structures that may, or may not, be aneurysmal). Type IIIa (multiple arteries-arterioles into an enlarged aneurysmal vein with an enlarged single outflow vein). Type IIIb (multiple arteries-arterioles into an enlarged aneurysmal vein with multiple dilated outflow veins). Type IV AVM is a type of AVM showing innumerable arterio-venous connections at the arteriolar level (typified by ear AVMs that infiltrate the entire cartilage structure of the pinna). The difference of this type of AVM from other types is that there are admixed among the innumerable fistulae capillary beds within the affected tissue. If the affected tissue only had AVFs, the tissue could not survive as capillary beds are required for tissue viability. No other AVM angioarchitecture has this duality. This angioarchitecture is not described in the world's literature except for Yakes et al.'s recent publications [1, 2].

Comparing Houdart's CNS Classification and the Do Peripheral Vascular Classification to the Yakes Classification has some parallels, as has been described, but has several distinct differences. Houdart Type A and Do Type I are the same and compared to the Yakes Type IIIa. Houdart Type B and Do Type II are the same and again are placed in the Yakes Type IIIa. Whether the arteriovenous (Type A/Type I) or arteriolar-venular connections (Type B/Type II) are present is not important as the same arterial physiology is present with the "nidus" being present in the aneurysmal vein wall itself. Regardless of the size of AVF on the vein wall, they are both treated endovascularly in the same way. Therefore, the AVF size is irrelevant. Further, even when larger AVFs are present, microfistulae are present as well and mixed with the larger connections. It never is purely one microsize only or one macrosize only.

The Houdart Type C is the same as bundling the Do Types IIIa (arteriovenous) and IIIb (arteriolar-venular). This is similar to the Yakes Type II. Both authors do not explain the Yakes Type IV

in their classifications. The angioarchitecture of arteriovenous shunting through arteriolar-venular innumerable fistulae, totally infiltrating a particular tissue, is another vascular phenomenon which is present that is not explained by the Houdart nor the Do Classifications. When these microfistulae infiltrated into the tissue on an angiogram, we can consider it as microfistulous arterio-venous fistulae mixed with normal capillaries of the tissue. Normal capillaries must be present and admixed with the innumerable AVF in the infiltrated tissue, or it would not be viable and could not survive. Venous hypertension is usually the culprit in the injury that occurs in that infiltrated tissue. This phenomenon of arterialized veins (venous hypertension) as a vascular etiology for pathologic tissue changes was first elucidated by Jean-Jacques Merland, M.D., and Marie Claire Riche, M.D. [8]. Thus, the "normal" vascularity with capillary beds in the infiltrated tissue to allow it to exist is not discussed in the Houdart or in the Do AVM Classifications, nor are the infiltrative AVM angioarchitecture characteristics described.

The Yakes Type I AVM is a direct AV macro-connection that is characteristic of pulmonary AVF and renal AVF but can also occur in other tissues. This direct AV connection is not described in the Houdart Classification or in the Do Classification. The Yakes Type I AV connection can also be present and interspersed in other AVM types as well.

The Yakes Type II AVM Classification possesses an angioarchitecture synonymous with the classical "nidus" pattern commonly seen in AVMs with multiple inflow arteries of varying sizes coursing toward a "nidus" (a complex tangle of vascular structures without any intervening capillaries and exiting from this "nidus" into multiple veins). The Houdart Type C and the Do Type IIIa/Type IIIb most resemble this angioarchitecture pattern.

As an aside, the term "nidus" is rampant in the medical literature (AVM nidus, nidus of infection, etc.). Unfortunately, the initial author was only partially familiar with the Latin language. "Nidus" means "nest" in Latin, and indeed it does. However, "nidus" with the ending "us" denotes male gender. In the Latin language, the true term meaning "nest" is, in fact, "nidum." The ending "um" denotes the neuter gender which a "nest" truly is. Thus, the original author accurately describing "nest-like" conglomeration of vascular structure was woefully inaccurate penning the words as "nidus" (masculine) instead of the true word "nidum" (neuter). Being rife in the literature for decades (nidus of infection; AVM nidus), I do not foresee any correction of this term.

In summary, Yakes Type I is the simplest macro-direct AV connection. Yakes Type II is the common "nidum" (nest-like) AV connection. Yakes Type IIIa has multiple AV connections (arterial and arteriolar into an aneurysmal vein; "nidum" is in the vein wall itself) with single outflow vein physiology. Yakes Type IIIb has multiple arterial inflow connections (arterial and arteriolar) into an aneurysmal vein ("nidum" is in the vein wall) with multiple outflow veins that is more difficult but still treatable by retrograde vein approaches.

Yakes Type IV angioarchitecture has innumerable micro-AV connections (with lowered vascular resistance) infiltrating an entire tissue but with concurrent normal vascular structures possessing nutrient capillary beds (with normal vascular resistance) to supply and drain the tissue that is diffusely infiltrated to allow this tissue to survive and not be devitalized. The postcapillary veins compete with AVF outflow veins that are arterialized (hypertensive) and cause the resultant non-healing tissue pathology [8]. This infiltrative AVM entity was first described by Yakes in the recent literature (Fig. 11.1) [1, 2].

Therapeutic Implications of the Yakes Classification

Determining a classification system based on the AVM angioarchitecture is of little use without a practical application. For example, the Spetzler-Martin Brain AVM Classification is of importance to determine the surgical morbidity for treating brain AVMs [9]; the higher the Spetzler-Martin grade, the higher the morbidity. This allows the neurosurgeon to inform his patient accurately of the risks for treatment. The Schobinger AVM Classification for peripheral AVMs (non-neuro) is useful to quantify the degrees of symptomatology a patient possesses regardless of the AVM's angioarchitecture [10]. The Yakes AVM Classification System is utilized to determine endovascular approaches and the embolic agents that will be successful to ablate these AVMs.

Embolic Agents Employed in the Yakes AVM Classification

Yakes Type I direct AV connections, as typically seen in pulmonary AVF and renal AVF, can be permanently ablated by occluding the AVF with mechanical devices. Coils, Amplatzer plugs, occluders, detachable balloons, and the like are universally successful to cure Yakes Type I AVMs. Ethanol can also be curative in Yakes Type I AVMs if the AVF is of a small caliber.

Yakes Type II AVMs with the "nidum" nest-like angioarchitecture can be permanently ablated with absolute ethanol from a superselective transcatheter/transmicrocatheter arterial approach. Also, a direct puncture into the artery(ies) supplying the AVM immediately

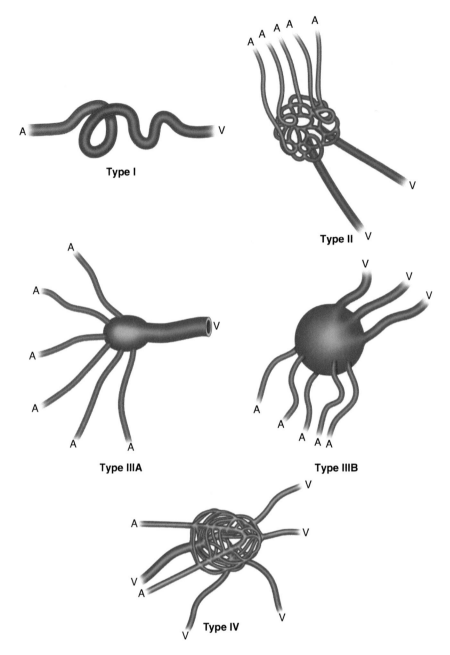

Fig. 11.1 Schematic drawing of Yakes classification of AVMs

Type I is a direct arteriovenous fistula, a direct artery to vein connection, typified by pulmonary AVF and renal AVF, for example. This angioarchitecture type is not specifically described in the Houdart or Do classification systems

Type IIa – AVM characterized usually by multiple inflow arteries into a "nidus" pattern with direct artery-arteriolar to vein-venular structures that may, or may not, be aneurysmal

Type IIb – AVM characterized by an AVM nidus that then drains into an aneurysmal vein

Type IIIa – multiple arteries-arterioles connecting microfistulae into the wall of an enlarged aneurysmal vein with an enlarged single outflow vein

Type IIIb – multiple arteries-arterioles connecting microfistulae into the wall of an enlarged aneurysmal vein with multiple dilated outflow veins

Type IV AVMs are microfistulous innumerable arteriolar structures shunting into innumerable venular connections that diffusely infiltrate a tissue (typified by ear AVMs that infiltrate the entire cartilage structure of the pinna)

proximal to the AVM "nidum" and distal to any parenchymal arterial branches, to then inject ethanol superselectively, can be employed to circumvent catheterization obstacles when a transcatheter/transmicrocatheter positioning to achieve the same position to deliver ethanol into the "nidum" is not possible. These two transarterial approaches allow ethanol to sclerose and permanently ablate the "nidum." Also the "nidum" itself can be direct-punctured, and ethanol (undiluted) can be injected to sclerose the "nidum" directly to effect cure in its multiple compartments as well.

Yakes Type IIIa AVMs (multiple inflow arteries shunting into an aneurysmal vein with a single enlarged outflow vein) and Yakes Type IIIb AVMs (multiple inflow arteries into an aneurysmal vein with multiple enlarged outflow veins) can be curatively treated by several endovascular approaches. The "nidum" in this type of angioarchitecture with an aneurysmal vein is within the vein wall itself. Superselective transarterial ethanol embolization distal to all parenchymal branches via transcatheter/transmicrocatheter and direct puncture endovascular approaches to the vein wall nidus can be curative. A simpler additional curative endovascular approach for Type IIIa AVMs is to coil embolize the aneurysmal vein itself with, or without, concurrent ethanol injection into the coils within the aneurysmal vein. This is also curative when the aneurysmal vein is totally and densely packed with coils. The aneurysmal vein can be accessed by direct 18 g needle puncture and by retrograde vein catheterization to achieve the same position within the aneurysmal vein to pack it with coils. The retrograde vein approach to curatively treat high-flow AVM vascular lesions was first published and illustrated in 1990 by Yakes et al. [11]. Yakes et al. described cures of post-traumatic and congenital high-flow lesions [5]. The second article articulating the vein approach to AVM treatment was subsequently published in 1996 by Jackson

et al. [6]. Cures were documented in these published patient series. Jackson et al. described cures of congenital AVMs by way of the retrograde vein approach in 1996 [6]. Cho and Do et al. also published the retrograde vein approach to curative Yakes Type IIIa/IIIb AVM treatment in 2008 [7].

In the Yakes Type IIIb, aneurysmal vein with enlarged multiple outflow veins can be cured by transarterial transcatheter ethanol embolization and can be cured by direct puncture and retrograde vein coiling techniques. However, the aneurysmal vein portion and the immediate adjacent segments of each outflow vein must also be packed with coils completely to achieve cure. Yakes Type IIIb AVMs are more challenging to coil and cure than the Yakes Type IIIa AVMs due to the more complex multiple outflow vein morphology requiring coil treatment in multiple vein compartments.

Yakes Type IV AVMs present a unique challenge to determine curative endovascular treatment strategies. AVMs, by definition, are direct AV connections without an intervening capillary bed (Yakes Types I–IV). Thus, superselective catheter and direct puncture needle positioning distal to *all* normal branches supplying parenchyma and immediately proximal to the AVM "nidum" itself will obviate tissue necrosis being that the capillary beds are not embolized and only the abnormal AV connections are sclerosed. However, Yakes Type IV AVMs infiltrate an entire tissue, thus termed as an "infiltrative" form of AVM. Being that the "infiltrated" tissue (e.g., auricular AVMs) is viable proves that capillary beds are undoubtedly interspersed along with the innumerable microfistulae throughout the involved tissue as well. Transarterial injection of ethanol by transcatheter/transmicrocatheter and direct puncture approaches will sclerose the innumerable microfistulae but also would flood the capillary beds with ethanol devitalizing that infiltrated tissue. Necrosis of that tissue would then ensue with concurrent occlusion of the capillary beds. Thus, Yakes Type IV AVMs posited a profound conundrum to treat by endovascular approaches. Polymerizing agents would occlude AVFs but also occlude the capillary beds causing massive tissue necrosis of that embolized tissue as well.

Thinking through this conundrum, one could rightly conclude that the only option is total surgical resection of that entire tissue as the only treatment option. After further reflection, an endovascular option for curative treatment, not palliative treatment, was considered a strong possibility. Capillary beds have normal increased peripheral resistance which has a somewhat restrictive vascular flow pattern from artery to capillary to veins. AVMs/AVFs have abnormally lowered peripheral vascular resistance with rapid shunting into arterialized veins. The arterialized AVM outflow veins are arterialized and hypertensive and have arterialized pressures. The post-capillary outflow normotensive veins then compete with the higher arterialized pressure AVM outflow veins for outflow venous return. This vein hypertension then further restricts normal vein outflow, which in turn increases the systemic vascular resistance (SVR) of the normal arterioles immediately proximal to the capillary beds, now restricting arteriolar inflow to the capillary beds. The increased SVR into the capillaries coupled with abnormally low resistance shunting into the admixed innumerable AVF allows for preferential vascular flow into the AVFs.

Mixing nonionic contrast with absolute ethanol changes the viscosity and specific gravity of ethanol in this embolic mixture. Being "thickened" allows for preferential flow to the AVFs (lower resistance vessels) and further restricts flow into the capillaries (higher-resistance vessels). Despite being 50% diluted with contrast, the ethanol can still effectively sclerose the innumerable microfistulae due to the small luminal diameters. This combination of preferential flow into the innumerable AVFs, the increased SVR

into the capillaries restricting flow, the increased viscosity, and changing the specific gravity of the contrast with the ethanol 50% mixture all work to spare the capillaries and sclerose the innumerable AVFs. Using pure ethanol would diminish this capillary sparing effect, and the AVFs and capillaries would both be sclerosed and occluded. This would cure the AVFs but would devitalize the tissue itself with occlusion of the capillaries. The use of various polymerizing embolic occlusive agents (nBCA; Onyx) would also cause the same devitalization of the tissues with occlusion of the capillaries. Particulate embolic agents (PVA, Contour Embolic, Embospheres, etc.) cannot permanently occlude the AVFs and will make the capillaries ischemic with the proximal occlusion in the inflow arterioles but will not devitalize the tissues. Therapeutic implication of AVM based on Yakes classification will be described in detail in Chap. 30.

References

1. Yakes W, Baumgartner I. Interventional treatment of arterio-venous malformations. Gefässchirurgie. 2014;19:325–30.
2. Yakes WF, Yakes AM. Arteriovenous malformations: the Yakes classification and its therapeutic implications. Egyptian J Vasc Endovasc Surg. 2014; 10:9–23.
3. Houdart B, Gobin YE, Casasco A, Aymard A, Herbreteau D, Merland JJ. A proposed angiographic classification of intracranial arteriovenous fistulae and malformations. Neuroradiology. 1993;35:381–5.
4. Cho SK, Do YS, Shin SW, Kim DI, Kim YW, Park KB, et al. Arteriovenous malformations of the body and extremities: analysis of therapeutic outcomes and approaches according to a modified angiographic classification. Endovasc Ther. 2006;13:527–38.
5. Yakes WF, Luethke JM, Merland JJ, Rak KM, Slater DD, Hollis HW, Parker SN, Casasco A, Aymard A, Hodes JE, Hopper KD, Stavros AT, Carter TE. Ethanol embolization of arteriovenous fistulas: a primary mode of therapy. J Vasc Interv Radiol. 1990;1:89–96.
6. Jackson JE, Mansfield AO, Allison DJ. Treatment of high-flow vascular malformations by venous embolization aided by flow occlusion techniques. Cardiovasc Intervent Radiol. 1996;19:323–8.

7. Cho SK, Do YS, Kim DI, Kim YW, Shin SW, Park KB, Ko JS, Lee AR, Choo SW, Choo IW. Peripheral arteriovenous malformations with a dominant out-flow vein: results of ethanol embolization. Korean J Radiol. 2008;9:258–67.

8. Merland JJ, Riche MC, Chiras J. Intraspinal extra-medullary arteriovenous fistula draining into medul-lary veins. J Neuroradiol. 1980;7:271–320.

9. Spetzler RE, Martin NA. A proposed grading sys-tem for arteriovenous malformations. J Neurosurg. 1986;473(65):476–8.

10. Lee BB, Baumgartner I, Berlien HP, Bianchini G, Burrows P, Do YS, Ivancev K, Kool LS, Laredo J, Loose DA, Lopez-Gutierrez JC, Mattassi R, Parsi K, Rimon U, Rosenblatt M, Shortell C, Simkin R, Stillo F, Villavicenzio L, Yakes W. Consensus docu-ment of the International Union of Angiology; current concepts on the management of AVMs. Int Angiol. 2013;32:9–36.

11. Yakes WF, Huguenot M, Yakes AM, Continenza A, Kammer R, Baumgartner I. Percutaneous emboliza-tion of aretrio-venous malformations at the plantar aspect of the foot. J Vasc Surg. 2016;64(5):1478–82.

James Laredo and Byung-Boong Lee

Congenital vascular malformations (CVMs) remain a significant clinical challenge due to the nature and complexity of the vascular lesions encountered in clinical practice [1, 2]. CVMs are often confused with hemangiomas [3]. The term "hemangioma" is commonly used to name different types of vascular tumors and vascular malformations, despite the fact that these vascular anomalies are distinct vascular lesions. CVMs and hemangiomas not only have different etiologies, anatomy, and pathophysiology, but they also exhibit unique hemodynamic and embryologic characteristics [2–6]. Both of these vascular anomalies have entirely different clinical courses and long-term prognoses. Furthermore, the management strategies of both conditions are fundamentally different [2–6].

J. Laredo, MD, PhD (✉)
Division of Vascular Surgery, Department of Surgery,
George Washington University Medical Center,
Washington, DC, USA
e-mail: jlaredo@mfa.gwu.edu

B.-B. Lee, MD, PhD, FACS (✉)
Professor of Surgery and Director, Center for the
Lymphedema and Vascular Malformations, George
Washington University, Washington, DC, USA

Adjunct Professor of Surgery, Uniformed Services,
University of the Health Sciences, Bethesda, MD, USA
e-mail: bblee38@gmail.com

Hemangioma

A hemangioma is vascular tumor, the most common type being the infantile hemangioma [3, 6]. The hemangioma is a "self-limited" vascular tumor, while the CVM is a "self-perpetuating" embryologic tissue remnant. The hemangioma originates from endothelial cells and appears in the early neonatal period. Unlike CVMs, hemangiomas undergo self-limited growth followed by subsequent involution that usually occurs before the age of 5–10 years [3, 6].

Most hemangiomas are small and produce only minor clinical problems before they involute and become clinically silent. However, about 20 % become clinically significant and require treatment [3]. Indications for treatment include aggressive growth, tumor proximity to vital anatomic structures, ulceration, and bleeding. In addition, the disfiguring nature of certain lesions may prompt parents to seek early intervention [3, 6].

Congenital Vascular Malformation

A CVM is a vascular anomaly that presents at birth and continues to grow at a rate proportional to the growth rate of the body regardless of its type. Data reported by Tasnadi et al. show an overall incidence of CVMs to be 1.2 % [7]. These birth defects involving the vascular system are present at birth in over 90 % of cases, with a male to female ratio of 1:1 [7]. The majority of CVMs are either venous malformations (VMs) or lymphatic malformations (LMs) [7–9]. VMs represent approximately 2/3 of all CVMs [7–9].

CVMs are classified by vessel type according to the Hamburg classification (refer to Table 9.2) [9, 10]. In each class of vascular malformation, "extratruncular malformations" composed of small vessels intimately embedded in the host tissue and "truncular malformations," affecting individual large vessels, are recognized [1, 2, 4, 5].

Extratruncular vascular malformations arise when developmental arrest has occurred during the reticular stage of embryonic development [1, 2, 4, 5]. The mesenchymal cell properties persist, and the lesions retain the potential to proliferate when stimulated (e.g., menarche, pregnancy, hormone, surgery, and trauma).

Truncular vascular malformations arise when developmental arrest has occurred during vascular trunk formation at the later stage of embryologic development [1, 2, 4, 5]. These lesions no longer possess the potential to proliferate. Truncular lesions present as poorly developed, immature vessels (aplasia or hypoplasia) or as hyperplastic vessels (hyperplasia) [1, 2, 4, 5].

Arteriovenous Malformations

The incidence and prevalence of arteriovenous malformations (AVMs) is reported to be approximately one per 250,000 individuals in the USA based on cerebrospinal AVMs [11]. They present in the age range of 20–40 years with a male to female ratio of 1:1 or 1:2 [11]. Peripheral AVMs represent approximately 10–20 % of all clinically significant CVM lesions [12].

The AVM is the most challenging of all the CVMs due to the wide range of clinical presentations, unpredictable clinical course, complex anatomy and hemodynamics, pathophysiology, and high morbidity [13, 14]. The AVM anatomic defect results in shunting of arterial blood into the venous system [13, 14]. The majority of AVMs present as single component lesions but may have other CVM lesion components, complicating the diagnosis and treatment [13, 14]. These mixed CVMs often become a clinician's nightmare (e.g., Parkes-Weber syndrome) where management is difficult, and treatment results are often disappointing (e.g., micro-shunting AVM) [13, 14].

Extratruncular AVM lesions maintain the original reticular network resulting in AV shunting with no capillary check valve system [13, 14]. The "nidus" of the lesion retains its "nonfistulous" condition (in contrast to the truncular lesion with its "fistulous" condition). The extratruncular lesion produces significant hemodynamic alterations to both the arterial and venous systems. Extratruncular AVM lesions proliferate in response to stimulation (e.g., trauma, surgery, hormone, menarche, pregnancy), resulting in an increase in its size, extent, and severity. Suboptimal treatment of extratruncular AVMs often results in lesion recurrence [13, 14].

In contrast, the truncular AVM lesions affect individual large vessels and carry no risk of recurrence. However, these lesions often have more serious hemodynamic effects on the vascular system compared with the extratruncular form. Truncular AVMs persist as "fistulous" lesions with a direct connection between an artery and vein with no defined "nidus." This fistulous lesion produces significantly more serious hemodynamic sequelae such as cardiac failure, arterial insufficiency, and chronic venous insufficiency [13, 14].

Venous Malformations

Venous malformations clinically present as a single component lesion or combined with other CVMs: lymphatic malformation (LM), arteriovenous malformation (AVM), and/or capillary malformation (CM) [15, 16].

Extratruncular VMs often present as infiltrating lesions or as clusters of primitive venous tissue without direct involvement of the main venous trunk. Truncular VMs present as poorly developed, immature venous structures (aplasia or hypoplasia) or as hyperplastic venous vessels (hyperplasia) [15, 16]. Hypoplastic or hyperplastic truncular VM lesions produce venous obstruction or dilatation, respectively. Examples of truncular VMs include popliteal vein aneurysms, azygous vein stenosis, and intraluminal defects within the vein (e.g., vein webs or membrane) resulting in stenosis or obstruction [15, 16]. Truncular VM lesions may also present as a persistent fetal remnant vein that has failed to involute or regress normally (e.g., marginal and sciatic embryonic veins) [15, 16]. Truncular VM lesions have more significant hemodynamic consequences than do extratruncular VMs, due to the direct involvement of the lesion with the truncal venous system often producing venous stenosis or obstruction [15, 16].

Lymphatic Malformations and Capillary Malformations

Lymphatic malformations are made up of variously dilated lymphatic channels or cysts, lined with endothelial cells with a lymphatic phenotype [9, 17, 18]. The extratruncular LMs are classified as microcystic, macrocystic, and mixed subtypes. There is no uniform consensus regarding the definition of microcystic or macrocystic LMs [9]. A useful distinction is whether the cysts can be successfully aspirated/sclerosed, resulting in a decrease in LM size, with the smaller cysts being more challenging [19]. Radiographic features also can help to define the difference because macrocystic LMs often have discernible fluid-filled areas. The primary lymphedemas are considered truncular forms of LMs and are characterized by a poorly developed lymphatic system or agenesis of the lymphatic network. LMs are often associated with other CVMs [9, 17, 18].

Capillary malformations (CM), including fading capillary stains and port-wine stains, are among the most common vascular malformations affecting the skin and mucosa [9]. CMs occur in approximately three of 1000 infants, are present at birth, and have a male to female ratio of 1:1 [9]. They are of minimal clinical significance (mainly a cosmetic issue) and are most often associated with other CVMs [1, 2, 9].

Evaluation

CVMs commonly occur as mixed lesions presenting with AVM, VM, LM, and/or CM components [1, 2, 4, 5]. Therefore, the evaluation of any

suspected CVM should proceed in a logical, stepwise manner, bearing in mind that any suspected CVM lesion may actually prove to be a mixed lesion. Diagnosis of a suspected VM or AVM requires specific evaluation and confirmation as a single component lesion or mixed lesion.

As a general rule, the extent and severity of any CVM affecting the vascular system (anatomically and hemodynamically) usually determine the type of clinical manifestations observed [1, 2, 4, 5]. The history and physical examination should be followed by diagnostic imaging in order to determine the type of CVM suspected. When an AVM is suspected, workup should proceed to confirm the diagnosis and to distinguish the AVM from among the various CVMs (e.g., duplex ultrasonography and MRI). Most AVMs occur as single component lesions [1, 13, 14].

A mixed CVM with VM and LM components is classified as a hemolymphatic malformation (HLM) [1, 10]. Klippel-Trenaunay syndrome is an example of a HLM. When an AVM is present in a patient with Klippel-Trenaunay syndrome, it is also known as Parkes-Weber syndrome [20]. In this situation, the initial priority of investigation should be to confirm the presence of the AVM component.

Initial diagnostic imaging should be performed with a combination of baseline noninvasive imaging [2, 4, 5, 15, 16]. More specific diagnostic imaging should then follow for further assessment of the embryological subtype (extratruncular vs. truncular) of the AVM or VM. The recommended initial studies include duplex ultrasonography, magnetic resonance imaging (MRI) with T1- and T2-weighted imaging, and computed tomography (CT) angiography with three-dimensional reconstruction. The final diagnosis should be confirmed with angiography/phlebography to further define the lesion and plan appropriate treatment [2, 4, 5, 13, 15, 16].

Duplex ultrasonography allows hemodynamic assessment of the arterial and venous components involved with an AVM and VM. LMs often have discernible fluid-filled areas. Duplex ultrasound is extremely valuable for clinical follow-up and remains the initial study of choice for CVM evaluation [2, 4, 5].

MRI remains the major diagnostic study for the entire group of CVMs. MRI allows assessment of lesion extent, severity, and anatomic relationship with the surrounding tissues and organs [2, 4, 5]. MRI of an AVM, VM, or LM lesion is usually followed up with CT angiography as a confirmatory study.

References

1. Lee BB, Laredo J, Lee TS, Huh S, Neville R. Terminology and classification of congenital vascular malformations. Phlebology. 2007;22(6):249–52.
2. Lee BB. Critical issues on the management of congenital vascular malformation. Ann Vasc Surg. 2004;18(3):380–92.
3. Mulliken JB, Glowacki J. Hemangiomas and vascular malformations in infants and children: a classification based on endothelial characteristics. Plast Reconstr Surg. 1982;69:412–22.
4. Lee BB, Kim HH, Mattassi R, Yakes W, Loose D, Tasnadi G. A new approach to the congenital vascular malformation with new concept -Seoul Consensus. Int J Angiol. 2003;12:248–51.
5. Lee BB. Chapter 41. Vascular surgery – 2nd edition: cases, questions and commentaries. Geroulakos, van Urk, Hobson II, Calligaro, editors. Congenital vascular malformation. Great Britain: Springer-Verlag London Limited; 2005. p. 377–92.
6. Mulliken JB. Treatment of hemangiomas. In: Mulliken JB, Young AE, editors. Vascular birthmarks, hemangiomas and malformations. Philadelphia: WB Saunders; 1988. p. 88–90.
7. Tasnadi G. Epidemiology and etiology of congenital vascular malformations. Semin Vasc Surg. 1993;6:200–3.
8. Belov S. Anatomopathological classification of congenital vascular defects. Semin Vasc Surg. 1993;6:219–24.
9. Wassef M, Blei F, Adams D, Alomari A, Baselga E, Berenstein A, Burrows P, Frieden IJ, Garzon MC, Lopez-Gutierrez JC, Lord DJ, Mitchel S, Powell J, Prendiville J, Vikkula M, ISSVA Board and Scientific Committee. Vascular anomalies classification: recommendations from the International Society for the Study of Vascular Anomalies. Pediatrics. 2015 Jul;136(1):e203–14.
10. Enjolras O, Wassef M, Chapot R. Introduction: ISSVA classification. In: Color atlas of vascular tumors and vascular malformations. New York: Cambridge University Press; 2007. p. 1–11.
11. Al-Shahi R, Warlow C. A systematic review of the frequency and prognosis of arteriovenous malformations of the brain in adults. Brain. 2001;124(10):1900–26.
12. Cho SK, Do YS, Shin SW, Choo SW, Choo IW, et al. Arteriovenous malformations of the body and extremities: analysis of therapeutic outcomes and approaches according to a modified angiographic classification. J Endovasc Ther. 2006 Aug;13(4):527–38.
13. Lee BB, Laredo J, Deaton DH, Neville RF. Arteriovenous malformations: evaluation and treatment. In: Gloviczki P, editor. Handbook of venous disorders: guidelines of the American Venous Forum. 3rd ed. London: Hodder Arnold Ltd; 2009.
14. Lee BB. Chapter 76. Mastery of vascular and endovascular surgery. Zelenock, Huber, Messina, Lumsden, Moneta, editors. Arteriovenous malformation. Philidelphia: Lippincott, Williams and Wilkins publishers; 2006. p. 597–607.
15. Lee BB. Current concept of venous malformation (VM). Phlebolymphol. 2003;43:197–203.
16. Lee BB, Baumgartner I, Berlien P, Bianchini G, Burrows P, Gloviczki P, Huang Y, Laredo J, Loose DA, Markovic J, Mattassi R, Parsi K, Rabe E, Rosenblatt M, Shortell C, Stillo F, Vaghi M, Villavicencio L, Zamboni P. Diagnosis and treatment of venous malformations. Consensus document of the International Union of Phlebology (IUP): updated 2013. Int Angiol. 2015;34(2):97–149
17. Lee BB, Laredo J, Seo JM, Neville R. Chapter 29. Hemangiomas and vascular malformations. Mattassi, Loose, Vaghi, editors. Treatment of lymphatic malformations. Milan: Springer-Verlag Italia; 2009. p. 231–50
18. Lee BB, Kim YW, Seo JM, Hwang JH, Do YS, Kim DI, Byun HS, Lee SK, Huh SH, Hyun WS. Current concepts in lymphatic malformation (LM). J Vasc Endovasc Surg. 2005;39(1):67–81.
19. Fishman SJ, Young AE. Slow-flow vascular malformations. In: Mulliken JB, Burrows PE, Fishman SJ, editors. Mulliken & young's vascular anomalies, hemangiomas and malformations. 2nd ed. New York: Oxford University Press; 2013. p. 562–94.
20. Ziyeh S, Spreer J, Rossler J, Strecker R, Hochmuth A, Schumacher M, Klisch J. Parkes weber or klippel-trenaunay syndrome? Non-invasive diagnosis with MR projection angiography. Eur Radiol. 2004;14(11):2025–9.

Differential Diagnosis from Hemangioma

13

Francine Blei

Introduction

The term "vascular anomalies" represents a diverse range of vascular lesions. In order to properly manage patients, it is essential to understand the difference between a hemangioma and other vascular anomalies, as the clinical course and potential complications are very different. To date, many individuals are diagnosed as having "hemangiomas" irrespective of the clinical progression, patient age, appearance, and behavior of the vascular lesion. In one study which reviewed "hemangioma" publications in PubMed, "terminological imprecision is prevalent among both medical and surgical fields. Inaccurate designation of the vascular anomaly is associated with an increased risk of erroneous management" [1]. These authors also found that nearly 50% of patients directed to their multidisciplinary vascular anomalies program were referred with an incorrect diagnosis of hemangioma.

This chapter will focus on approaches to distinguish hemangiomas from vascular malformations. Selected citations represent updated reviews, when possible. Reference to the updated ISSVA classification is recommended (ISSVA classification of vascular anomalies ©2014 available at "issva.org/classification") as well as the manuscript elucidating this classification [2]. (Refer to Table 8.1) illustrates the basic ISSVA classification, and (refer to Table 8.3) Table 13.1 further define diagnoses of importance and representative clinical features contributing to the accurate characterization of vascular lesions.

Differentiation Between Vascular Tumor and Vascular Malformation

Refer to Table 8.1 illustrates the introductory and basic compartmentalization of vascular anomalies into malformations vs. tumors, the latter group exhibiting proliferation during all or part of the life cycle of the lesion. The benign and locally aggressive vascular tumors (further described in refer to Table 8.3) predominantly occur in the pediatric population. The categories in Table 13.1 simplify this stratification by age group and delve further into features to distinguish vascular tumors/hemangiomas vs. vascular malformations by answering relevant queries. These tables validate the axiom "not every vascular anomaly is a hemangioma" and provide a rationale for judiciously acquiring a meaningful history (initial appearance and clinical evolution of the vascular lesion) and physical examination to suitably individualize the evaluation and management of the patient. Figures 13.1 and 13.2 illustrate visual differences among these diagnoses.

F. Blei, MD, MBA
Co-Director, Vascular Anomalies Program of Lenox Hill Hospital, 210 East 64th Street - 7th Floor, New York, NY 10065, USA
e-mail: fblei@northwell.edu

© Springer-Verlag Berlin Heidelberg 2017
Y.-W. Kim et al. (eds.), *Congenital Vascular Malformations*, DOI 10.1007/978-3-662-46709-1_13

Table 13.1 Features of vascular tumors/hemangiomas vs. vascular malformations

Query	Vascular tumor/hemangioma	Vascular malformation
What is the age of the patient – infant, older child, adult?	Infant child	Infant, child adult
Was the lesion diagnosed in utero?	Congenital hemangioma RICH – rapidly involuting NICH – non-involuting PICH – partially involuting Kaposiform hemangioendothelioma	May be diagnosed prenatally
Was it present at birth?	Precursor lesion of infantile hemangioma Congenital hemangioma Tufted angioma Kaposiform hemangioendothelioma	May be evident at birth or later
Has it remained stable, proliferated, or improved with time?	Minimally proliferative or abortive hemangioma [10, 11]	May remain stable unless subjected to trauma, infection, hormonal changes, aging, etc.
Is there more than one vascular lesion (and did they all appear at the same time or are more appearing over time)?	Does not distinguish diagnosis	Does not distinguish diagnosis
Location and quality – cervicofacial, trunk, intraoral, etc.; superficial, subcutaneous, or both; soft/firm; transilluminates, fills in dependent position; red/blue/purple/flesh colored; segmental distribution, smooth surface vs. cobblestoned, etc.	Location does not distinguish diagnosis however several features may point in the direction of a specific syndrome Segmental distribution cues PHACE[a] or LUMBAR[b] evaluation [12, 13]	Location does not distinguish diagnosis; however, several features may point in the direction of a specific syndrome or diagnosis, e.g.: VVM: fills in dependent position AVM: thrill, bruit LM transilluminates, serous/serosanguinous oozing, blebs
Are there any associated problems? (e.g., pain, bleeding – epistaxis/intraoral/other – oozing of clear or serosanguinous fluid, ophthalmologic issues, swelling, limb girth/length discrepancies?)	Location does not distinguish diagnosis; however, several features may point in the direction of a specific syndrome or diagnosis	Location does not distinguish diagnosis; however, several features may point in the direction of a specific syndrome or diagnosis, e.g., HHT: Recurrent epistaxis [14] Macrocephaly: PTEN or other vascular malformation syndrome [15–19]
Is there a family history of similar lesions, macrocephaly, cancers, other symptoms?	Rare in vascular tumors	Important to determine in many vascular malformations/vascular malformation syndromes [15, 20–24]

[a]Posterior fossa structural malformations, hemangiomas (segmental), arterial anomalies, cardiac defects, eye anomalies, and sternal and other midline deformities
[b]Lower body hemangioma, urogenital anomalies, ulceration, myelopathy, bony deformities, anorectal malformations, arterial anomalies, and renal anomalies

Features of Hemangiomas

Hemangiomas of infancy are considered the most common tumor of childhood. They exemplify benign growths of endothelial cells and have a unique natural history, distinguished by a rapid growth phase usually beginning during the first few weeks of life and continuing until 9–12 months of age. The typical growth curve of hemangiomas is noted in Fig. 13.1. Note that in addition to the more typical hemangiomas of infancy, congenital hemangiomas represent a distinct hemangioma subtype of that proliferates in utero and is thus present as an obvious mass at birth. Congenital hemangiomas may be diagnosed by prenatal ultrasound and may become symptomatic in utero due to arterial flow which can result in a high output state in the fetus. There

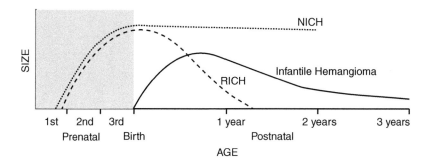

Fig. 13.1 Growth curves for infantile hemangioma, RICH and NICH (Mulliken and Enjolras [7]). *RICH* rapidly involuting congenital hemangioma, *NICH* non-involuting congenital hemangioma, *PICH* partially involuting congenital hemangioma

may be an associated transient, spontaneously resolved modest thrombocytopenia during the first week of life. Rapidly involuting congenital hemangiomas have a characteristic circumferential halo. Without treatment, most will undergo gradual involution. Often, the end result is a wrinkly and/or discolored area. Figure 13.2 depicts a representative RICH lesion, which was present at birth, had a circumferential halo, and improved without intervention. Partially involuting congenital hemangiomas (PICH) and non-involuting congenital hemangiomas will have the features of a RICH; however, the end result will differ based on the degree of improvement. In comparison, a hemangioma of infancy is minimally noted during the first week of life and proliferates postnatally. "Beard" distribution hemangiomas should alert the practitioner to possible airway involvement [3]. When hemangiomas are located in a segmental distribution, syndromes such as PHACE or LUMBAR should be considered [4]. Immunohistochemical differentiation between these lesions is represented by the absence of GLUT-1 staining in congenital hemangiomas and strong expression of GLUT-1 in hemangiomas of infancy. While they are histologically benign, hemangiomas may cause substantial psychosocial morbidity; thus, treatment during the initial growth phase aims to prevent further growth and associated morbidity, stimulate an earlier and more complete involution, and allow for an acceptable esthetic result. An updated, comprehensive guideline and executive summary published by the American Academy of Pediatrics provides a detailed review of hemangiomas, including clinical features, pathogenesis, and management [5, 6].

Kaposiform Hemangioendothelioma

Another relatively vascular lesion seen in the pediatric and neonatal age group is kaposiform hemangioendothelioma. This diagnosis and tufted angioma may be associated with Kasabach-Merritt phenomenon, with profound thrombocytopenia, hypofibrinogenemia, and elevation of D-dimers [8, 9]. Kaposiform hemangioendothelioma often appears boggy. The radiologic feature is stranding of the lesion into adjacent muscle tissue.

In contrast, *congenital vascular malformations* are present in utero and at birth (although not always detected until later in life) and do not undergo the proliferation and involution seen with hemangiomas of infancy. Observations and research in recent years have defined vascular malformations by the predominantly affected vessel type and potential associated symptoms and/or skeletal or other developmental anomalies. Depending on the location and extent of anatomic involvement and/or associated symptoms, patients may require early therapies. Those with significant cervicofacial and airway compromise may warrant heightened in utero monitoring and modified means of delivery[1]. However, some patients with

---

[1] e.g., EXIT procedure: *ex* utero *i*ntrapartum *t*reatment – cesarean section with partial delivery of the infant and establishment of a secure airway prior to detaching the infant from the umbilical cord.

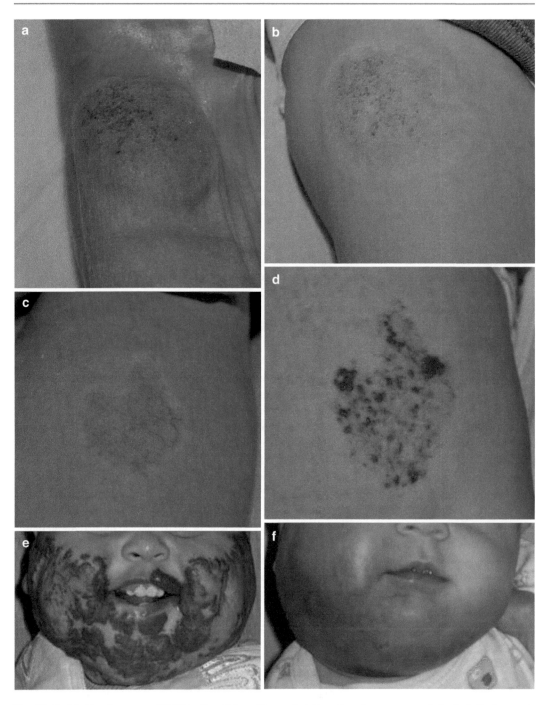

Fig. 13.2 (**a**) Vascular mass (RICH) of a 9-day-old infant. Lesion was present at birth. Note circumferential halo. (**b**) Vascular mass of same patient at 9 months of age, with spontaneous improvement. (**c**) Vascular lesion at 6 days of age. (**d**) Vascular lesion in C at 2 months of age. (**e**) Segmental vascular lesion with postnatal proliferation and stridor. Bronchoscopy revealed subglottic hemangioma. Imaging demonstrated arteriopathy compatible with PHACE syndrome. (**f**) Kaposiform hemangioendothelioma, with boggy fullness. Patient had profound thrombocytopenia, hypofibrinogenemia, and elevation of D-dimers (Kasabach-Merritt phenomenon)

less acute areas of involvement can be monitored over time, with treatments timed to associated or impending symptoms. Identification of the correct diagnosis is essential to guide the appropriate monitoring. This information is included in Table 13.1. It is now recognized that some vascular malformations are syndromic and an expanding list of causal germline and somatic mutations has been identified as reviewed in Chap. 4.

Conclusion

Differentiation of vascular malformations from hemangiomas is important in order to provide appropriate care and inform patients and families of realistic expectations. Fortunately, there is a mounting interest in vascular anomalies in the medical community, which ideally will translate into a heightened awareness of the differences among these diagnoses and improved clinical care.

Acknowledgments The author is grateful for the patients with vascular anomalies, their families, and colleagues who participate in the care of and research in this field.

References

1. Hassanein AH, Mulliken JB, Fishman SJ, Greene AK. Evaluation of terminology for vascular anomalies in current literature. Plast Reconstr Surg. 2011;127(1):347–51.
2. Wassef M, Blei F, Adams D, Alomari A, Baselga E, Berenstein A, et al. Vascular anomalies classification: recommendations from the International Society for the Study of Vascular Anomalies. Pediatrics. 2015; 136(1):e203–14.
3. Orlow SJ, Isakoff MS, Blei F. Increased risk of symptomatic hemangiomas of the airway in association with cutaneous hemangiomas in a "beard" distribution. J Pediatr. 1997;131(4):643–6.
4. Haggstrom AN, Lammer EJ, Schneider RA, Marcucio R, Frieden IJ. Patterns of infantile hemangiomas: new clues to hemangioma pathogenesis and embryonic facial development. Pediatrics. 2006;117(3):698–703.
5. Darrow DH, Greene AK, Mancini AJ, Nopper AJ, Section On Dermatology SOO-H, Neck S, et al. Diagnosis and management of infantile hemangioma. Pediatrics. 2015;136(4):e1060–104.
6. Darrow DH, Greene AK, Mancini AJ, Nopper AJ, Section On Dermatology SOO-H, Neck S, et al. Diagnosis and management of infantile hemangioma: executive summary. Pediatrics. 2015;136(4):786–91.
7. Mulliken JB, Enjolras O. Congenital hemangiomas and infantile hemangioma: missing links. J Am Acad Dermatol. 2004;50(6):875–82.
8. Sarkar M, Mulliken JB, Kozakewich HP, Robertson RL, Burrows PE. Thrombocytopenic coagulopathy (Kasabach-Merritt phenomenon) is associated with Kaposiform hemangioendothelioma and not with common infantile hemangioma. Plast Reconstr Surg. 1997;100(6):1377–86.
9. Enjolras O, Wassef M, Mazoyer E, Frieden IJ, Rieu PN, Drouet L, et al. Infants with Kasabach-Merritt syndrome do not have "true" hemangiomas. J Pediatr. 1997;130(4):631–40.
10. Corella F, Garcia-Navarro X, Ribe A, Alomar A, Baselga E. Abortive or minimal-growth hemangiomas: immunohistochemical evidence that they represent true infantile hemangiomas. J Am Acad Dermatol. 2008;58(4):685–90.
11. Suh KY, Frieden IJ. Infantile hemangiomas with minimal or arrested growth: a retrospective case series. Arch Dermatol. 2010;146(9):971–6.
12. Metry D, Heyer G, Hess C, Garzon M, Haggstrom A, Frommelt P, et al. Consensus statement on diagnostic criteria for PHACE syndrome. Pediatrics. 2009;124(5):1447–56.
13. Iacobas I, Burrows PE, Frieden IJ, Liang MG, Mulliken JB, Mancini AJ, et al. LUMBAR: association between cutaneous infantile hemangiomas of the lower body and regional congenital anomalies. J Pediatr. 2010;157(5):795–801 e1–7.
14. Yin LX, Reh DD, Hoag JB, Mitchell SE, Mathai SC, Robinson GM, Merlo CA. The minimal important difference of the epistaxis severity score in hereditary hemorrhagic telangiectasia. Laryngoscope. 2016; 126(5):1029–32.
15. Vanderver A, Tonduti D, Kahn I, Schmidt J, Medne L, Vento J, et al. Characteristic brain magnetic resonance imaging pattern in patients with macrocephaly and PTEN mutations. Am J Med Genet A. 2014; 164A(3):627–33.
16. Mester JL, Tilot AK, Rybicki LA, Frazier 2nd TW, Eng C. Analysis of prevalence and degree of macrocephaly in patients with germline PTEN mutations and of brain weight in Pten knock-in murine model. Eur J Hum Genet. 2011;19(7):763–8.
17. Vogels A, Devriendt K, Legius E, Decock P, Marien J, Hendrickx G, et al. The macrocephaly-cutis marmorata telangiectatica congenita syndrome. Long-term follow-up data in 4 children and adolescents. Genet Couns. 1998;9(4):245–53.
18. Williams CA, Dagli A, Battaglia A. Genetic disorders associated with macrocephaly. Am J Med Genet A. 2008;146A(15):2023–37.
19. Tosi LL, Sapp JC, Allen ES, O'Keefe RJ, Biesecker LG. Assessment and management of the orthopedic and other complications of Proteus syndrome. J Child Orthop. 2011;5(5):319–27.
20. Bubien V, Bonnet F, Brouste V, Hoppe S, Barouk-Simonet E, David A, et al. High cumulative risks of cancer in patients with PTEN hamartoma tumour syndrome. J Med Genet. 2013;50(4):255–63.
21. Pilarski R, Burt R, Kohlman W, Pho L, Shannon KM, Swisher E. Cowden syndrome and the PTEN hamartoma tumor syndrome: systematic review and revised

diagnostic criteria. J Natl Cancer Inst. 2013;105(21): 1607–16.

22. Mahdi H, Mester JL, Nizialek EA, Ngeow J, Michener C, Eng C. Germline PTEN, SDHB-D, and KLLN alterations in endometrial cancer patients with cowden and cowden-like syndromes: an international, multicenter, prospective study. Cancer. 2014.

23. Tan WH, Baris HN, Burrows PE, Robson CD, Alomari AI, Mulliken JB, et al. The spectrum of vascular anomalies in patients with PTEN mutations: implications for diagnosis and management. J Med Genet. 2007;44(9):594–602.

24. Alomari AI, Spencer SA, Arnold RW, Chaudry G, Kasser JR, Burrows PE, et al. Fibro-adipose vascular anomaly: clinical-radiologic-pathologic features of a newly delineated disorder of the extremity. J Pediatr Orthop. 2014;34(1):109–17.

Venous Malformation of the Head and Neck and Extremities

14

Patricia E. Burrows

Venous malformation [VM] is the most common symptomatic vascular malformation. Most are sporadic. Familial mucocutaneous VM is caused by germline mutations in the gene for the endothelial tyrosine kinase receptor TIE2, while 50% of sporadic VM has somatic TIE2 mutations [1]. These genetic changes result in poor development of the basement membrane and smooth muscle layer, irregular formation of the endothelial cell monolayer, and dysregulation of plasminogen/ plasmin proteolytic pathway enzymes. As a result, the affected veins are enlarged and irregularly shaped and tend to form thrombi. Intralesional thrombosis can result in further expansion and deformity. VM can involve the main conducting venous channels, termed truncal VM, or smaller veins within the various tissues, termed extratruncal VM [2, 3]. They can be focal, multifocal, or diffuse and occur in most of the human tissue planes, especially the skin and subcutaneous tissue, mucosa, and musculoskeletal structures.

Clinical Presentation of VM

VMs involving the skin have a blue color, while those in the deeper soft tissues cause swelling (Figs. 14.1 and 14.2). The swelling can be focal or symmetrical, the latter in the case of diffuse VM. Typically, skin temperature is normal and lesions are not pulsatile. Most VMs are compressible, due to communication with draining veins. Some focal VM without major draining veins can be more cyst-like in consistency. Typically, VM will expand or swell with dependency or increased venous pressure. In the head and neck, Valsalva maneuver or crying can cause swelling. Intralesional thrombi are frequently palpable; calcified thrombi or phleboliths are typical. Extensive VMs are associated with increased systemic levels of d-dimers and reduced fibrinogen levels, often referred to as localized intravascular coagulation [LIC] [4]. This usually does not cause symptoms, unless the patient is undergoing surgery or has traumatic injury. VMs are usually present at birth but may be diagnosed later in life, especially if the skin is not involved. Most VMs progress over time, especially during adolescence [5].

In the head and neck, symptomatology depends upon the location and extent of VM. Orbital involvement leads to proptosis with dependency and enoptosis in the upright position. VM within or adjacent to the airway causes airway obstruction and difficulty with breathing, swallowing, and speech, also worse with dependency [6]. Spontaneous bleeding is not common but can occur with intubation or other instrumentation. VM is usually associated with underdevelopment of the underlying bones, and in the head and neck, this can lead to dental bite abnormalities and erosion of the skull base

P.E. Burrows, MD
Medical College of Wisconsin, Children's Hospital of Wisconsin, Milwaukee, WI, USA
e-mail: PBurrows@chw.org

© Springer-Verlag Berlin Heidelberg 2017
Y.-W. Kim et al. (eds.), *Congenital Vascular Malformations*, DOI 10.1007/978-3-662-46709-1_14

leading to encephalocele and sinus pericranii. A high percentage of patients with diffuse facial VM have intracranial developmental venous and dural sinus anomalies [7]. VM of the face and scalp frequently presents with pain, related to swelling and intralesional clots.

In the extremities, VM typically presents with painful swelling, often worse with standing and activity. Pain is usually relieved with elevation. Many patients complain of severe pain on awakening in the morning, likely due to intralesional thrombosis. Diffuse VMs are often associated with undergrowth of the affected limb (Fig. 14.2). Bones may be thin, deformed, and easily fractured. VM of the lower extremity is usually associated with intrasynovial VM of the knee joint, which progresses to severe arthropathy due to the presence of cartilage damage, over time [8]. Intramuscular VM is often associated with joint contractures, partly caused by chronic decreased movement related to pain. Many females notice

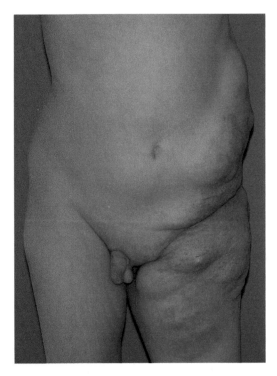

Fig. 14.1 Extensive diffuse VM of the left flank and thigh with subcutaneous and cutaneous involvement. Lesion is soft and compressible, with palpable clots. Blue color is typical

increased swelling and pain around the time of menses, as well as during pregnancy or with the use of estrogen containing oral contraceptives.

Uncommon Forms of Venous Malformation

Mucocutaneous venous malformations can be familial, caused by TIE2 mutations. As the name implies, these involve the skin and mucous membranes and tend to be multifocal, involving multiple sites in the same patient. Most of the lesions represent focal blebs that respond well to sclerotherapy or resection. However, patients can also have focal varices of major conducting veins.

Blue rubber bleb nevus syndrome [Bean syndrome] can be sporadic or familial and appears to be caused by TIE2 mutations. Affected patients have multifocal VM involving the skin, muscles, and gastrointestinal (GI) tract. Cutaneous lesions are usually small and dome-shaped and develop progressively over the life of the patient. Muscular lesions are also focal but can occur in clumps to form a large mass. They present with pain. They usually have minimal communication with draining veins and respond well to sclerotherapy. Many patients present at birth with a large dominant venous malformation that can be extremely deforming (Fig. 14.3). Gastrointestinal lesions are usually small and numerous, often reaching more than 100 and extending throughout the GI tract. They cause bleeding, often leading to transfusion requirements, and are treated by resection. They are often diagnosed by a combination of upper and lower endoscopy and capsule endoscopy. Occasionally, they can be associated with abdominal pain due to intussusception. Successful treatment with rapamycin has been reported.

Glomuvenous malformations are familial, autosomal dominant, and caused by mutations in glomulin. They typically involve the skin and subcutaneous tissues and appear as small, often confluent nodules. They are often not completely compressible due to the presence of solid components and are quite tender and painful. These lesions develop progressively over the life of the patient. They do not respond well to sclerother-

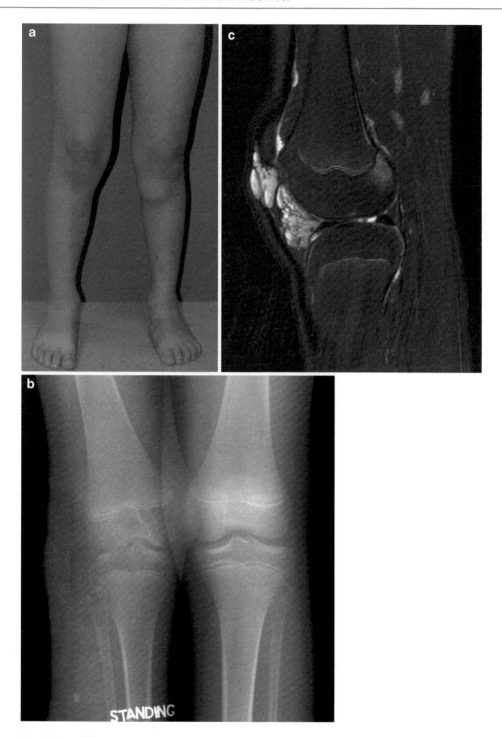

Fig. 14.2 Diffuse VM of the lower extremity. (**a**) A 5-year-old with diffuse VM of the left lower extremity. Note the blue color, underdevelopment with significantly smaller left foot, subcutaneous varicosities, and focal swelling below the medial knee. (**b**) Radiograph of a patient with diffuse VM of the right lower extremity, including the knee, shows decreased size and density of the bones and severe narrowing of the joint space. Note swelling and phleboliths in the soft tissues. (**c**) Sagittal STIR image shows VM in Hoffa's fat pad in another patient, impinging on the articular surfaces of the femur and patella

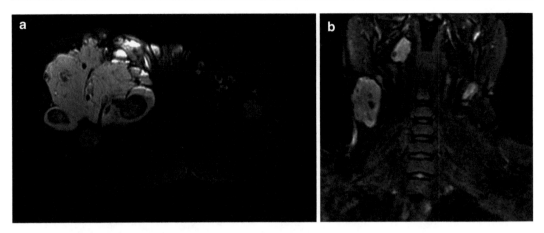

Fig. 14.3 Blue rubber bleb nevus syndrome with large dominant and multiple smaller focal intramuscular VMs. Patient had multiple GI lesions resected for severe GI bleeding. (**a**) Axial STIR image of the thighs shows a large dominant focal VM with numerous phleboliths and thrombi. (**b**) Coronal T2-weighted image showing multiple focal VMs in the neck of the same patient

apy and are often too extensive to resect completely. However, resection is often effective in treating focal painful lesions.

Fibroadipose vascular anomaly [FAVA] is an intramuscular lesion, often involving the gastrocnemius muscles, that contains a combination of fibroadipose tissue, lymphatic malformation, and dysplastic venous channels [9]. It is associated with pain and often does not respond well to sclerotherapy.

Laboratory Evaluation

Patients with extensive VM should have a coagulation profile, including PT, PTT, INR, fibrinogen level, and d-dimers. If it is normal, it does not need to be repeated frequently. If fibrinogen levels are low and INR is elevated, the patient should be treated with low molecular weight heparin prior to any invasive procedures in order to improve coagulation.

Imaging of VM

While clinical evaluation is adequate to diagnose superficial VMs, ultrasonography is useful to confirm the diagnosis and magnetic resonance [MR] imaging is best to assess the extent of dis-

ease and secondary effects (Figs. 14.4 and 14.5). Computed tomography [CT] is usually not a good modality to evaluate VM, since they have similar Hounsfield units to normal soft tissues and enhance unevenly. CT is helpful however in studying bone involvement and clearly demonstrates calcified phleboliths.

Magnetic resonance [MR] imaging is the best imaging modality because of the high contrast resolution [10]. VMs produce a similar signal [isointense] to muscle on T1-weighted sequences but are strongly hyperintense compared with the muscle on fluid-sensitive sequences such as T2-weighted images with fat suppression or STIR. After the administration of gadolinium, they enhance slowly, depending on the degree of arterial supply, communication with conducting veins, and the time delay between intravenous contrast injection and imaging. VMs typically enhance inhomogeneously, often leading to the erroneous diagnosis of "venolymphatic malformation" (Fig. 14.4b). VMs usually contain signal voids due to the presence of intralesional clots or phleboliths. The structure of VM varies from patient to patient. They may appear as focal, septated masses in the subcutaneous tissue or muscle. Alternatively, diffuse VM may appear as large collections of T2 hyperintensity corresponding to affected tissue planes. Diffuse lesions often

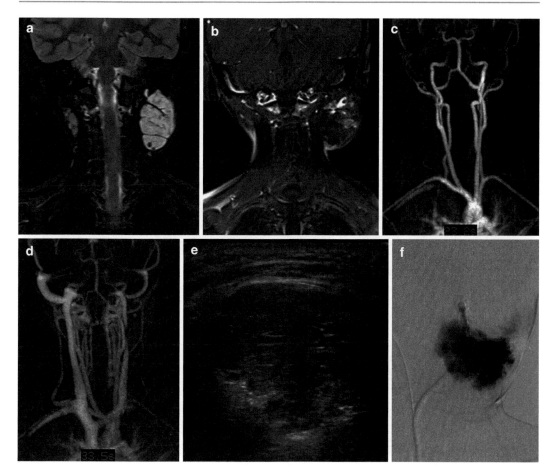

Fig. 14.4 Imaging of focal VM of the left neck in a child. (**a**) Coronal STIR image shows a smooth walled, septated, hyperintense mass containing phleboliths. (**b**) Coronal T1-weighted image with IV contrast enhancement and fat saturation shows only partial enhancement of the mass, due to slow filling. This is a pure VM, not LVM. (**c, d**) Time-resolved contrast-enhanced MR angiography of the neck shows normal arteries and conducting veins. The VM does not fill. (**e**) Ultrasonography shows a focal septated sponge-like mass. (**f**) Percutaneous contrast injection with road map technique shows the typical internal architecture of a focal VM, without significant drainage

contain non-truncal and truncal components, the latter seen as deep or superficial varicosities (Fig. 14.5). Lesions may involve the bones or periosteum as well as joints (Fig. 14.2).

MR angiography may be useful to demonstrate the anatomy of the main conducting veins but can also lead to misdiagnosis of AVM. In many cases, dilated cutaneous or muscular arterial branches may appear to shunt into the malformation. However, on close inspection, the bulk of the VM is not opacified, and the small channels that are visualized appear only slightly earlier than normal veins. However, misdiagnosis as AVM has led to improper treatment by arterial

embolization, which typically results in severe tissue necrosis.

Typical findings on conventional angiography are similar. The lesions may not be visible, but usually, small curvilinear channels are opacified slightly before the normal veins. To visualize the main components or channels making up the VM, direct injection of contrast medium into the lesion is necessary. As with MRI, findings on contrast injection are variable. Some focal lesions are circumscribed and have no, or minimal, venous drainage. It may be difficult to distinguish VM without venous drainage from lymphatic malformation with

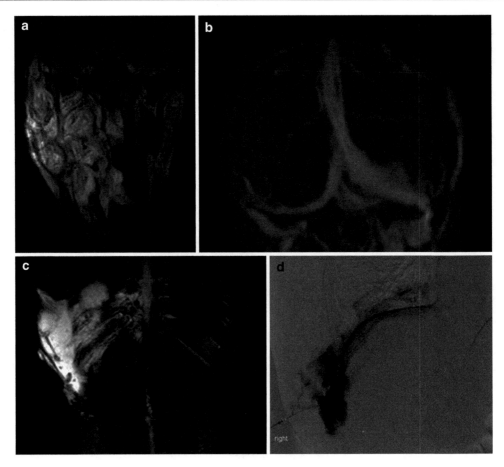

Fig. 14.5 Examples of diffuse VM. (**a**) Coronal T2-weighted image of the neck shows a diffuse VM involving the right face and neck, including all of the anatomical structures, with some airway narrowing. (**b**) MR venogram of the brain in a patient with diffuse VM of the face and neck showing anomalies of the dural sinuses and scalp veins. The patient also had sinus pericranii. (**c**) Coronal STIR image of the abdomen shows diffuse VM of the abdominal and thoracic wall including the ribs and intercostal veins. (**d**) Contrast injection into lesion shown in (**b**), confirming the presence of large varices and direct drainage into dysplastic intercostal veins

intralesional hemorrhage. With adequate contrast injection, however, some draining veins can almost always be demonstrated. Puig et al. reported a classification of VM based on venous drainage patterns, which is helpful in predicting the safety and effect of intralesional sclerosant injection [11].

MR imaging of glomuvenous malformations demonstrates enhancing T2 hyperintense nodules in the subcutaneous tissue and skin, with multiple nodules often connected by tiny venous channels. Occasionally, underlying muscle can be involved as well. On ultrasonography, individual nodules often have solid, as well as compressible components.

MR imaging of blue rubber bleb nevus syndrome shows multiple focal lesions, sometimes clustered, without extensive dilated venous channels (Fig. 14.3). All of the muscles can be involved, but some common sites include the submandibular areas, neck muscles, and gluteal muscles. Minor involvement of the liver and spleen is common. Large dominant lesions often appear septated and contain clots or phleboliths. Bowel lesions may be difficult to image. Radionuclide blood pool imaging can be used to assess the extent, but capsule endoscopy is usually adequate.

References

1. Soblet J, Limaye N, Uebelhoer M, Boon LM, Vikkula M. Variable somatic TIE2 mutations in half of sporadic venous malformations. Molecular Syndromol. 2013;4(4):179–83.
2. Lee BB, Baumgartner I, Berlien P, Bianchini G, Burrows P, Gloviczki P, et al. Diagnosis and treatment of venous malformations. consensus document of the international union of phlebology (iup): updated-2013. Int Angiol. 2015; 34:97–149.
3. Wassef M, Blei F, Adams D, Alomari A, Baselga E, Berenstein A, et al. Vascular anomalies classification: recommendations from the International Society for the Study of Vascular Anomalies. Pediatrics. 2015;136(1):e203–14.
4. Mazoyer E, Enjolras O, Laurian C, Houdart E, Drouet L. Coagulation abnormalities associated with extensive venous malformations of the limbs: differentiation from Kasabach-Merritt syndrome. Clin Lab Haematol. 2002;24(4):243–51.
5. Boon LM, Brouillard P, Irrthum A, Karttunen L, Warman ML, Rudolph R, et al. A gene for inherited cutaneous venous anomalies ("glomangiomas") localizes to chromosome 1p21-22. Am J Hum Genet. 1999;65(1):125–33.
6. Ohlms LA, Forsen J, Burrows PE. Venous malformation of the pediatric airway. Int J Pediatr Otorhinolaryngol. 1996;37(2):99–114.
7. Konez O, Burrows PE, Mulliken JB. Cervicofacial venous malformations. MRI features and interventional strategies. Inter Neuroradiol J Peritherapeutic Neuroradiol Surgical Procedures Related Neurosci. 2002;8(3):227–34.
8. Enjolras O, Ciabrini D, Mazoyer E, Laurian C, Herbreteau D. Extensive pure venous malformations in the upper or lower limb: a review of 27 cases. J Am Acad Dermatol. 1997;36(2 Pt 1):219–25.
9. Limaye N, Wouters V, Uebelhoer M, Tuominen M, Wirkkala R, Mulliken JB, et al. Somatic mutations in angiopoietin receptor gene TEK cause solitary and multiple sporadic venous malformations. Nat Genet. 2009;41(1):118–24.
10. Mulliken JB, Burrows PE, Fishman SJ, Mulliken JB. Mulliken and young's vascular anomalies: hemangiomas and malformations. 2nd ed. Oxford: Oxford University Press; 2013.
11. Puig S, Aref H, Chigot V, Bonin B, Brunelle F. Classification of venous malformations in children and implications for sclerotherapy. Pediatr Radiol. 2003;33(2):99–103.

Venous Malformation: Truncular Form

15

Young-Wook Kim and Raul Mattassi

Subtyping of venous malformation (VM) into truncular and extra-truncular form derives from the embryological background in Hamburg classification of CVM (see Chap. 9). In the International Society for the Study of Vascular Anomalies (ISSVA) classification, it is classified as "vascular anomaly of major named vessels" which is referred to "truncular form" malformations [1].

To understand the truncular congenital vascular malformation (CVM), it is important to know the pathogenesis of truncular VM. Primitive vascular tissue in the limb bud first appears in the third week of gestation. During the first stage (undifferentiated stage) of vasculogenesis, only a capillary network appears. In the second stage (retiform stage), large plexiform structures can be seen. In the third stage (maturation stage), it developed to larger channels and differentiate to the arteries, veins, and lymphatics [2].

Truncular VM lesions are believed to occur as a result of developmental arrest in the "later"

Y.-W. Kim, MD (✉)
Sungkyunkwan University, School of Medicine, Seoul, South Korea

Vascular Surgery, Samsung medical Center, Seoul, South Korea
e-mail: young52.kim@samsung.com; ywkim52@gmail.com

R. Mattassi (✉)
Department of Vascular Surgery, Center for Vascular Malformations "Stefan Belov", Clinical Institute Humanitas "Mater Domini" Castellanza, Varese, Italy
e-mail: raulmattassi@gmail.com

stage of the vasculogenesis. Since this developmental arrest occurs after an early stage (reticular stage) of the vasculogenesis, these lesions are also known as "post-truncal lesions." In contrast to "pre-truncal or extra-truncular lesion, truncular VM lesions do not have characteristics of an early embryonic vascular tissues, which can proliferate after birth by certain stimuli [3].

An International Interdisciplinary Consensus Committee on Venous Anatomical Terminology [4] defined venous abnormality as follows in Table 15.1.

It is reported that VM is the most common type of CVM, and deep vein anomaly presents in 47% of VM patients including various types of deep vein anomalies: *venomegalia* (phlebectasia) (36%), aplasia or hypoplasia (8%), venous aneurysm (8%), and avalvulia (congenital absence of valves in the venous trunks, 7%) [6].

The prevalence of deep venous anomalies is reported even higher in patients with mixed form of CVM which affects extremity veins, skin capillary (CM), lymphatic system (LM), and rarely arteriovenous malformation (AVM) [7].

The prevalence can be variable depending on the type of investigation and the definition of the anomaly. According to a study with fresh, non-embalmed cadavers by Jean-François Uhl et al. [8], they found that femoral venous system was unitruncular in 91% and bitruncular in 9%. Unitruncular femoral vein includes normal configuration (88%), deep femoral trunk (2%), and axio(sciatico)-femoral trunk (1%). Human

© Springer-Verlag Berlin Heidelberg 2017
Y.-W. Kim et al. (eds.), *Congenital Vascular Malformations*, DOI 10.1007/978-3-662-46709-1_15

Table 15.1 Terminology regarding abnormal caliber of the extremity vein

Anomaly	Definition
Dysplasia [4]	Complex abnormality of development of a vein or of a group of veins that greatly differ from the normal conditions in size, structure, and connections
Atrophy [4]	Decrease in size or wasting away of a normally developed vein or segment of a vein, following a degenerative process
Venous aneurysm [4]	Localized dilation of a venous segment, with a caliber increase ≥50% compared with normal
Venomegalia [4]	Diffuse dilation of one or more veins with a caliber increase ≥50% compared with normal
Agenesis [5]	Complete absence of a vein or of a segment of a vein
Aplasia [5]	Lack of development of a vein or of a segment of a vein. The vein is present but diminutive in size, and its structure is similar to that in the embryo
Hypoplasia [5]	Incomplete development of a vein or of a segment of a vein

Caggiati et al. [4]

Table 15.2 Frequency of truncular VM and various deep venous anomalies (at SMC, 1994–2015)

All CVM patients	$N = 3063$
Venous malformation	1576 (51.5%)
Pure VM	1378 (87%)
Venous predominant mixed CVM	198 (13%)
VM affecting the extremity	1019 (65%)
Extra-truncular VM	949 (93%)
Truncular[a] VM	146 (14%)
Venous aplasia	25 (17%)
Venous hypoplasia	18 (12%)
Venous aneurysm	1 (0.6%)
Venomegalia (phlebectasia)	12 (8%)
Persistent marginal vein	108 (74%)

VM venous malformation, *CVM* congenital vascular malformation

[a]Diagnosis of truncular VM was made with duplex ultra-sonography, MRI, whole-body blood pool scintigraphy, and/or venography

leg venous system finishes their embryologic development through the evolution and involution. In the case of axio(sciatico)-femoral and deep femoral trunk, the femoral vein is hypoplastic, and the axial (sciatic) vein or deep femoral vein works as the main draining trunk of the thigh. The venous duplication itself (e.g., double femoral veins) or patent but variant venous anatomy such as axio-femoral or deep femoral trunk does not cause hemodynamic abnormality in clinical practice.

According to the SMC database, venous predominant CVM accounts for 51.5% of all CVMs, and truncular VM accounts for 14% of all VM lesions affecting the extremity (Table 15.2).

Persistent marginal vein (MV) is not uncommon in patients with a lower extremity VM. It is an atypical truncular vein that failed to regress and characterized by superficially located dilated vein along the lateral aspect of the lower extremity with variable extension from the calf to the buttock.

Port-wine skin lesion (capillary malformation) and limb hypertrophy often coexist with MV as a combined type CVM. In addition to cosmetic problem due to varicosity and associated skin lesion, the clinical significance of MV is chronic venous insufficiency due to congenital absence of a venous valve in the MV. Besides, MV remains as a source of pulmonary embolism. MV is often associated with varying range of deep venous anomalies from aplasia or hypoplasia to intrinsic defects such as webs, stenosis, or defective valves of deep vein system. Weber et al. [9] classified marginal vein in five types with venographic study (Fig. 15.1).

As described above, the main clinical features of the truncular VM are venous hemodynamic consequences due to steno-occlusive (aplasia, hypoplasia), dilated lesions (venous aneurysm, venomegalia) of deep venous system in the extremity and venous reflux due to congenital absence of venous valve.

Since truncular VM is often combined with other forms of CVM such as capillary malformation (CM, skin red spot), lymphatic malformation (LM, lymphedema due to aplasia or hypoplasia of the main lymphatic trunks, lymphatic cyst or bleb, lymphorrhea), limb hypertrophy, or limb length discrepancy, the patients may present with

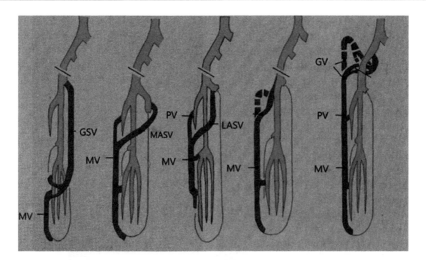

Fig. 15.1 Venographic classification of the marginal vein (Reprinted with permission [9]). *MV* marginal vein, *GSV* great saphenous vein, *MASV* medial accessory saphenous vein, *PV* perforator vein to deep femoral vein, *LASV* lateral accessory saphenous vein, *GV* gluteal vein

clinical features of complications of VM and LM such as cellulitis, venous thrombosis or pulmonary embolism, and stasis ulcer.

According to the extent and anatomic site of the VM lesion and combined CVM or its complication, clinical features are variable.

Because of sluggish blood flow through the anomalous venous channels, venous thrombosis is frequently formed causing local pain and tenderness. When the thrombus is superficially located, it may be palpable on physical examination and detectable on CT or MRI. Constant leg heaviness or acute intermittent episodes of pain may be a prominent feature of the VM patients. Various causes of leg pain are suggested in patients with mixed-type veno-lymphatic malformation (Klippel-Trenaunay syndrome), which include chronic venous insufficiency, cellulitis, growing bone pain, thrombophlebitis or venous thrombosis, phlebolith, intraosseous VM, arthritis, and neuropathic pain [10].

Phlebolith is a calcified organized venous thrombus, which is a characteristic feature of extra-truncular VM lesion. Diagnosis of VM in general is usually made with physical finding and either MRI or duplex ultrasonography. Deep vein anomaly (truncular VM) can be easily detected with duplex ultrasonography (US). Duplex US gives us an excellent morphological (caliber, depth, extent of deep vein abnormality or marginal vein) and hemodynamic information (connections with perforators and deep veins, flow direction) and presence of coexisting extra-truncular VM lesion.

For more detailed assessment of the associated VM lesion, MRI can be recommended. MRI is the most informative tool in the diagnosis and follow-up examinations of VM patients. Its advantages over duplex US are its capability to visualize the anatomic relationships between VM lesion and adjacent tissue (nerve, soft tissue, organ, bone, and joint). T2-weighted images are mainly used to evaluate the extent of the VM lesion, while gradient recalled echo (GRE) images are used to identify the lesion's flow characteristics. Gadolinium-enhanced MRI is used to determine the extent of the VM lesion and to distinguish slow-flow VM from lymphatic malformation (LM). And 3D, T1-weighted, contrast-enhanced MR image is similar to a venogram and readily identifies feeding and draining vessels [11].

Catheter venogram is not routinely performed as a diagnostic tool for patients with VM. However, venography is an essential road map during an embolo-sclerotherapy of an associated VM lesion because adjacent MV can provide a pathway of

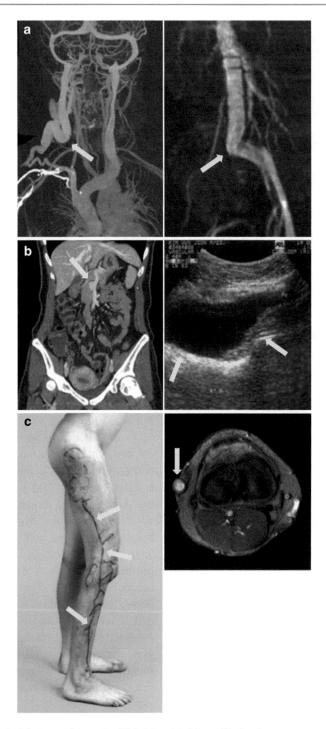

Fig. 15.2 Various clinical features of truncular VM. (**a**) Agenesis (aplasia): (*left*) right brachiocephalic vein agenesis on MR venogram and (*right*) right iliac vein agenesis on MR venogram. (**b**) Aneurysmal dilatation: (*left*) superior mesenteric vein aneurysm on CT venogram and (*right*) popliteal vein aneurysm on ultrasonography. (**c**) Persistent marginal vein along the lateral aspect of the right leg: (*left*) medical photo of the marginal vein in the right leg and (*right*) marginal vein in the right leg on contrast-enhanced CT scan

It can provide not only an abnormal blood pooling or lack of normal blood filling in the whole body (Fig. 15.3) but also interval changes of VM lesions with semiquantitative assessment of the amount of abnormal blood pooling in the VM lesion. Furthermore, WBBPS can also be an excellent tool to distinguish VM lesion from LM in patients with mixed form CVM.

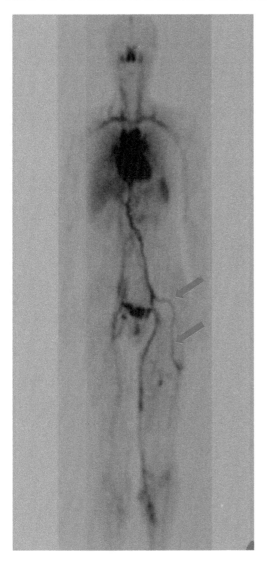

Fig. 15.3 Tc-99 m RBC whole-body blood pool scintigraphy (WBBPS). WBBPS in a 44-year-old male patient with venous malformation (VM) in the left leg, which shows uptake defect in the deep vein and increased uptake in the great saphenous vein and marginal vein (*arrow*)

pulmonary embolism from the preexisting venous thrombus in VM or embolization material.

We perform whole-body blood pool scintigraphy (WBBPS) to confirm the distribution of all VM lesions. WBBPS is a whole-body imaging obtained with dual-head gamma camera after intravenous injection of the radiolabeled erythrocytes (99mTc-RBC). High sensitivity (97%) is reported in the diagnosis of VM [12].

References

1. Wassef M, Blei F, Adams D, Alomari A, Baselga E, Berenstein A, Burrows P, Frieden IJ, Garzon MC, Lopez-Gutierrez JC, Lord DJ, Mitchel S, Powell J, Prendiville J, Vikkula M. Vascular anomalies classification: recommendations from the International Society for the Study of Vascular Anomalies. Pediatrics. 2015;136(1):e203–14. doi:10.1542/peds. 2014-3673.
2. Belov S. Anatomopathological classification of congenital vascular defects. Semin Vasc Surg. 1993; 6(4):219–24.
3. Lee BB, Baumgartner I, Berlien P, Bianchini G, Burrows P, Gloviczki P, Huang Y, Laredo J, Loose DA, Markovic J, Mattassi R, Parsi K, Rabe E, Rosenblatt M, Shortell C, Stillo F, Vaghi M, Villavicencio L, Zamboni P (2014) Guideline. Diagnosis and treatment of venous malformations. consensus document of the international union of phlebology (iup): updated-2013. Inter Angiol J Inter Union Angiol. International Angiology. 2015;34(2):97–149.
4. Caggiati A, Bergan JJ, Gloviczki P, Eklof B, Allegra C, Partsch H. Nomenclature of the veins of the lower limb: extensions, refinements, and clinical application. J Vasc Surg. 2005;41(4):719–24. doi:10.1016/j. jvs.2005.01.018.
5. Churchill's Medical Illustrated Dictionary. New York: Publisher Churchill Livingstone; 1994.
6. Eifert S, Villavicencio JL, Kao TC, Taute BM, Rich NM. Prevalence of deep venous anomalies in congenital vascular malformations of venous predominance. J Vasc Surg. 2000;31(3):462–71. doi:10.1067/ mva.2000.101464.
7. Lee BB, Laredo J, Lee SJ, Huh SH, Joe JH, Neville R. Congenital vascular malformations: general diagnostic principles. Phlebol Venous Forum Royal Soc Med. 2007;22(6):253–7.
8. Uhl JF, Gillot C, Chahim M. Anatomical variations of the femoral vein. J Vasc Surg. 2010;52(3):714–9. doi:10.1016/j.jvs.2010.04.014.
9. JH W. Invasive diagnostics of congenital vascular malformations. In: Mattassi R, DA L, Vaghi M, editors. Hemangiomas and vascular malformations. 1st ed. Milan: Springer; 2009. p. 139.
10. Lee A, Driscoll D, Gloviczki P, Clay R, Shaughnessy W, Stans A. Evaluation and management of pain in patients with Klippel-Trenaunay syndrome: a

review. Pediatrics. 2005;115(3):744–9. doi:10.1542/peds.2004-0446.

11. Rosenblatt M. Endovascular management of venous malformations. Phlebol Venous Forum Royal Soc Med. 2007;22(6):264–75. doi:10.1258/026835507782655290.

12. Kim YH, Choi JY, Kim YW, Kim DI, Do YS, Choe YS, Lee KH, Kim BT. Diagnosis and whole body screening using blood pool scintigraphy for evaluating congenital vascular malformations. Ann Vasc Surg. 2014;28(3):673–8. doi:10.1016/j.avsg.2013.02.025.

Hemolymphatic Malformation: Mixed Form Congenital Vascular Malformation

16

James Laredo and Byung-Boong Lee

Definition and Classification

Congenital vascular malformations (CVMs) are classified by vessel type according to the Hamburg classification (refer to Table 9.2) [1–4]. In each class of vascular malformation, "extra-truncular malformations" composed of small vessels intimately embedded in the host tissue and "truncular malformations" affecting individual large vessels are recognized [1–4].

Extratruncular vascular malformations arise when developmental arrest has occurred during the reticular stage of embryonic development [1, 2]. The mesenchymal cell properties persist and the lesions retain the potential to proliferate when stimulated (e.g., menarche, pregnancy, hormone, surgery, and trauma).

J. Laredo, MD, PhD (✉)
Division of Vascular Surgery, Department of Surgery, George Washington University, Washington, DC, USA
e-mail: jlaredo@mfa.gwu.edu

B.-B. Lee, MD, PhD, FACS (✉)
Professor of Surgery and Director, Center for the Lymphedema and Vascular Malformations, George Washington University, Washington, DC, USA

Adjunct Professor of Surgery, Uniformed Services, University of the Health Sciences, Bethesda, MD, USA
e-mail: bblee38@gmail.com

Truncular vascular malformations arise when developmental arrest has occurred during vascular trunk formation at the later stage of embryologic development [1, 2]. These lesions no longer possess the potential to proliferate. Truncular lesions present as poorly developed, immature vessels (aplasia or hypoplasia), or as hyperplastic vessels (hyperplasia) [1, 2].

The hemolymphatic malformation (HLM) is a combined CVM that has both venous malformation (VM) and a lymphatic malformation (LM) components [2]. This complex vascular malformation is found in Klippel-Trenaunay syndrome (KTS) [2, 5, 6]. These patients present with HLM lesions in addition to capillary malformations (CMs). Also known as a lympho-venous malformation, the HLM is one of the most well-studied combined CVMs that is almost exclusively found in KTS patients [2, 5, 6]. Another clinical entity classified as a HLM is Parkes-Webber syndrome, where patients with this combined CVM present with an arteriovenous malformation (AVM) in addition to the VM and LM [2].

Klippel-Trenaunay Syndrome

With its classic triad of port wine stains, lower-extremity soft tissue and bone hypertrophy and lower-extremity varicose veins, this clinical condition was originally described by French physicians, Maurice Klippel and Paul Trenaunay in 1900, based on observations in two patients with hemangiomatous lesions of the skin associated with asymmetric soft tissue and bone hypertrophy – "naevus variqueux osteohypertrophique" [5].

KTS is in general a sporadic occurring entity, with equal gender distribution and infrequent familial occurrence. No chromosomal localization or linkage with a causative gene has been reported, and its etiology remains unknown [5].

Clinical Presentation

KTS patients typically present with CMs (port wine stains), a usually longer and larger lower extremity because of soft tissue and bone hypertrophy and atypical mostly lateral superficial varicosities [5, 6]. Occasionally, a shorter and smaller limb may be present instead of hypertrophy. Patients with at least two of the three cardinal features have been classified as having an incomplete form of KTS [5, 6].

VM lesions frequently encountered in KTS patients include deep infiltrating venous malformations (extratruncular VMs), deep vein hypoplasia, atresia, or agenesis, deep vein dilatations, or aneurysms, and persistent embryonic veins (truncular VMs) [6, 7]. Persistent embryonic veins observed in KTS patients include the lateral marginal vein, which is the most common VM lesion found in KTS patients and the sciatic vein [8].

The lateral marginal vein originates from the lateral foot and courses upwards along the lateral border of the leg and thigh [6, 8]. The vein is usually thick walled, superficial, and incompetent due to the absence of venous valves [6, 8]. Drainage of the vein is usually into the internal iliac vein or a lateral branch of the profunda femoral vein [6, 8]. The vein may also cross anterior in the thigh and drain into the femoral vein adjacent to a normal great saphenous vein [6, 8]. The sciatic vein when present, may provide the main venous drainage of the limb from the popliteal vein up to the internal iliac vein [6, 8].

Varicose veins and VM lesions can also involve abdominal and pelvic organs [6, 7]. Bleeding from capillary or venous malformations or persistent embryonic veins may occur through defects in the skin or mucosa [6, 7]. Intramuscular and retroperitoneal bleeding may also occur in these patients in addition to hematuria, rectal bleeding, intracerebral, or intraspinal bleeding [6, 7].

LM lesions observed in KTS patients include primary lymphedema and lymphangiectasia (truncular LMs), as well as skin vesicles draining lymph fluid and cystic hygromas (extratruncular LMs) [6, 9, 10].

The severity of vascular lesions and symptoms observed in KTS patients can vary widely from those with an incomplete form of KTS with mild, asymptomatic port wine stains, and few varicose veins causing only minor cosmetic problems to patients with severe disability associated with massive limb overgrowth, chronic pain syndrome, skin infections, thromboembolism, and life-threatening pelvic or recurrent rectal bleeding from symptomatic VMs [5–7].

Diagnosis

HLMs are mixed congenital vascular lesions presenting with VM, LM, and/or CM components [1–4]. Therefore, the evaluation of a patient with a suspected HLM should proceed in a logical stepwise manner to confirm the presence of VM and LM lesions and to exclude the presence of an AVM lesion.

As a general rule, the extent and severity of any CVM affecting the vascular system (anatomically and hemodynamically) usually determines the type of clinical manifestations observed [1–4]. This is particularly true in patients with HLM and KTS. The diagnosis of KTS may often be made based on history and physical examination alone [5]. Confirmatory diagnostic imaging should follow in order to determine the type and extent of the VM and LM lesions present.

Physical examination of the affected limb and pelvic lesions should be followed by duplex ultrasound scanning of the venous system to define and determine the patency of the deep and superficial venous systems and characterize any aberrant anatomy such as hypoplasia, atresia, aneurysms, and persistent embryonic veins. Assessment of thrombosis and valvular incompetence of the deep, superficial, and perforating venous systems should also be performed. The presence of an AVM can also be determined with duplex ultrasound examination. Duplex ultrasound scanning should also be performed to determine the extent of the VM lesions present, specifically whether there is involvement of the subcutaneous tissues, fascia, muscle, and bone and the relationship to vascular structures.

Magnetic resonance imaging (MRI) and magnetic resonance angiography (MRA) remain the major diagnostic studies for all vascular anomalies including the entire group of CVMs. MRI allows assessment of lesion extent, severity, and anatomic relationship with the surrounding tissues and organs [2, 3]. It can differentiate between muscle, bone, fat, and vascular tissue without the need of radiation or nephrotoxic intravenous contrast. Axial, coronal, and sagittal images can be generated and gadolinium enhancement produces high-resolution angiography. Lymphedema also has a typical appearance on MRI [6, 9, 10].

Computed tomography (CT) imaging with high-resolution three-dimensional reconstruction allows assessment of vascular lesion extent, severity, and anatomic relationship with the surrounding tissues and organs. The quality of the imaging is usually adequate for planning treatment.

Contrast venography of the lower extremity allows complete evaluation of the venous system and assessment of patency, venous stenosis, occlusion, aberrant anatomy, and the presence of collateral venous circulation [2, 3]. Direct puncture phlebography of the venous malformation allows the diagnosis or exclusion of an AVM and assessment of the lesion and its relationship to the lower-extremity venous and arterial vasculature. When treatment is indicated, endovascular therapy can also be performed at the time of venography and direct puncture phlebography [2, 3].

Treatment of Hemolymphatic Malformation Lesions

The treatment strategy for mixed VM and LM lesions has changed significantly based on observations regarding their embryology [2, 11]. Incomplete lesion excision is usually followed by recurrence and may become a potential source of significant complication and morbidity [11]. The role of traditional surgical excision has changed in the treatment of HLM and in the context of a multidisciplinary treatment approach. Surgical excision is no longer considered first-line therapy or a preferred single treatment modality. When indicated, conventional surgical excision is combined with preoperative and postoperative endovascular therapy [2, 11].

The treatment of a patient with HLM is best individualized and treated via a multidisciplinary team approach [11]. The treatment strategy should involve input from all specialists involved in the patient's care and include a vascular surgeon, orthopedic surgeon, plastic surgeon, head and neck surgeon, interventional radiologist, physiatrist, and physical therapist. The VM and LM components of HLMs are rarely life- or limb-threatening; therefore, invasive treatment modalities should only be considered after conservative treatments have failed.

Precise assessment of each vascular malformation component is essential for prioritizing treatment among the different lesions and to allow appropriate treatment selection when therapy is indicated. Absolute indications for treatment of HLM lesions in KTS patients include hemorrhage, infection, acute thromboembolism, and refractory venous ulcers [2, 6, 7, 11]. Relative indications for treatment include pain, functional impairment, chronic venous insufficiency, limb asymmetry due to vascular bone syndrome, or cosmetic reasons [2, 6, 7, 11].

Conservative Treatment

The treatment and management of HLMs and KTS has been largely conservative [6, 7, 10]. Compression therapy, in the form of elastic, graduated compression garments, remains the mainstay of treatment in patients with HLMs and KTS [6, 10]. Compression therapy is beneficial in treating both lymphedema and chronic venous insufficiency associated with LM and VM lesions. Compression garments should be initiated at an early age to improve later compliance and should be tailored for the patient by an experienced practitioner, with close attention to areas of the malformation that are symptomatic [6, 7,

10]. Patients require new garments at least twice per year to ensure adequate fit and therapeutic benefit. Garments are also an important adjunct post sclerotherapy. In addition, compression bandaging, manual lymphatic drainage, and intermittent pneumatic compression therapy have all been shown to be effective treatments in the management of both lymphedema and swelling due to chronic venous insufficiency [6, 10].

Endovascular Therapy

Endovascular therapy is preferred over traditional surgical excision alone in the treatment of HLM and KTS [11, 12]. Sclerotherapy with absolute alcohol, sodium tetradecyl sulfate, polidocanol, and OK-432 and embolotherapy with endovascular coils, n-butyl cyanoacrylate, and Onyx have been used alone or in combination for the treatment of VM and LM lesions [12–14]. In addition, endovenous thermal ablation utilizing radiofrequency or laser energy in the treatment of venous insufficiency in KTS patients has been reported [15–18].

Sclerotherapy Agents

Sclerotherapy involves the injection of a sclerosant into the lumen of a vascular malformation. This chemical causes destruction of endothelium resulting in inflammation with thrombosis and fibrosis within the vascular lesion [12–14].

OK-432 is a lymphatic sclerosant and is the preferred initial treatment for LM lesions [12]. Also known as Picibanil, OK-432, is the lyophilized exotoxin of the low-virulence Su strain of type III group A *Streptococcus pyogenes*. It is produced after removing streptolysin S-producing activity and has a specific affinity for lymphatic endothelium resulting in selective injury via a relatively benign inflammatory process.

OK-432 can easily be injected into a macrocystic lesion or cavity [12]. Outcomes are excellent, with minimal morbidity in the majority of cases. Microcystic cavernous lesions, on the other hand, are virtually impossible to treat/ inject. In addition, these honey-combed lesions are more likely to communicate with the lymph-transporting system, posing the additional risk of injury to the lymphatic system and perilymphatic tissues (e.g., nerves and blood vessels). Nevertheless, OK-432 is relatively safe, even when extravasation occurs, compared to other sclerosing agents. OK-432 is much less effective than more powerful sclerosing agents, such as ethanol, but carries a lower risk of complications with minimal potential for collateral damage and acceptable recurrence rates [12, 13].

Absolute alcohol is a powerful sclerosant with curative potential in the treatment of all vascular malformation types [12–14]. However, ethanol sclerotherapy carries a significant risk of cardiopulmonary complications to warrant appropriate measures to be taken during its administration including close monitoring with a Swan-Ganz catheter under the general anesthesia [12–14]. Pulmonary hypertension is a potentially fatal complication caused by pulmonary arterial spasm when a significant amount of ethanol reaches the pulmonary circulation. The pulmonary hypertension can lead acute right heart failure and progress to cardiopulmonary arrest [12–14].

A total dose of ethanol of 1 ml/kg of body weight is generally accepted as the maximum volume that can be safely administered during a treatment session in order to prevent pulmonary hypertension [14]. The safe use of ethanol in vascular malformation sclerotherapy requires precise delivery into the lesion with the use of microcatheters. The minimally effective amount and concentration of ethanol should be administered whenever possible to reduce the risk of complications [14]. Absolute ethanol may be diluted to 60% when used to treat superficial VM and LM lesions with a high risk of skin necrosis and lesions in close proximity to nerves [12–14]. Because of its associated risks, many clinicians have limited the use of absolute alcohol in the treatment of VM and LM lesions to lesions that have failed treatment with sodium tetradecyl sulfate and polidocanol [12–14].

Sodium tetradecyl sulfate and polidocanol are detergent sclerosants that are most commonly used in the treatment of lower-extremity varicose veins [12–14]. Compared to absolute alcohol, these sclerosants have significantly lower risks of skin breakdown, nerve injury, and systemic complications [12–14]. Both sclerotherapy agents have become the preferred sclerosants in the treatment of VM lesions [7, 12]. In addition to being administered as liquid sclerosants, both sodium tetradecyl sulfate and polidocanol can be delivered as a foam preparation increasing its effectiveness in the treatment of these lesions [7, 12].

Embolotherapy Agents

Combining conventional sclerotherapy with coil and/or chemical embolization therapy may improve the efficacy of HLM treatment. Sclerotherapy and embolization is often performed as an adjunct to surgical excision of large venous malformations [12–14]. N-butyl cyanoacrylate and Onyx are the two most commonly used liquid embolization agents [14].

N-Butyl cyanoacrylate (NBCA) is a liquid glue that polymerizes on contact with any ionic solution [14]. Following the immediate mechanical effect to occlude the malformation lumen, NBCA causes an inflammatory response to the polymer [14]. NBCA has been used as single-agent therapy with acceptable results in limited specific situations (e.g., inoperable pelvic AVMs) [14]. It should not be used as single-agent therapy in the vast majority of VM lesions requiring therapy for significant symptoms and is often combined with sclerotherapy and/or surgical excision [14]. Furthermore, NBCA appears to be "resorbed" over time resulting in lesion recurrence [14].

Onyx is a new, less adhesive, liquid polymerizing embolic agent consisting of ethylene copolymer and vinyl alcohol dissolved in dimethyl sulfoxide [14]. Onyx has several advantages over NBCA as an embolization agent. It is less adhesive and polymerizes more slowly [14]. During administration of Onyx, the microcatheters are rarely glued into the lesion and delivery of the agent is more easily controlled [14]. Like NBCA, Onyx is often combined with sclerotherapy and/or surgical excision for treatment of VM lesions [14].

Embolization coils are designed to focally occlude blood vessels and vascular structures [14]. The mechanism of action of coil embolization is limited to the vessels in which it is placed. Therefore, coil embolization produces only a mechanical effect to occlude blood flow and induce thrombosis within the malformation. Coils do not have any direct effect on the endothelium and do not prevent recanalization of the malformation. Subsequent recanalization and recovery of the endothelium will result in recurrence of the lesion. Therefore, coil embolization therapy is often combined with sclerotherapy and/or surgical excision in the treatment of VM and LM lesions [12–14].

Endovenous Thermal Ablation

Endovenous thermal ablation has been used in the treatment of symptomatic venous insufficiency in KTS patients [15–18]. Frasier et al. reported their treatment results of radiofrequency ablation of the great saphenous vein performed in three female KTS patients with symptomatic lower-extremity varicose veins and venous insufficiency [15]. There were no complications and all three patients experienced improvement in their varicose veins and improvement in pain and leg edema.

King et al. reported their treatment results in four pediatric KTS patients with symptomatic, incompetent lateral marginal veins that were treated with endovenous laser ablation [16]. Five incompetent lateral marginal veins were treated in two boys and two girls aged 13–26 months. The procedures were performed under general anesthesia with contrast venography. Ultrasound guidance was used to access the marginal vein followed by instillation of tumescent anesthetic prior to delivery of laser energy to the vein. All four patients had excellent outcomes without complication [16].

Combination therapy utilizing foam sclerotherapy with endovenous thermal ablation in KTS patients for the treatment of symptomatic varicose veins and venous insufficiency has been reported [17, 18]. Radiofrequency ablation of incompetent anterior accessory great saphenous veins and incompetent perforating veins was performed in symptomatic KTS patients [17, 18]. This was followed by foam sclerotherapy of symptomatic lower-extremity varicose veins. All of the treated patients experienced improvement in pain, cramping, limb swelling and bulging of varicose veins, and had no complications [17, 18].

Surgical Therapy

Surgical treatment of patients with HLM and KTS is reserved for symptomatic patients where endovascular therapy is not available, has failed, or is not indicated [6, 7, 11, 19, 20]. Prior to planning surgical excision, the presence of a patent deep venous system must be confirmed with preoperative radiologic studies, as KTS patients may present with deep venous system hypoplasia, atresia, or agenesis [6, 11].

Surgical procedures that are commonly performed in symptomatic KTS patients are for the treatment of varicose veins and venous insufficiency. These procedures include excision of the lateral marginal vein, phlebectomy of lower-extremity varicose veins, perforating vein ligation, great saphenous vein stripping, excision of persistent sciatic vein, and excision of venous and lymphatic malformations [6, 19, 20].

In a recent study by Malgor et al., 27 female and 22 male KTS patients had surgical treatment of varicose veins and venous malformations [19]. The mean age of patients was 26.5 years (range 7.7–55.8). The most frequent symptom was pain (N=43, 88%). Forty-nine patients underwent operations on 53 limbs. Stripping of the great saphenous vein (17 limbs), small saphenous vein (10 limbs), accessory saphenous vein (9 limbs), and lateral embryonic vein (15 limbs) was performed, and complications observed included two patients with postoperative deep vein thrombosis, one with pulmonary embolism and one patient with a peroneal nerve palsy. Freedom from disabling pain at 1, 3, and 5 years was 95%, 77%, and 59%, respectively, and the venous clinical severity score had decreased from 9.48 to 6.07 at follow-up visit [19].

Another study by Baraldini et al. where 29 KTS patients underwent surgical treatment of varicose veins, venous malformations, lymphatic malformations, and capillary malformations [20]. Sixteen patients had stripping of the lateral marginal vein, 10 patients had ligation of varicose veins, 14 patients had sclerotherapy treatments, 5 patients had excision of lymphatic malformations, and 13 patients had laser photocoagulation therapy of capillary malformations. Surgery was well tolerated and patients had minimal morbidity and no mortality [20].

Conclusion

The hemolymphatic malformation is a combined congenital vascular malformation that has both venous malformation and lymphatic malformation components. This complex vascular malformation is found in Klippel-Trenaunay syndrome patients. These patients typically present with the classic triad of port wine stains, lower-extremity soft tissue and bone hypertrophy, and lower-extremity varicose veins. The treatment of hemolymphatic malformation and Klippel-Trenaunay syndrome patients is mainly conservative where compression therapy has been shown to be effective in the treatment and management of both lymphedema and swelling due to chronic venous insufficiency. When treatment is indicated, both endovascular therapy and surgical therapy performed alone or in combination has been shown to be effective in the treatment of symptomatic hemolymphatic malformation and Klippel-Trenaunay syndrome patients.

References

1. Lee BB, Laredo J, Lee TS, Huh S, Neville R. Terminology and classification of congenital vascular malformations. Phlebology. 2007;22(6):249–52.
2. Lee BB. Critical issues on the management of congenital vascular malformation. Ann Vasc Surg. 2004;18(3):380–92.
3. Enjolras O, Wassef M, Chapot R. Introduction: ISSVA classification. In: Color atlas of vascular tumors and vascular malformations. New York: Cambridge University Press; 2007; p. 1–11.

4. Wassef M, Blei F, Adams D, Alomari A, Baselga E, Berenstein A, Burrows P, Frieden IJ, Garzon MC, Lopez-Gutierrez JC, Lord DJ, Mitchel S, Powell J, Prendiville J, Vikkula M, ISSVA Board and Scientific Committee. Vascular anomalies classification: recommendations from the international society for the study of vascular anomalies. Pediatrics. 2015;136(1):e203–14.

5. Oduber CE, van der Horst CM, Hennekam RC. Klippel-Trenaunay syndrome: diagnostic criteria and hypothesis on etiology. Ann Plast Surg. 2008 Feb;60(2):217–23.

6. Gloviczki P, Driscoll DJ. Klippel-Trenaunay syndrome: current management. Phlebology. 2007;22(6):291–8.

7. Dasgupta R, Patel M. Venous malformations. Semin Pediatr Surg. 2014;23(4):198–202.

8. Oduber CE, Young-Afat DA, van der Wal AC, van Steensel MA, Hennekam RC, van der Horst CM. The persistent embryonic vein in Klippel-Trenaunay syndrome. Vasc Med. 2013;18(4):185–91.

9. Elluru RG, Balakrishnan K, Padua HM. Lymphatic malformations: diagnosis and management. Semin Pediatr Surg. 2014;23(4):178–85.

10. Lee BB, Laredo J, Neville RF, Mattassi R. Chapter 52. Lymphedema and Klippel-Tenaunay Syndrome. In: Lee BB, Bergan J, Rockson SG, editors. Lymphedema: a concise compendium of theory and practice. London: Springer; 2011.

11. Lee BB, Laredo J, Kim YW, Neville RF. Congenital vascular malformations: general treatment principles. Phlebology. 2007;22:258–63.

12. Gurgacz S, Zamora L, Scott NA. Percutaneous sclerotherapy for vascular malformations: a systematic review. Ann Vasc Surg. 2014;28(5):1335–49.

13. Aronniemi J, Castrén E, Lappalainen K, Vuola P, Salminen P, Pitkäranta A, Pekkola J. Sclerotherapy complications of peripheral venous malformations. Phlebology 2016;31(10):712–722.

14. Lee BB, Laredo J, Neville RF, Sidawy AN. Chapter 56. Arteriovenous malformations: evaluation and treatment. In: Gloviczki P, editor. Handbook of venous disorders: guidelines of the American Venous Forum. 4th ed. London: A Hodder Arnold; 2016 .In press

15. Frasier K, Giangola G, Rosen R, Ginat DT. Endovascular radiofrequency ablation: a novel treatment of venous insufficiency in Klippel-Trenaunay patients. J Vasc Surg. 2008;47(6):1339–45.

16. King K, Landrigan-Ossar M, Clemens R, Chaudry G, Alomari AI. The use of endovenous laser treatment in toddlers. J Vasc Interv Radiol. 2013;24(6):855–8.

17. Sermsathanasawadi N, Hongku K, Wongwanit C, Ruangsetakit C, Chinsakchai K, Mutirangura P. Endovenous radiofrequency thermal ablation and ultrasound-guided foam sclerotherapy in treatment of klippel-trenaunay syndrome. Ann Vasc Dis. 2014; 7(1):52–5.

18. Harrison C, Holdstock J, Price B, Whiteley M. Endovenous radiofrequency ablation and combined foam sclerotherapy treatment of multiple refluxing perforator veins in a Klippel-Trenaunay syndrome patient. Phlebology. 2014;29(10):698–700.

19. Malgor RD, Gloviczki P, Fahrni J, Kalra M, Duncan AA, Oderich GS, Vrtiska T, Driscoll D. Surgical treatment of varicose veins and venous malformations in Klippel-Trenaunay syndrome. Phlebology. 2015;31(3):209–15. pii: 0268355515577322. [Epub ahead of print]

20. Baraldini V, Coletti M, Cipolat L, Santuari D, Vercellio G. Early surgical management of Kippel-Trenaunay syndrome in childhood can prevent long-term haemodynamic effects of distal venous hypertension. J Pediatr Surg. 2002;37:232–5.

Young Soo Do, Young-Wook Kim,
Byung-Boong Lee, and Wayne F. Yakes

Introduction

Arteriovenous malformation (AVM) is a type of congenital vascular malformations (CVM) that result from birth defects involving the vessels of both arterial and venous origins, resulting in direct communications between the different size vessels or a meshwork of primitive reticular networks of dysplastic minute vessels which have failed to mature to become "capillary" vessels termed "nidus." As described in previous chapter, development of AVM attributes to an embryonal defect in the earlier stage of the angiogenesis than other forms of CVM. Therefore, the components of AVMs are more primitive than other types of CVM. In other words, it means AVM has higher potential to change after birth during growth of the patients. These lesions are defined by shunting of high-velocity, low-resistance flow from the arterial vasculature into the venous system in a variety of fistulous conditions.

AVMs differ from other types of CVM in the clinical features and natural course of the lesion. In addition to its biologic property, high flow and high pressure in the venous system result in more frequent complications and sequelae in the cardiovascular system even life- or limb-threatening complications. Among all CVMs, peripheral AVM is the least common type and accounts for 15–20% of CVMs [1]. However, numerous arteriovenous connections make it difficult to eradicate by means of endovascular or open surgical treatment in these patients.

In this chapter, clinical features and evaluation of AVMs will be described.

Y.S. Do, MD (✉)
Department of Radiology, Samsung Medical Center,
Sungkyunkwan University School of Medicine,
Seoul, South Korea
e-mail: ys.do@samsung.com

Y.-W. Kim, MD
Department of Vascular Surgery, Samsung Medical
Center, Sungkyunkwan University School of
Medicine, Seoul, South Korea

B.-B. Lee, MD, PhD, FACS
Professor of Surgery and Director,
Center for the Lymphedema and Vascular
Malformations, George Washington University,
Washington, DC, USA

Adjunct Professor of Surgery, Uniformed Services,
University of the Health Sciences, Bethesda,
MD, USA
e-mail: bblee38@gmail.com

W.F. Yakes, MD
Vascular Malformation Center, Swedish Medical
Center, Eaglewood, CO, USA

Clinical Features

AVM lesion involving the skin shows a red-colored skin spot with surrounding soft tissue swelling. Skin temperature at the lesion is usually warmer than other site and can feel pulsatile thrill or pulsation. Many patients complain of intermittent episodes of pain.

© Springer-Verlag Berlin Heidelberg 2017
Y.-W. Kim et al. (eds.), *Congenital Vascular Malformations*, DOI 10.1007/978-3-662-46709-1_17

In patients with AVMs at the extremity, abnormal venous dilatation (varicosity), palpable pulse or thrill on the superficial veins, or dark skin color or venous ulcer by the long-standing venous hypertension can be observed (Fig. 17.1). Unlike a common varicose vein, varicosity in AVM patient distributes unusual sites (e.g., lateral aspect of the leg) and frequently shows skin red mark and length or size discrepancy of the limbs (Fig. 17.2).

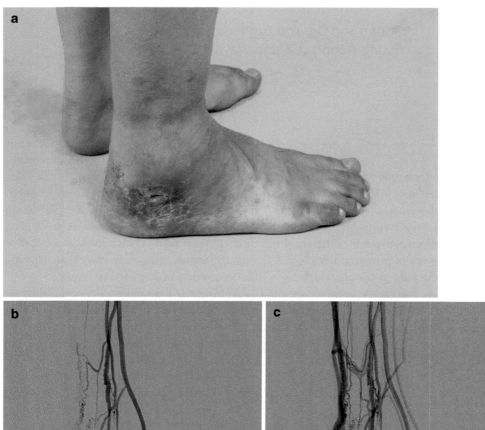

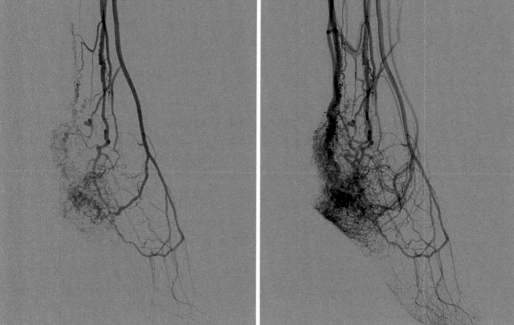

Fig.17.1 A 58-year-old female with AVMs at the ankle and heel of the right foot. (**a**) Note the stasis venous ulcer at the heel and surrounding skin pigmentation due to venous hypertension (**b**) and (**c**). Oblique angiograms in arterial (**b**) and venous (**c**) phases show AVMs at the ankle and heel of the right foot

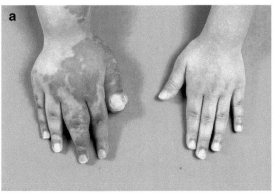
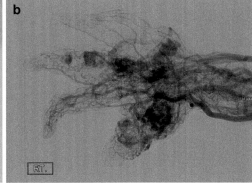

Fig. 17.2 An eight-year-old girl with bone AVMs in the right hand. (**a**) Note hypertrophic and deformed right hand. Skin spot at the dorsum and palpable thrill were also noted. (**b**) Angiogram shows multiple AVMs involving carpal and metacarpal bones in the right hand

Patients with hand or foot AVMs more frequently shows ischemic pain, ischemic ulcer, or tissue necrosis. Intermittent arterial bleeding from the skin lesion are not rare in patients with the hand or foot AVMs. About 20% of patients with AVMs in extremity are associated with intraosseous AVMs. In addition to the abnormality of the limb growth, bone AVMs can cause pathologic fracture of the affected bone.

In patients with head and neck AVMs, symptoms vary with the location and extent of AVMs. Disfiguring and pulsating mass is the most common clinical feature, and intermittent episodes of arterial bleeding from the gum, scalp, or ear are another serious problem (Fig. 17.3). AVM lesions rarely affect visceral organs. AVM lesions around the kidney and renal artery are a rare cause of gross hematuria. The clinical manifestations of pelvic AVMs are diverse ranging from asymptomatic to massive rectal, urethral, or vaginal bleeding requiring emergency treatment. In our experience, around 40% of patients with pelvic have no symptoms despite of the presence of huge dilated vascular lesions in the pelvis (Fig. 17.4).

Among the AVM patients, around 5% have symptoms of heart failure and show enlarged both ventricles due to long-standing overwork of the heart due to high-flow arteriovenous shunting. When there is a cardiac enlargement on a plain chest P-A film, specific cardiac evaluation is recommended.

Most AVMs progress over time with growing of body mass, characteristically shows more rapid progression during adolescence, pregnancy, or after local blunt trauma on it. A thorough physical examination and history taking are important to make a diagnosis of AVMs [2–7].

Imaging of AVMs

Simple Radiography

Chest and simple bone radiographies are useful in an evaluation of cardiac enlargement and bone length discrepancy or intraosseous involvement of AVMs.

Color Doppler Imaging

Color Doppler imaging (CDI) is an essential and simple tool in the diagnosis and follow-up of AVMs. Both highflow type (AVMs, AVF) and low-flow type (venous malformations, lymphatic malformations) CVM lesions can be accurately diagnosed with CDI. Furthermore, CDI is also an important noninvasive method for following patients undergoing therapy. Documentation of decreased arterial flow rates can be accurately assessed [8].

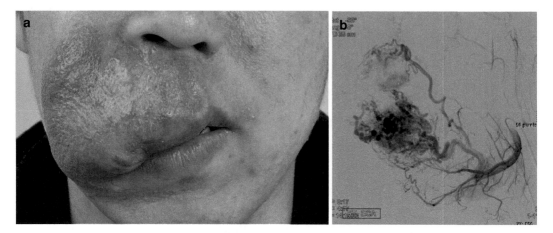

Fig. 17.3 A 23-year-old male with AVMs lesion at the right upper lip and face. (**a**) Note disfiguring soft tissue swelling with red skin spot at the right upper lip and face. (**b**) Lateral angiogram shows AVMs lesion supplied by the fascial artery in the cheek

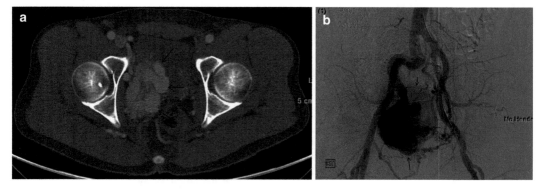

Fig. 17.4 A 47-year-old male with asymptomatic huge AVMs in the pelvis. (**a**) CT axial image shows AVM lesion (arrows) in the pelvis. (**b**) Posteroanterior angiogram shows aneurysmal dilatation (*arrows*) of AVMs

CT Scan

Contrast-enhanced computed tomography (CT) and 3-D reconstruction CT angiography images are really helpful in the diagnosis, planning of treatment, and follow-up of after treatment. Current technique with 3-D reconstruction CT image provide informations regarding extension of AVM lesion, feeding artery, shunting points, draining vein, and involvement of surrounding organ or tissue (Fig. 17.5). CT is also quite helpful for the diagnosis of intraosseous AVMs. However, it has limitation in pediatric patients or in pregnant women because of radiation hazard.

MRI

In initial assessment of CVM patients, MRI demonstrates anatomic relationship of the CVM lesion to adjacent tissues (nerves, muscles, tendons, bone, and subcutaneous fat) or organs and renders a total assessment of the CVM lesions. MR is also an excellent noninvasive method for following patients to determine the efficacy of therapy and can obviate repetitive arteriography or venography in CVM patients [9].

MRI can distinguish high-flow type from the low-flow type in CVM patients with ease.

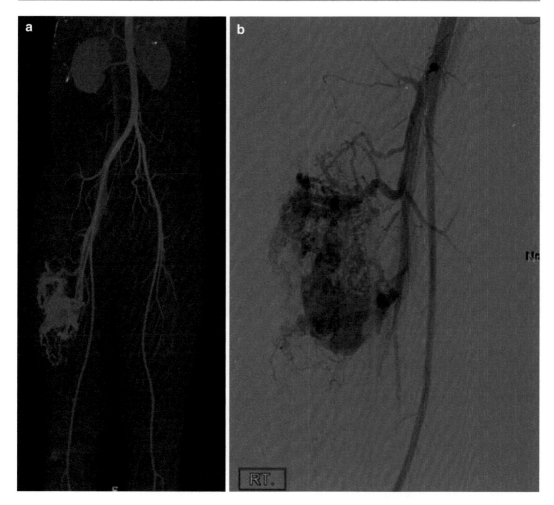

Fig. 17.5 A 24-year-old male with thigh AVMs. (**a**) CT angiography shows enlarged deep femoral artery, dilated AVM nidus, and early opacification of the draining veins. (**b**) Posteroanterior angiogram shows the same findings as those of CT angiography

High-flow type CVM typically demonstrates signal voids on most sequences (Fig. 17.6), which is due to time-of-flight phenomenon with turbulence-related rephasing also contributing to signal loss. An additional feature to differentiate highflow lesions from low-flow lesions is the presence of enlarged feeding arteries and dilated draining veins. Gradient echo sequences show AVM as bright signal serpiginous vascular structures. Furthermore, various MR imaging sequences make it available to determine relationships to adjacent anatomic structures (muscles, bone, nerve) or organs.

Angiography

For the diagnosis of AVM and to determine treatment strategy, angiography is the most accurate diagnostic option. In addition to the primary AVM lesion, it can provide findings of secondary changes (e.g., enlargement, tortuosity) of artery and veins around the AVM lesion. Particularly, it provides us hemodynamic information of AVM lesion which is critical to establish treatment plan. In case of microshunting AVM lesion, we cannot see arteriovenous fistula tracts on the angiogram but can see an earlier

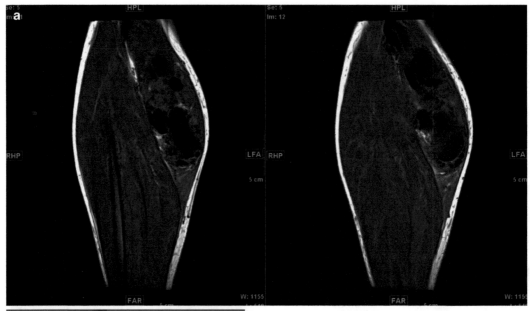

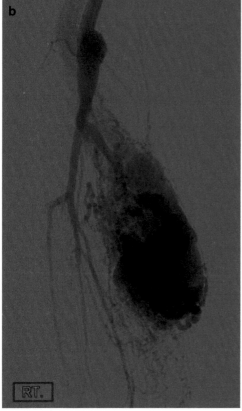

Fig. 17.6 A 31-year-old male with calf AVMs. (**a**) Coronal images of MRI show AVMs lesion in the calf shows signal voids on T1-weighted images. (**b**) Posteroanterior angio-gram shows dilated feeding artery, aneurysmal change of AVM nidus, and enlarged draining vein

visualization of venous phase, enlargement of feeding arteries, and draining veins. Though angiography can provide most valuable anatomic and hemodynamic informations for AVM patients, its invasiveness and contrast or radiation-associated hazard deter frequent use of it. In practice, angiography is often used during endovascular treatment not for the diagnosis of AVM. Above-described noninvasive tools replaced the role of angiography in the diagnosis of AVMs.

For the endovascular treatment of AVM lesion, angiographic feature is critically important. Angiographic features and types of AVM were described in detail in other chapters (see Chap. 10A and 10B).

Transarterial Lung Perfusion Scintigraphy (TLPS)

TLPS is a radionuclide scintiscanning of lung perfusion utilizing Tc-99m macroaggregated albumin (MAA). Its application is particularly helpful for patients having suspected AVM lesion in the extremity. With this technique, we can measure the arteriovenous shunt fraction through the AVM lesion with a semiquantitative method. TLPS is useful not only for the detection of gross or microshunting AVM lesions in the extremity but for the follow-up assessment of AVM lesions (see Chap. 25 for details).

References

1. Lee BB, Baumgartner I, Berlien HP, Bianchini G, Burrows P, Do YS, et al. Consensus document of the international union of angiology (IUA)-2013. Current concept on the management of arterio-venous malformations. Int Angiol. 2013;32(1):9–36.
2. Park KB, Do YS, Kim DI, Kim YW, Shin BS, Park HS, et al. Predictive factors for response of peripheral arteriovenous malformations to embolization therapy: analysis of clinical data and imaging findings. J Vasc Interv Radiol. 2012;23:1478–86.
3. Do YS, Kim YW, Park KB, Kim DI, Park HS, Cho SK, et al. Endovascular treatment combined with embolosclerotherapy for pelvic arteriovenous malformations. J Vasc Surg. 2012;55:465–71.
4. Park HS, Do YS, Park KB, Kim DI, Kim YW, Kim MJ, et al. Ethanol embolotherapy of hand arteriovenous malformations. J Vasc Surg. 2011;53:725–31.
5. Do YS, Park KB, Park HS, Cho SK, Shin SW, Moon JW, et al. Extremity arteriovenous malformations involving the bone: therapeutic outcomes of ethanol embolotherapy. J Vasc Interv Radiol. 2010;21:807–16.
6. Hyun D, Do YS, Park KB, Kim DI, Kim YW, Park HS, Shin SW, Song YG. Ethanol embolotherapy of foot arteriovenous malformations. J Vasc Surg. 2013;58:1619–26.
7. Zhang B, Jiang ZB, Huang MS, Zhu KS, Guan SH, Shan H. The role of transarterial embolization in the management of hematuria secondary to congenital renal arteriovenous malformations. Urol Int. 2013;91:285–90.
8. Yakes WF, Stavros AT, Parker SH, Luethke JM, Rak KM, Dreisbach JN, Slater DD, Burke BJ, Chantelois AE. Color doppler imaging of peripheral high flow vascular malformations pre- and post-ethanol embolotherapy. Published in the Program of the 76th Scientific Assembly of the Radiological Society of North America; November 25–30, 1990; Chicago; Radiology. 1990; 177(P): 156.
9. Rak KM, Yakes WF, Ray RL, et al. MR imaging of peripheral vascular malformations. AJR. 1992;159:107–12.

Lymphatic Malformation (LM) (Extratruncular): Lymphangioma

18

Jovan N. Markovic and Cynthia K. Shortell

Introduction

Lymphatic malformations (LMs) as a subgroup of congenital vascular malformations (CVMs) are localized or diffused abnormalities of lymphogenesis which lead to true structural and/or functional anomalies of the lymphatic system [1, 2]. Most clinicians – from primary care doctors to subspecialists (including vascular surgeons) – consider the management of LMs a difficult task reserved for referral centers with specialized expertise in this area. The main reason why expertise for LMs management is centralized to major clinics is the low frequency at which CVMs occur in general, the confusing nomenclature, and the lack of a uniform classification system which traditionally characterized majority of the literature discussing LMs, as well as the absence of established guidelines for their management [3, 4]. Consequently, a significant number of LM patients have been discouraged by the lack of correct diagnosis and proper treatment despite numerous visits to different clinics.

Classification

Historically, numerous attempts have been made to properly classify CVMs based on anatomic, clinical, and/or embryologic criteria, and no real consensus existed regarding nomenclature and management of these lesions. Based on a classification of "vascular birthmarks," initially proposed by Mulliken and Glowacki in 1982 [1], the International Society for the Study of Vascular Anomalies (ISSVA) introduced a classification system in which all vascular anomalies were divided into two categories: vascular malformations and vascular tumors. The differentiation of vascular anomalies into tumors and CVMs permitted more effective communication between different medical specialists. Unfortunately, the eponym-based terminology which characterized the ISSVA classification, as well as the lack of clinical applicability of this classification with regard to pretreatment planning, was believed by significant majority of practitioners to be the main limitation for widespread acceptance and utilization of this classification system. Consequently, the ISSVA classification has been modified numerous times to address concerns about clinical applicability, especially with regard to the differentiation between truncular and extratruncular subtypes of all CVMs and LMs in particular. This differentiation, based on the embryonic stage of developmental arrest, is clinically important because these two groups of LMs are significantly different with regard to

J.N. Markovic, MD (✉) • C.K. Shortell, MD, FACS (✉)
Duke University Medical Center, Durham, NC, USA
e-mail: jovan.markovic@duke.edu;
Cynthia.shortell@dm.duke.edu

© Springer-Verlag Berlin Heidelberg 2017
Y.-W. Kim et al. (eds.), *Congenital Vascular Malformations*, DOI 10.1007/978-3-662-46709-1_18

morphology, clinical severity, response to treatment, and recurrence rates presumably because of their preserved mesenchymal characteristics of independent growth potential [5, 6]. To address ISSVA classification limitations, the authors of "Hamburg" and subsequently "modified Hamburg classification" developed a classification system by incorporating CVM flow characteristics (i.e., arterial, venous, capillary) and defining CVMs based on the stage of developmental arrest during embryogenesis into truncular and extratruncular lesions which is as mentioned earlier important for treatment selection and prognosis of treatment outcomes. The "modified Hamburg classification" system has been considered to be "a more clinician-friendly classification for CVM management" as outlined in the 2009 Consensus Document for the treatment of venous malformations of the International Union of Phlebology (IUP) [7]. Malformations were categorized according to hemodynamic characteristics, either as high flow or low flow, with further subdivision into anatomic subgroups designated by the predominant vascular element (arterial, venous, capillary, or lymphatic). In this scheme, venous, lymphatic, and capillary malformations are all low-flow lesions. Arterial malformations are considered high-flow lesions. Malformations are furtherly classified either as extratruncular or truncular. Extratruncular lesions are categorized as diffuse/infiltrating or localized, whereas truncular lesions are categorized as obstruction/narrowing or dilatation. The current chapter will deal with the diagnosis and management of CVMs that are considered to be predominantly extratruncular LMs – "lymphangiomas."

Pathophysiology

Although the exact pathophysiologic mechanism responsible for development and progression of LMs remains to be elucidated, data from biomolecular studies showed that several members of the PI3K/mTOR pathway have been implicated in the pathogenesis and progression of vascular anomalies. Vascular endothelial growth factor

(VEGF) is a key regulator in lymphangiogenesis and angiogenesis and acts as both a potential upstream stimulator of and a downstream effector in the mTOR signaling pathway [8]. Data from animal studies demonstrated that another metabolic pathway involving Akt (just upstream of mTOR) has been found to be overexpressed in the endothelial cells of cutaneous LMs [9]. More recently, increasing volume of data from genetic studies is becoming available to suggest that LM development is caused by gene mutations. In 2015, Luks et al. evaluated genetic aberration responsible for LM pathogenesis in patient with LM ($n = 17$) and/or syndromes in which LM is present including patient with CLOVES ($n = 33$), KTS ($n = 21$), and FAVA ($n = 8$) [10]. Data from this study showed that somatic mosaic mutations in PIK3CA genetic locus represent genetic mechanisms underlying development of LM and associated syndromes. However, it remains to be elucidated why the same genetic PIK3CA gene mutation causes an isolated LM in one patient and a different syndrome associated clinical presentation in another patient. One of the explanations can be based on the stage of the embryonic development when the genetic mutation arises as well as the location of the first mutated embryonic cell and the stem cells that arise from that particular cell linkage. Mammalian target of rapamycin (mTOR) is a serine/threonine kinase regulated by phosphoinositide 3-kinase (PI3K). mTOR acts as a master switch of numerous cellular processes, including cellular catabolism and anabolism, cell motility, angiogenesis, and cell growth and is becoming a target of relatively novel pharmaceutical agents being tested for the LM treatment [11].

Clinical Presentation

In most of the patients, LMs are present at birth or before the patient reaches the age of 2 years. However, these lesions may not become evident until later childhood or adolescence when the malformation size increases enough to become a visible deformity or to cause symptoms

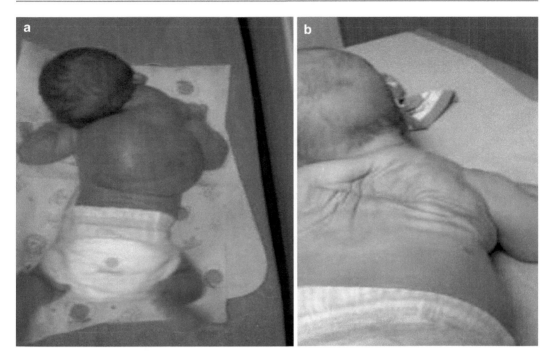

Fig. 18.5 (**a**) Extensive lymphatic malformation affecting majority of the back and posterior neck. (**b**) Staged surgical resection of defined anatomic regions can be used for extensive and/or diffuse lymphatic malformations

patients with LMs. Biomolecular and genetic research, development of clinically applicable classification system, utilization of diagnostic modalities that avoid noncontributory imaging, and introduction of novel treatment options all represent advancements in the management of these lymphatic lesions. However, further research is warranted to contribute to additional refining of diagnostic and treatment algorithm(s) for the management of this traditionally underserved patient population.

References

1. Mulliken JB, Glowacki J. Hemangiomas and vascular malformations in infants and children. A classification based on endothelial characteristics. Plast Reconstr Surg. 1982;69:412–22.
2. Young AE. Pathogenesis of vascular malformations. In: Mulliken JB, Young AE, editors. Vascular birthmarks: hemangiomas and malformations. Philadelphia: W.B. Saunders Co; 1988. p. 107–13.
3. Villavicencio JL, Scultetus A, Lee BB. Congenital vascular malformations: when and how to treat them. Semin Vasc Surg. 2002;15(1):65–71.
4. Lee BB, Laredo J, Lee TS, Huh S, Neville R. Terminology and classification of congenital vascular malformations. Phlebology. 2007;22(6):249–52.
5. Belov S. Classification, terminology, and nosology of congenital vascular defects. In: Belov S, Loose DA, Weber J, editors. Vascular malformations. Reinbek: Einhorn-Presse; 1989. p. 25–30.
6. Belov S. Anatomopathological classification of congenital vascular defects. Semin Vasc Surg. 1993;6:219–24.
7. Lee BB, Bergan J, Gloviczki P, Laredo J, Loose DA, Mattassi R, Parsi K, Villavicencio JL, Zamboni P. Diagnosis and treatment of venous malformations - Consensus Document of the International Union of Phlebology (IUP)-2009. Int Angiol. 2009;28(6):434–51.
8. Ferrara N. Vascular endothelial growth factor: basic science and clinical progress. Endocr Rev. 2004;25: 581–611.
9. Bissler JJ, McCormack FX, Young LR, et al. Sirolimus for angiomyolipoma in tuberous sclerosis complex or lymphangioleiomyomatosis. N Engl J Med. 2008;358:140–51.
10. Luks VL et al. Lymphatic and Other Vascular Malformative/Overgrowth Disorders Are Caused by Somatic Mutations in PIK3CA. J Pediatr. 2015;166: 1048–54.
11. Vignot S, Faivre S, Aguirre D, et al. mTOR-targeted therapy of cancer with rapamycin derivatives. Ann Oncol. 2005;16:525–37.
12. Padwa BL, Hayward PG, Ferraro NF, et al. Cervicofacial lymphatic malformation: clinical course,

surgical intervention, and pathogenesis of skeletal hypertrophy. Plast Reconstr Surg. 1995;95:951e60.

13. AM H et al. Sirolimus for the treatment of complicated vascular anomalies in children. Pediatr Blood Cancer. 2011;57:1018–24.

14. OzekI M, Fukao T, Kondo N. Propranolol for intractable diffuse lymphangiomatosis. N Engl J Med. 2011;364:1380–2.

15. Annabel M, Shanna B, Gerard L, Soizick PL, Denis H, Allan E. Lack of effect of propranolol in the treatment of lymphangioma in two children. Pediatr Dermatol. 2013;30(3):383–5.

16. Swetman GL, Berk DR, Vasanawala SS, Feinstein JA, Lane AT, Bruckner AL. Sildenafil for severe lymphatic malformations. N Engl J Med. 2012;366:384–6.

17. Villavicencio JL. Primum non nocere: is it always true? The use of absolute ethanol in the management of congenital vascular malformations. J Vasc Surg. 2001;33:904–6.

18. Smith MC, Zimmerman B, Burke DK, et al. Efficacy and safety of OK-432 immunotherapy of lymphatic malformations. Laryngoscope. 2009;119:107e15.

19. Burrows PE, Mitri RK, Alomari A, et al. Percutaneous sclerotherapy of lymphatic malformations with doxycycline. Lymphat Res Biol. 2008;6:209e16.

20. Bai Y, Jia J, Huang XX, et al. Sclerotherapy of microcystic lymphatic malformations in oral and facial regions. J Oral Maxillofac Surg. 2009;67:251e6.

Truncular Lymphatic Malformation (LM): Primary Lymphedema

Ningfei Liu

Primary lymphedema is defined as edema caused by lymphatic dysplasia and/or dysfunction due to congenital [1, 2] or unknown factors. Primary lymphedema occurs in 1 of every 10,000 people in the general population [3]. A recent study in the author's clinic showed that primary lymphedema accounted ~27% of the 3252 lymphedema cases in the last 2 years in the author's lymphology clinic in Shanghai Ninth People's Hospital.

Classification

1. According to the onset time, primary lymphedema is classified as:
   (a) Congenital: lymphedema occurs at birth or a few months after birth, which accounts for 10% of total incidence.
   (b) Praecox: the onset of the disease during early childhood and adolescence before the age of 35, which accounts for 71% of total incidence.
   (c) Tarda: lymphedema occurs after the age of 35, which accounts for 19% of total incidence.
2. According to the clinical manifestations:
   The clinical manifestations of primary lymphedema are variable. It most commonly occurs in one lower extremity but may affect both lower limbs. The relatively rare types of primary lymphedema are edema in the unilateral upper extremity, semi-face, and external genitals alone. In general, external genital lymphedema is mostly associated with edema of the lower limb(s). In very rare cases, lymphedema occurs in multiple sites as the ipsilateral face, upper and lower limbs, or contralateral upper and lower extremities. However, even in the familial hereditary lymphatic edema with known genetic mutations, lymphedema only appears in part of the body and does not affect the whole body. The pathological mechanisms underlying the "selective location" in primary lymphedema are unclear.

In the lower limb, edema usually starts at the distal part of the limb, at the dorsum of the foot, and around the ankle. But edema can start from the thigh when the inguinal lymph node anomalies are the etiology. At the early stage, edema may disappear spontaneously in the morning and become evident during the night. The insidious onset and slow progression of symptoms usually result in delayed diagnosis. Along with the progress of the disease, the volume of the affected limb becomes evident like elephantiasis.

N. Liu, MD, PhD (✉)
Lymphology Center of Department of Plastic and Reconstructive Surgery, Shanghai Ninth People's Hospital, Shanghai Jiao Tong University School of Medicine,
639 Zhi Zao Ju Road, Shanghai 200011, China
e-mail: Liuningfei@126.com

© Springer-Verlag Berlin Heidelberg 2017
Y.-W. Kim et al. (eds.), *Congenital Vascular Malformations*, DOI 10.1007/978-3-662-46709-1_19

3. According to the family history:

There are two types of inherited lymphedema:

(a) The hereditary lymphedema type I. Milroy reported in 1892. Milroy disease (MD; MIM# 153100) is a rare autosomal, dominantly inherited primary lymphedema. Patients with MD generally present bilateral lower leg lymphedema at birth or shortly after birth [1–3]. The FLT4 gene (also known as VEGFR-3), which encodes vascular endothelial growth factor receptor 3, was identified as being responsible for the majority of MD cases [4]. Clinical studies have found that not all the members of the same family with VEGFR-3 gene variants have clinical symptoms. So far, 60 mutations in FLT4 have been reported [4–6], with most reported as missense mutations. All the mutations are located in exons 17–20 and 22–26 of FLT4, within the tyrosine kinase domain of the receptor. A study found that mutations within the tyrosine kinase domains of FLT4 are sufficient to reduce tyrosine kinase activity [7], thereby affecting lymphatic development. Typical lymphoscintigraphy image of MD is absence of observable lymphatic collector and inguinal lymph node in the affected limb. Some studies believe that MD is a disease caused by lymphatic dysfunction because (a) there are primary lymphatic vessels in the skin of the affected feet by immunohistochemical staining and (b) the main functional lymphatic tract is displayed on lymphoscintigrams in a few MD patients [8]. If so, a more complicated mechanism may underlie the pathology of MD, and more genes, other than VEGFR-3, may be involved in MD as modifier genes.

(b) The hereditary lymphedema type II, also known as Meige's syndrome (MIM# 153200). Meige first reported in 1898. Meige's lymphedema accounts for about 65–80% of hereditary diseases. It is a chromosome dominant inheritance and begins sometime during puberty. Some may occur after 35 years old. Lymphedema is often accompanied by infection and mostly located in the lower extremity but also occurs in the upper limbs and face. Other abnormalities are cardiovascular system abnormality, cleft palate, deafness, pleural lymphatic leakage, varicose veins, and double row eyelash, and spinal deformities.

More than 90% of primary lymphedema cases do not have a family history.

4. According to the lymphatic system malformation based on MR lymphangiography:

The lymphatic system malformations in primary lymphedema have not been intensively studied until recent improvements of imaging technique with use of MR lymphangiography [9, 10]. Dynamic and real-time observation of contrast enhancement of lymphatic vessels and drainage nodes with high-resolution images provides comprehensive information concerning both the structural and functional abnormalities of the lymphatic system in primary lymphedema [11]. The changes of lymphatic system in primary lymphedema may occur either in the lymph vessels or in the nodes, or in both. On the MRL images, lymphatic abnormalities fell into two major categories, aplasia/hypoplasia or hyperplasia. Lymph node abnormalities fell into three major categories, aplasia/hypoplasia, hyperplasia, or structural abnormalities. The MRL findings of lymphatic system anomalies in primary lymphedema could be divided into three major patterns. Evident defects of the inguinal lymph node with moderate dilatation of afferent lymph vessels were found in 17% of patients. Lymphatic anomalies, including lymphatic aplasia, hypoplasia, or hyperplasia with no obvious defect of the drainage lymph nodes, were observed in 28% of patients. The abnormalities of both lymph vessels and lymph nodes in the affected limb were exhibited in 55% of cases [12]. Thus, a classification of lymphatic system in primary lymphedema based on MRL imaging is proposed as follows (Figs. 19.1, 19.2 and 19.3):

1. Lymph nodes affected only with nodal structural abnormality

2. Lymph vessel affected only
   (a) Lymphatic aplasia/hypoplasia
   (b) Lymphatic hyperplasia

3. Lymph vessel and lymph node affected with subgroups
   (a) Lymphatic and nodal aplasia/hypoplasia
   (b) Lymphatic aplasia/hypoplasia + nodal hyperplasia
   (c) Lymphatic aplasia/hypoplasia + nodal structural abnormalities
   (d) Lymphatic and nodal hyperplasia
   (e) Lymphatic hyperplasia + nodal aplasia/hypoplasia
   (f) Lymphatic hyperplasia + nodal structural abnormalities

There was no significant difference concerning the severity of the disease between lymphatic hypoplasia and hyperplasia groups. In general, edema was more extensive, and tissue fibrosis progressed as the course of the disease progressed in all groups. Edema in the ankle and foot was most common in lymphatic hypoplasia-only group. Edema in the thigh and/or extragenital and/or buttocks and lower abdomen wall was more common in inguinal lymph node aplasia/hypoplasia and nodal affected only types. The malformations of lymph vessels were not always concordant with those of the lymph nodes in primary lymphedema. The lymph vessel and node may be involved together or affected alone and may express different types of anatomical anomalies. This updated classification clearly defines the location and pathological characteristics of the disease to provide a clear and more useful definition.

The imaging of lymphatic system with MR lymphangiography revealed the importance of the lymph nodes, as opposed to the peripheral vessels, in primary lymphedema. Nodal defects alone might be the cause of the disease or involved in both the lymphatic hypoplasia and hyperplasia groups. Similar to lymph vessels, diseased lymph nodes may be expressed as the aplasia, hypoplasia, and hyperplasia types; the most common form of lymph node pathology was nodal structural anomalies.

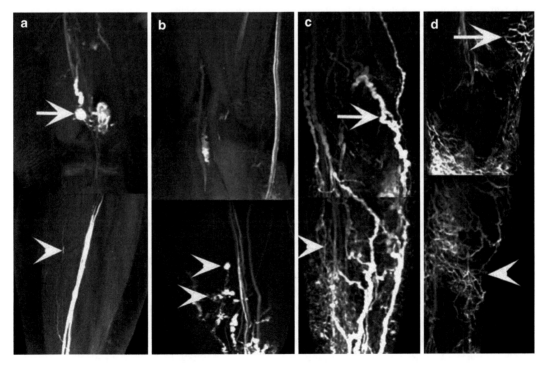

Fig. 19.1 Composition images of MR lymphangiogram show various lymphatic drainage pathways in primary lymphedematous limbs. (**a**) Single deep lymph vessel (*arrowhead*) and popliteal nodes (*arrow*) were enhanced with the absence of superficial lymph vessel. (**b**) Enhanced lymph vessels with cystic dilatation (*arrow-* *head*) in the distal part of the leg. (**c**) Both superficial lymphatics (*arrowhead*) and deep lymph vessels and popliteal nodes (*arrow*) were involved. (**d**) A crisscross network of hyperplastic vessels in the thigh (*arrow*) and the calf (*arrowhead*)

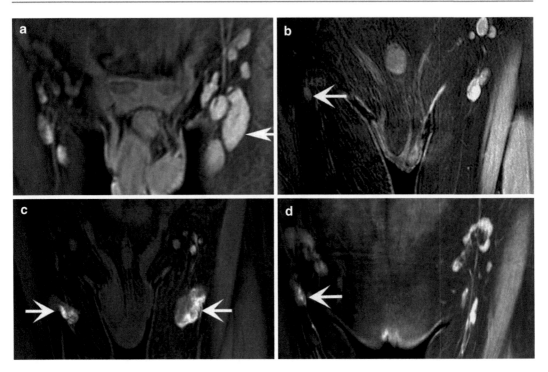

Fig. 19.2 Diverse inguinal node abnormalities of primary lymphedematous displayed on MR lymphangiograms. (**a**) Enlarged inguinal lymph nodes (*arrow*) with homogeneous texture in the left side in contrast with lymph nodes of normal size in the right side. (**b**) Single small node in a limb (*arrow*) with lymphatic hypoplasia and lymphedema is compared with lymph nodes in a limb without lymphedema. (**c**) Partially contrast-enhanced inferior inguinal nodes (*arrow*) in bilateral lymphedema with secondary lymphatic dilatation. (**d**) Small nodes that are irregularly shaped (*small arrow*) in a limb with lymphangiectasia (*large arrow*)

Lymphedema in Syndromes

The primary lymphedema may be one of the symptoms of various syndromes, as Klippel-Trenaunay syndromes, lymphedema-distichiasis syndromes, yellow nail syndromes, Turner's syndromes, Hennekam syndromes, and hypotrichosis-lymphedema-telangiectasia syndrome. Among them, Klippel-Trenaunay syndrome is the most common one in the clinic. Edema and repeated erysipelas are frequently accompanied with the progress of the disease. However, the role of lymphatic system dysplasia in the initiation and progression of Klippel-Trenaunay syndromes has long been overlooked. Recent study with the use of MR lymphangiography demonstrated that lymphatic system malformation is a common component of Klippel-Trenaunay syndromes [13], as about 97% of the patients have lymphatic

malformations and lymphedema. The lymphatic system dysplasia observed in Klippel-Trenaunay syndromes was similar to that seen in congenital primary lymphedema, such as lymphatic hyperplasia (34%), hypoplasia or aplasia (63%) of lymph vessels and/or lymph node hyperplasia (34%), or hypoplasia (9%). The coexistence of venous and lymphatic malformations in the extremities affected by Klippel-Trenaunay syndromes that was found in the majority of the patients implies again a close embryonic structure or developmental relationship between the two circulation systems. It is, therefore, essential to consider lymphatic system dysplasia in the diagnosis of Klippel-Trenaunay syndromes besides vascular system anomalies (Fig. 19.4).

Lymphedema-distichiasis syndromes are relatively rare disease. The clinical manifestations of the patients with lymphedema-distichiasis

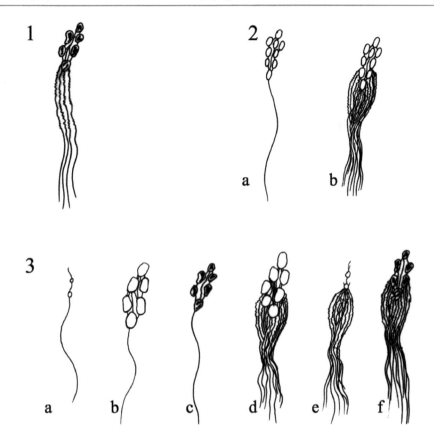

Fig. 19.3 Schematic drawing of the updated classification of primary lymphedema. (**1**) Lymph node affected only. (**2**) Lymphatic affected only: (*a*) lymphatic aplasia/hypoplasia and (*b*) lymphatic hyperplasia. (**3**) Both lymphatic and lymph nodes affected: (*a*) lymphatic and nodal aplasia/ hypoplasia, (*b*) lymphatic aplasia/hypoplasia + nodal hyperplasia, (*c*) lymphatic aplasia/hypoplasia + nodal structural abnormalities, (*d*) lymphatic and nodal hyperplasia, (*e*) lymphatic hyperplasia + nodal aplasia/hypoplasia, and (*f*) lymphatic hyperplasia + nodal structural abnormalities

syndromes are similar as hereditary lymphatic edema type II – Meige's syndrome. Foxc2 is one of the pathogenic genes [14]. The variation of FOXC2 gene can be different. The most prominent symptoms are double eyelashes but usually not easy to find. Edema may affect single or bilateral lower limbs. The imaging of MR lymphangiography revealed a significantly dilatation of superficial lymph collectors with valvular insufficiency. Some patients show varicose veins; color Doppler ultrasound examination showed a deep venous reflux.

Yellow nail syndrome is a very rare disease and can be hereditary or non-hereditary. FOCX2 mutation is identified in patients with yellow nail syndromes [15]. The three main symptoms of the disease were yellow nail of the hand and foot (89%), lymph edema (80%), and pulmonary lesions (63%). The cause of the formation of the lymphatic edema is the aplasia or hypoplasia of development of the lymphatic vessels.

Special Types of Primary Lymphedema

1. Chylous reflux lymphedema is caused by malformation of the thoracic duct, chylocyst, and lymphatic in the intestine and extremity. Lymph stasis in chylocyst can spread to the entire intestinal branch drainage area. Mesenteric lymph duct with chylous fluid may result in chylous lymphoma and rupture and chylous ascites. Chylous reflux can also spread to the

joint, often leading to joint pain and/or fever. There are complex connections of lymphatic and lymph nodes in between the thoracic and abdominal cavity; the stasis of chylous fluid can therefore spread to axillary, subclavicle, posterior sternum, and inguinal lymph nodes.

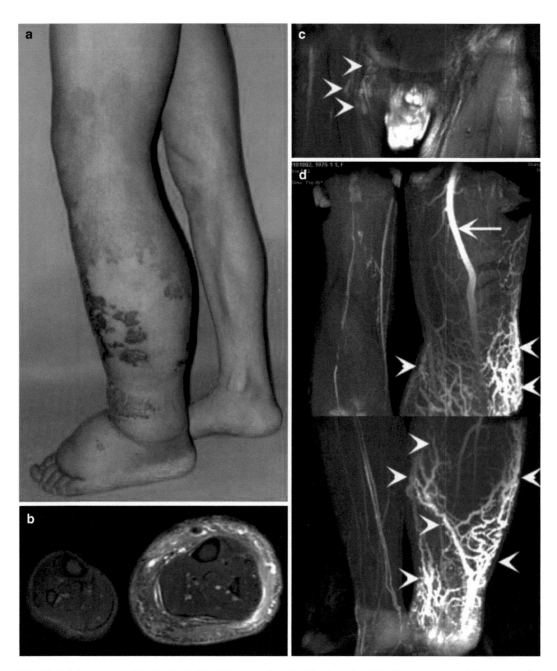

Fig. 19.4 (a) A man age 34 with chief clinical features of KTS as skin port-wine stain and hypertrophy of the left lower limb. (b) Transverse section of T2-weighted MR image shows hypertrophy of subcutaneous tissue and edema fluid (high signal intensity) dispersing in the subcutaneous layer. (c) No inguinal lymph nodes were clearly visualized on the left side in contrast with lymph nodes (*arrowhead*) visualized on the contralateral side on coronal T2-weighted image. (d) Composition image of MR lymphangiogram shows numerous dilated lymphatic vessels (*arrowheads*) and enlarged deep vein (*arrow*)

The common clinical symptoms of chylous reflux are the vesicles on the surface of the skin with white chyle due to stagnant chylous in the dermal lymphatic, skin chylous leakage, ulceration formed after skin chylous leakage, and edema in the inguinal region and extragenital and/or lower limb. Primary chylous reflux may occur in children of less than 1 year old. Most of the patients with chylous reflux were in the late stage as they are diagnosed and had been associated with frequent lymph leakage and/or infection of the affected region and limb for a long time. MR image is the best protocol for the diagnosis of chylous reflux lymphedema to localize the lymphatic malformations in both the superficial and deep systems (Fig. 19.5).

2. Protein-losing enteropathy: protein-losing enteropathy is characterized by edema, abdominal pain, diarrhea, hypoproteinemia, and anemia associated with plasma protein leakage from the intestinal lymphatic duct to the intestinal lumen. The symptoms become more evident after high-fat meal. It is common in children. Majority of primary protein-losing enteropathy is due to intestinal wall lymphedema that resulted from intestinal lymphatic mechanical dysfunction and often associated with lymphangiectasia [16]. The thoracic duct and chylocyst dysplasia may be the pathogenesis of some cases. The lymphatic backflow of the extremity may also be impaired, and patient may associate with a primary lower limb lymphedema. The diagnosis is based on the clinical signs of edema and blood test of protein, globulin, calcium, and vitamin D and iron deficiency. Image tests with lymphoscintigraphy may detect the leakage of isotopic tracer into the lumen of the intestine in ~ 30% of cases. Capsule endoscopy may also help in observation of lesions in the intestinal wall. MR imaging is capable of demonstrating malformations (dilatation) of thoracic duct and enlarged mesenteric lymphatics [17].

3. Lymphangiomatosis: it is a syndrome of the lymphatic system malformation, that is, lymphangioma or cystic lesions of the lymphatic vessels [18]. There is no standard definition of the disease. The cause of lymphangiomatosis is a congenital malformation that arises from abnormal lymphatic system during embryologic formation. The lymphangioma is isolated and localized, while lymphangiomatosis is multiple located. The lymphangiomatosis originates in the lymphatic system and is benign in

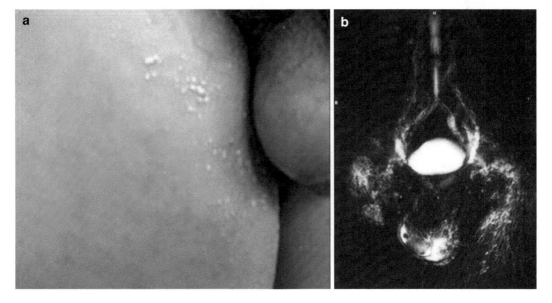

Fig. 19.5 (**a**) A 45-year-old man with perineal skin chylous leakage for 30 years. (**b**) 3D MRI clearly shows a dense mesh of the dilated lymphatic vessels in the groin, the scrotum, and the left thigh and the dilated bilateral lumbar trunk

nature, but it can invade multiple parts and multiple organs of the body, showing progressive development. It commonly occurs in the lung, bone, kidney, chest, connective tissue, and spleen. The tumor tissue will cause osteolysis when violating the bone, most commonly in the long bones, vertebrae, and ribs. It is also called "Gorham's" syndrome when massive osteolysis and vanishing bone disease occur. The disease can occur at any age but most often in infants and young children, especially before the age of 20, with no familial heredity. The incidence is unclear. The diagnosis of the disease is based on the clinical, imaging, and histological analysis.

References

1. Kinmonth JB. The lymphatics, disease, lymphography, and surgery. London: Arnold; 1982. p. 128–9.
2. Ferrell RE, Levinson KL, Esman JH, Kimak MA, Lawrence EC, Barmada MM, Finegold DN. Hereditary lymphedema: evidence for linkage and genetic heterogeneity. Hum Mol Genet. 1998;7:2073–8.
3. Petrek JA et al. Lymphedema: current issues in research and management. CA Cancer J Clin. 2000; 50(5):292–307.
4. Gordon K, Spiden SL, Connell FC, Brice G, Cottrell S, Short J, Taylor R, Jeffery S, Mortimer PS, Mansour S, Ostergaard P. FLT4/VEGFR-3 and Milroy disease: novel mutation, a review of published variants and database updated. Hum Mutat. 2013;34(1):23–31.
5. DiGiovanni RM, Erickson RP, Ohlson EC, Bernas M, Witte MH. A novel FLT4 gene mutation identified in a patient with Milroy disease. Lymphology. 2014;47(1):44–7.
6. Liu N, Yu Z, Luo Y, Sun D, Yan Z. A Novel FLT4 Gene Mutation and MR lymphangiography in a Chinese Family with Milroy Disease. Lymphology. 2015;48(2):93–6.
7. Karkkainen MJ, Ferrell RE, Lawrence EC, Kimak MA, Levinson KL, McTigue MA, Alitalo K, Finegold DN. Missense mutation interfere with VEGFR-3 signaling in primary lymphedema. Nat Genet. 2000;25(2): 153–9.
8. Mellor RH, Hubert CE, Stanton AWB, Tate N, Akhras V, Smith A, Burnand K, Jeffery S, Makinen T, Levick JR, Mortimer PS. Lymphatic dysfunction, not aplasia, underlines Milroy disease. Microcirculation. 2010; 17(4):281–96.
9. Liu NF, Wang CG, Sun MH. Noncontrast three-dimensional magnetic resonance imaging vs lymphoscintigraphy in the evaluation of lymph circulation disorders: a comparative study. J Vasc Surg. 2005;41:69–75.
10. Liu NF, Lu Q, Wu XF. Comparison of radionuclide lymphoscintigraphy and dynamic magnetic resonance lymphangiography for investigating extremity lymphoedema. Br J Surg. 2010;97:359–65.
11. Liu NF, Lu Q, Jiang ZH. Anatomic and functional evaluation of lymphatics and lymph nodes in diagnosis of lymphatic circulation disorders with contrast magnetic resonance lymphangiography. J Vasc Surg. 2009;49:980–7.
12. Liu NF, Yan ZX. Classification of lymphatic system malformations in primary lymphoedema based on MR lymphangiography. Eur J Endovasc Surg. 2012;44:345–9.
13. Liu NF, Lu Q, Yan Z. Lymphatic malformation is a common component of Klippel-Trenaunay syndrome. J Vasc Surg. 2010;52:1557–63.
14. Fang J, Dagenais SL, Erickson RP, et al. Mutations in FOXC2 (MFH-1), a forkhead family transcription factor, are responsible for the hereditary lymphedema – distichiasis syndrome. Am J Hum Genet. 2000;67:1382–8.
15. Paradisis M, Asperen PV. Yellow nail syndrome in infancy. J Paediatr Child Health. 1997;33:454–7.
16. Földi M, Földi E, Kubik S, editors. Textbook of lymphology: for physicians and lymphoedema therapists. San Francisco: Urban and Fischer; 2003.
17. Liu NF, Lu Q, Zhou JG. Magnetic resonance imaging as a new method to diagnose protein losing enteropathy. Lymphology. 2008;41:111–5.
18. Kelly J. Moss J:Lymphangioleiomyomatosis. Am J Med Sci. 2001;321:17–25.

Clinical Features and Evaluation of Superficial & Deep Capillary Malformation (CM)

20

Peter Berlien

A distinct classification of congenital vascular anomalies is necessary because there is a broad list of lesions with variability in signs, symptoms, and clinical behavior. Vascular malformations may have any combination of capillary, venous, arterial, and lymphatic components, with or without fistulae (Table 20.1). There are truncular and extratruncular forms [1–3]. Often one can find a combination of both. An irregular structure of the vessel wall, position anomaly as a result of an irregular origin and course, or a persistent fetal vessel can be the reason for this. The vascular system results in a differentiation from mesodermal steam cells into Hemangioblasts [4]. They later differentiate to the primitive vascular system – the Vasculogenesis. This has to be discriminate from the Angiogenesis, the formation of vessels from existing vascular system. In which embryological phase the defect happens determines the kind of vascular malformation – the later in the phase after differentiation to the vascular system the more truncular malformations happens. Typical example for this are congenital heart defects. The more in the vasculogenesis phase or before the differentiation to hemangioblasts the more extratruncular malformations or combined other mesenchymal malformations

happens. This explains the findings in Phakomatosis e.g. in overgrowth syndromes [5]. Furthermore this explains why the use of syndrome names make sense: They are typical combinations of defects in different organ systems. Capillary Vascular Malformations results from an early defect in the vasculogenesis. This means that Capillary Vascular Malformations mostly are part of a mixed Vascular Malformation. Furthermore this explains why Capillary Vascular Malformation never can heal but have progress. For several forms there is a tumor like growing behavior, the so called Hamartoma. In some cases, the vascular malformation remains preformed and latent and grows as a result of a lesion, trauma, or a hormonal effect. This can happen during adolescence or even during adulthood. The most vascular anomalies are well known with their eponymous conditions [6].

Port-Wine Stains

The term port-wine stain (PWS) or nevus flammeus is historically an old term and has to be replaced by the correct classification as Capillary Vascular Malformation. On the other hand this type is the typical finding for a capillary vascular malformation so in the daily clinical routine these terms are further in use. A port-wine stain (PWS) is a congenital malformation of the superficial cutaneous vascular plexus, involving venules, capillaries, and possibly perivenular nerves.

P. Berlien
Wissenschaft und Forschung, Lasermedizin,
Elisabeth Klinik, Berlin, Germany
e-mail: lasermed.elisabeth@pgdiakonie.de

© Springer-Verlag Berlin Heidelberg 2017
Y.-W. Kim et al. (eds.), *Congenital Vascular Malformations*, DOI 10.1007/978-3-662-46709-1_20

Table 20.1 The "ISSVA" and the "Hamburg" classifications are not contradictionry but the ISSVA is in the Hamburg. The ISSVA classification describes the findings ("What") the Hamburg additionally the embryological origin and the biological behavior ("What", "Why", "Where", "How"). So the Hamburg gives the indication for further diagnostic or treatment like the "Schobinger" for A-V-malformations

Hamburg mod. ISSVA-Classification Congenital Vascular Anomalies

	I.S.S.V.A.		Hamburg		
	Vascular Tumors (VT)		**Vascular Malformations (VM)**		
WHAT I.S.S.V.A. Hamburg	Classical Infantile Hemangioma (iH) Glut1+ Stage • I Prodromal phase • II Initial phase • III Proliferation phase • IV Maturation phase • V Regression phase	Congenital Hemangio(endothelio)ma (cHE) Glut1- Type • Rapidly involuting (RICH) • Non involuting (NICH) • "Tufted" Angioma • Kaposiforme (KHE)	Fault in Embryological Determination • Vasculogenesis („Extratruncular") • Angiogenesis („Truncular")	Predominantly Origin • Capillary • Venous • Lymphatic • Arterial • Arterio-venous • Mixed	Embryological Defect • Aplasia • Hypoplasia • Dysplasia • Hyperplasia • Hamartoma • Mixed
WHY I.S.S.V.A.	No reason	Embryopathic -placental -toxic -infectious		Genetic -sporadic -somatic -germ cell -familial	
WHERE Hamburg	Organ -intracutaneous/-mucous -subcutaneous/- mucous -intramuscular intraosseous/intraarticular -intracranial -parenchymatous -intracavitary -mesenterial				-
	Localization -peri-/intraorbital -peri-/intraauricular -peri-/enoral -laryngo/tracheal -remaining face -head/neck -peri-/mammary -anogenital/intraanal/intestinal -remaining Trunk -acral/Hand/Foot -remaining Extremities				
	Number -singular —multiple -disseminated				
HOW Hamburg I.S.S.V.A.	Growth -limited —moderate infiltrating —highly infiltrating Perfusion -slow —moderate —high				
Schobinger	Complications -ulceration -infection -bleeding -cardiac failure -intravasal coagulopathy -associated defects -excessive growth -vent. obstruction -feeding problems -intestinal obstruction -visual Obstruction				

It first appears as a pale pink macule that evolves with time and becomes dark red to purple. In 65% of these patches nodularities and a cobblestone puffy pattern may develop, and severe hypertrophy of the soft tissue with facial asymmetry or deformity occurs by the fifth decade of life. Particularly, eruptive angiomas (tiny bleb lesions) are a frequent complication of port-wine stains. Port- wine stains are usually unilateral and segmental, though they may be bilateral, and they most commonly occur on the face (Fig. 20.1).

Naevus Unna

The transient macular stains so called "*stork bite*" or "*salomon patch*" belong in a seperate category from the permanent capillary malformations. They are usually located on the glabellar region, eyelids, and nape. In contrast to port-wine stains,

these lesions are more pale, fade and disappear. Mulliken suggested that a small percentage may persist, although diminished in intensity, and he would classify this subgroup as vascular malformations [7]. This can explain the recurrence in adult during increased microcirculation and in elderly persons.

Cutis Marmorata Telangiectatica Congenita (Van Lohuizen Syndrome)

The characteristic lesion of cutis marmorata telangiectatica congenita (CMTC) has a distinctive deep purple color and is depressed in a serpiginous reticulated pattern One can understand the CMTC as the hypoplasia forme of CVM in contrast to the Klippel-Trenaunay which is the hyperplasia forme. In some cases of CMTC asso-

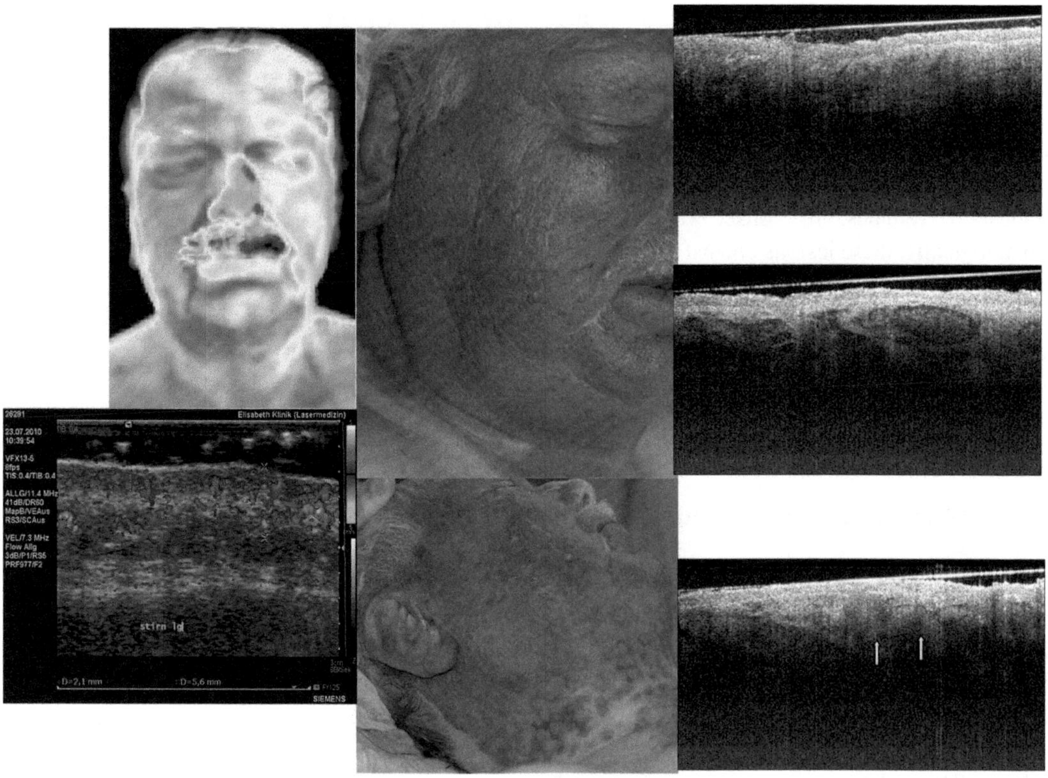

Fig. 20.1 Centro-facial port-wine stains may be only an overlying symptom of a deep vascular malformation. As a screening method thermography is an important investigation. The simple PWS shows normotemperature, whereas a hyperthermia is a sign for an a-v malformation. In this case no embolization was possible, so transcutaneous Nd:YAG laser therapy with ice cube-cooling was started to occlude the microfistulas. The result is seen in the CCDS investigation with a decrease in perfusion

ciated deep venous anomalies, ulceration of the reticulated purple areas and hypotrophy of the involved limb and subcutaneous tissue have been reported. The skin atrophy and deep vascular staining can persist into adulthood, along with diffuse ectasia of the veins in the involved extremities. If the steal effect of this these pathological vessels causes the skin atrophy, a coagulation can enhance the microcirculation to avoid further trophic defects.

ished levels of immunoglobulins. Cutaneous and ocular teleangiectases occur at 3–6 years of age, first noted in the temporal and nasal area of the bulbar conjunctiva, later bright red cutaneous teleangiectases appear on the eyelids, nasal bridge, cheeks, ears, neck, upper chest, and flexor surfaces of the forearms. The course is foudroyant and lethal, and death occurs in the second decade, because of recurrent pulmonary infections and bronchiectasis, or from lymphoreticular malignancy.

Ataxia-Telangiectasia (Louis-Bar Syndrome)

The ataxia-teleangiectasia is a rare syndrome, autosomal recessive disorder, consist of cerebellar ataxia, ocular and cutaneous teleangiectasis, frequent severe respiratory tract and sinus infections caused by immunologic deficiency with dimin-

Generalized Essential Telangiectasia (Angioma Serpiginosum)

The aquired, idiopathic vascular ectasia is characterized by multiple, minute, red to purple pinsized vascular punctata, appearing in groups that extend over a period of months or years in serpiginous and gyrate patterns. Frequently, there is a background of diffuse erythema. The condition is asymptomatic and usually does not hemorrhage. The may occur anywhere on the extremities, but the lower limbs are the sites most commonly affected. These lesions typically appear in females; the onset varies widely. Histologically, these lesions consist of clusters of dilated capillaries housed in dermal papillae and lined by thick walls with no signs of inflammation or hyperplasia. The lesions usually remains stable in adult life and sometimes partially regess, but it is never complete.

Spider Nevus (Nevus Araneus)

The acquired spider nevus can be part of late manifestation of a congenital vascular malformation or as a secondary hyperproliferation then named as a Pyogenic granuloma. This is an extremely common lesion of the skin, that is present in up to 15% of children and young adults. These lesions occur more frequently between 7 and 10 years of age, with no significant difference between boys and girls, while there is increased frequency of spider marks in pubertal females, more so than in males, suggests a hormonal mechnanism. Spontaneous disappearance has been seen in childhood, and does not occur after puberty.

Other Telangiectasias

Patients with diffuse teleangiectasias as a component of the Rothmund-Thompson syndrome (Fig. 20.2) or Teleangiectasia Macularis Eruptiva Perstans demonstrate other spider vascular lesions with a central artery.

Capillary-Lymphatic Malformations

In the strong sense Capillary-Lymphatic Malformations doesn't exist because the lymphatic vascular system has no capillaries but only lymphatic spaces. Pure lymphatic malformations are only found in the newborn period, but even here the majority of patients show additional venous malformations as a mixed malformation. The older the patient the more the venous part will be important for the complications; e.g., bleeding and overgrowth. The isolated single cystic lymphangioma of the neck is a truncular lymphatic malformation – If there is an early recurrence after surgery, the lesion was not an isolated truncular lymphatic malformation but an extratruncular malformation. In extratruncular lymphatic malformations the discrimination between micro- and macrocystic is not precise, but rather and is only like a screen shot. By changing of resorption or production, the size of the cysts can change within in short time period. Furthermore, due to sponta-

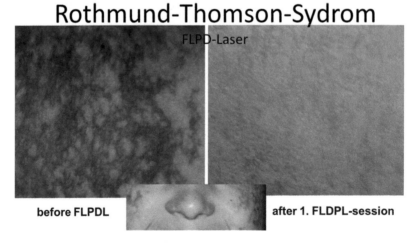

Fig. 20.2 The Rothmund-Thompson syndrome shows as one clinical symptom characteriscally teleangiectasias

Table 20.2   Not all vascular malformations show their symptoms at birth. The primary diagnosis is given by the clinical evaluation and the examination of history. Technical investigations are only necessary for specific questions

Differential Diagnostic Algorythm of Vasc. Tumors/ Vasc. Malformation

	time														color									consistence							
	prepartal	partal	postpartal	1M	3M	6M	9M	12M	2Y	4Y	8Y	16Y	25Y	35Y	pale red	dark red	livid	bluish	petechial	stained	mappy	grey	no changes	Chalasia	atrophied	bulging elastic	bulging tough	pasty	squeezeable	buzzing	hypertherme
vascular Tumors																															
infantile Hemangioma IH																															
Prodromal phase															X											X					
Initial phase															X											X		X			X
Proliferation phase																X										X					X
Maturation phase																X									X			X			
Regression phase																X						X			X				X		
cong. Hemangioendothelioma HE																															
RICH																	X		X		X		X	X							
NICH																		X									X				
"tufted Angioma"																				X							X				
kaposi forme KHE																	X			X	X						X				X
vasc. Malformation																															
Hamartoma																															
Glomangioma																X											X				X
Angioma racemosum																		X		X							X			X	X
Lymph-angiokeratoma																		X	X	X							X	X			
extratrunkular																															
PWS															X					X			X			X					
cutis marmorata															X					X						X					
trunkular																															
Lymphangioma																	X	X				X							X		
venous Malformation																		X												X	
AV-Malformation																	X			X							X			X	

time of first clinical signs, not the course of the treated or untreated anomaly

neous rupture of the interseptal pathologic veins massive bleeding can occur.

Capillary-lymphatic malformations may be discriminated from the classical PWS by light staining, and can be bluish-red to black in color (Table 20.2). Due to the lower erythrocyte concentration, the basic absorption is reduced. However, in these lesions the birthmark is only the tip if the iceberg. In nearly all cases there is a mixed venous-lymphatic malformation in the underlying organs.

Hyperkeratotic Capillary Malformation

Angiokeratomas are usually known by their eponyms, matched with the predilection of the lesions: Mibelli for lesions on the hands or feet, Fordyce for lesions on the scrotum, and Fabry for lesions on the trunk or thighs. If only the lymphatic spaces are affected, this is known as "lymphangioma circumscriptum ", but the subcutis may also be affected. Histologic examination demonstrates a collection of subcutaneous lymphatic cisterns with a thick muscle coat that communicates through dilated lymphatic cannels with the superficial vesicles. A combination of venous and lymphatic malformations mostly affects the extremities. These combined lesions are often associated with skeletal elongation and hypertrophy. When there is also a port-wine stain, the eponym Klippel-Trenaunay syndrome is applicable. Often these lesions bleed easily and weep, either spontaneously or following trauma. Another risk is the high rate of spontaneous erysipelas.

Lymphedema

The lymph vessels can also show structeral abnormalities or predispostion in the sense of a vascular malformation. The *lymphedema* caused by an hypoplasia or hyperplasia of the lymph vessels is a well-known example. So the primary origin is a truncular vascular malformation with an extratruncular manifestation.

Venous Malformations

Similar to the extratruncular lymphatic malformation, all tissues can be affected by extratruncular venous malformations like Soft Tissue Phlebectasias Cutaneous/Subcutaneous Malformation and Mucous Membrane Affection. The main localization for a mucous membrane affection is the oropharynx, followed by the vagina and the rectum. Beside this one has to differentiate the Glomuvenous Malformation ("Glomangioma"). Here one find cases of large raised, soft, and compressible glomangiomas have been mistakenly diagnosed as blue rubber bleb nevus syndrome [8]. Glomangiomas are less likely to be painful than solitary glomus tumors. Venous malformations are developmental abnormalities of veins, dysmorphic in configuration and structure. They usually occur in truncular or extratruncular form or they may be combined. Furthermore, the may be coexist as capillary-venous or lymphatic-venous anomalies. Combined capillary-venous malformation of the skin have a dark red to purple color. Phleboliths may be palpated within the lesion and confirmed by plain-film radiography and sonography [9]. Multiple venous malformations rarely associated with bleeding from similar vascular anomalies of the gastrointestinal tract, so-called "*blue rubber bleb nevus (Bean) syndrome*". Even other organs such as the lung, liver, muscle, bones, kidneys, brain, spleen, gall-bladder, adrenals, pleura and peritoneum can be affected. Therefore, hemoptysis, hematuria, epistaxis, and menorrhagia have been described in these patients. The lesions tend to enlarge with time and may be painful. In case of diffuse venous malformation of the rectum and perirectal tissue the eponym *Barker-Kausch syndrome* is used. In *Esau-Bensaude Malformation* diffuse venous malformation of rectum and perineum is associated with involvement of the ureterovesical mucosa. A generalized intestinal involvement by venous-lymphatic malformations is called *Kaijser syndrome*. Are the spinal cord affected, with enlargement in caliber and thickness of the vessels and varicose postspinal vein, the disease is called *Foix-Alajouanine syndrome*. Venous or venous-lymphatic type of vascular malformations associated with other lesions like enchondromas and dyschondroplasia of a limb or limbs, is a pathological entity, first described by Maffucci in 1881 and now known by the term *Maffucci syndrome* (syn. *Kast syndrome, Ollier-Klippel syndrome*). Pleboliths and expansive bone lesions can be seen on plain films. Multiple organ involvement has been reported. Different lesions may be confused with venous malformations like the *mongolian blue spot*, the *blue nevus* and the *nevus of Ota* are characteristically purple-blue or gray patches usually involving the extremities, in the first case the lesion has a predilection for the sacrum and buttocks, and are melanocytic, not vascular.

Arterial Malformations

Arterial malformations include coarctation, ectasia, aneurysm, truncal arteriovenous fistulae, and arteriovenous malformation. These arterial anomalies are characterized by increased skin temperature, a bruit, and thrill in contrast to capillary, lymphatic, venous, and combined malformations. Arteriovenous malformations of the head and neck region are quite rare in contrast to venous malformations. Otherwise frequently in the extremities Arteriovenous malformations will show an inexorable progression.

Angioma racemosum (of Virchow) became synonymous with a hamartoous arteriovenous malformations, especially for the head and neck region, for lesions where the course of the lesion is progressive. Biopsy of arteriovenous malformation characteristically shows close juxtaposition of medium sized arteries and veins and vessels of indeterminate nature. This explains the infiltrative destructive growing even in a normal non-tumorous replication rate. Frequently are so-called arterialized veins, caused by intimal thickening of veins, suggests by elevated pressure within the vasculature.

In *Wyburn-Mason syndrome/Bonnet-Decaume-Blanc syndrome* the facial PWS (Fig. 20.3) may be the sign of unilateral arteriovenous malformation of the retina and the intracranial optic pathway. Manifestations can be cerebral or ocular or both. Headaches, seizures, or subarachnoid haemorrhage are the usual indicators of involvement of the central nervous system, although the specific symptoms and signs will vary depending on the location and extent of the arteriovenous malformations. The retinal lesions, generally unilateral, range from ophthalmoscopically barely visible vessels covering a substantial portion of the retina and can cause cystic retinal degeneration between the dilated vessels, and impaire vision, to optic atrophy, enlargement of the optic

foramen, and occasionally exophthalmos. Some authors supposed that retinal involvement is not essential for the diagnosis of the Wyburn-Mason syndrome.

Rendu-Osler-Weber Syndrome (Hereditary Hemorrhagic Telangiectasia)

This disease is classified as a extratruncular arterial-capillary malformations and can appear as telangiectasias in the skin and arteriovenous malformations widely distributed throughout the body with a predilection for the gums, lips, mucosa of the nose, face and fingers. The major complication is recurrent bleeding, especially of the nasopharyngeal cavity and the gastrointestinal tract with secondary iron deficiency. Beside this manifestation the most important secondary involvement is the lung and the liver with a-v shunts. Cardiac failure, hepatic portosystemic

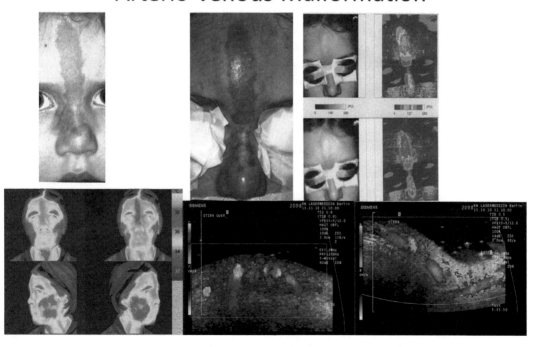

Fig. 20.3 Usually the simple Port Wine Stain shows normal temperature. In cases with hyperthermia is the diagnosis of a mixed capillary-av.-malformation in a

Wyborn-Mason syndrome. This is shown in CCDS with high spontaneous flow and soft tissue hypertrophy. The OCT shows enlarged vessels

Table 20.3 With increasing knowledge about genetics and molecular biology several vascular malformations have a defect in the RAS-signal way. So they have some similarities to other phakomatosis which means that e.g. systemic procedures are even indicated in extratruncular malformations

RAS-associated diseases		
	RASopatias "Phakomatosis"	Other reasons
Vascular malformations	Noonan-Syndrom Parks-Weber-Syndrome Sturge Weber Crest Glomangiomatose Lymphangioleiomyomatosis(LAM)	KTS Gorham Stout BRBS Proteus
Tumours	M. Bourneville Pringle (TSC) M. v. Recklinghausen (NF 1 & 2 Gorlin-Goltz-Syndrome Leopard (cardio-cutaneous S) Peutz-Jeghers-Syndrome	Infant Hemangioma cong. Hämangioendothelioma erupt. Angioma
Other malformations	Mafucci Costello Legius	

encephalopathy, embolic abscesses, and a variety of neurologic symptoms are complications, resulting in the need for some of these patients to have organ transplantation.

Arteriovenous malformations at the extremities are usually symptomatic at time of first presentation. Increased warmth of the limb, pain, paresthesia, and hyperhidrosis are common symptoms. They are frequently associated with bone distortion and overgrowth, in the past called *Parkes-Weber syndrome*. This syndrome exhibits bony overgrowth with capillary-lymphatic-venous malformations, but there is arteriovenous shunting. The later distinguishes it from Klippel-Trenaunay syndrome (Table 20.3).

Capillary Vascular Malformation with Associated Mesenchymal Malformations (Neurocutaneous and Dysplasia Syndromes/ Phakomatois)

Capillary or dermal vascular malformations are occasionally associated with deeper vascular anomalies. The key point is that these cutaneous signs permit early diagnosis, thus helping in further recognition of more complex syndromes [10].

Capillary malformations of face may be associated with choroidal and leptomeningeal vascular malformations, well known is the eponymous condition: Sturge-Weber syndrome. This syndrome, is commonly found among those patients with port-wine stains involving the distribution of the first and second branch of the trigeminal nerve. It has a high incidence of congenital glaucoma of the ipsilateral eye, intracranial vascular malformation of the brain with calcification and atrophy of the underlying cerebrum, associated seizure disorders, and, in some cases mental retardation and hemiparesis. The same malformation affects the soft tissue of the face with the risk of subsequent hypertrophy. This can be detected early by color-coded duplex sonography (CCDS) and especially by thermography with hyperthermy. The *Jahnke syndrome* describes a Sturge-Weber syndrome without ocular involvement. In case of Sturge-Weber syndrome with choroidal involvement but no glaucoma the eponym *Milles syndrome* is used. Brushfield-Wyatt Syndrome is a capillary malformation in the trigeminal area may be the sign of a associated vascular malformation and calcificied cerebral cortex. In von Hippel-Lindau syndrome, facial port-wine stain is associated with retinal capillary malformation, non-calcified vascular malformation of the brain and the spinal cord. Polyzystic tumors affecting other viscera, especially the kidneys, are also a diagnostic clinical feature.

In contrast to N. Ota the Phakomatosis Pigmentovascularis (PPV) is a combined mesodermal malformation with bilateral PWS and Hyperpigmentation [11, 12].

Port-wine stains of the extremities may be associated with systemic abnormalities such as Klippel-Trenaunay syndrome. The Klippel-Trenaunay syndrome (combined capillary-venous-lymphatic malformation with skeletal overgrowth) is characterised by a large port-wine stain of the extremities, malformation of the venous system associated with hypertrophy of the soft tissue and skeletal tissue. The lymphatic system could be involved as well. It is also not uncommon to see a PWS overlying an arteriovenous malformation.

Furthermore there is a great variety of other Overgrowth syndromes. In Proteus syndrome diffuse patchy port-wine stains also may be associated with partial gigantism of hands or feet, usually bilateral and asymmetrical, and hemihypertrophy. Numerous systemic abnormalities such as macrocephaly, skull exostoses, lipomas, and sometimes café au lait patches are notable.

The *Riley-Smith syndrome* is probably part of Proteus syndrome, that characteristically consist of capillary and/or venous malformations associated with lymphatic anomalies, macrodayctyly, macrocephaly, chylous cysts and pseudopapilledema. Another association that partly subsumed by the term Proteus syndrome, is called *Bannayan syndrome*, which consist of macrocephaly with subcutaneous lipomas and vascular malformations. A port-wine stain of the posterior thorax, especially at the lumbar skin, may also indicate an underlying arteriovenous malformation of the spinal cord, called *Cobb syndrome*. In this syndrome, the vascular malformation is in the lumbar skin or vertebrae and underlying spinal meninges, causing neuological damage by the bulk of the malformation. In a great number one can find a genetical defect [13] (Tables 20.4 and 20.5).

Table 20.4 Infantile hemangioma and vascular malformation

Infantile hemangiomas and other benign vascular tumors
- Induction of regression through inflammatory processes after intravascular absorption and larger vessel occlusion
(downgrading)
Vascular malformation
- Destruction of pathologic capillarization (extratruncular VM)
- Occlusion of cavernous vessels and small AV fistulas (truncular VM)
(avoid secondary complications)

Table 20.5 Therapeutic algorithm of congenital vascular malformations

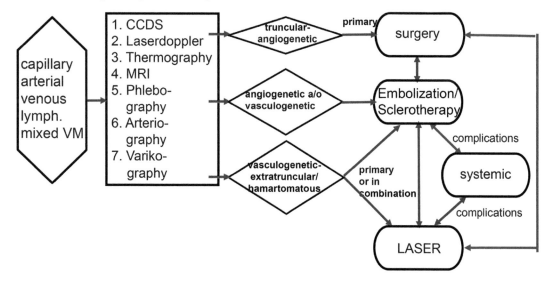

Literature

1. Belov ST. Classification, terminology and nosology of congential vascular defects. In: Belov ST, Loose D, Weber J, editors. Vascular malformations, Periodica angiologica, vol. 16. Reinbek: Einhorn Presse Verlag; 1989. p. 25–8.
2. Lee BB, Baumgartner I, Berlien HP, et al. Consensus document of IUP diagnosis and treatment of venous malformations. Int Angiol. 2014;34(2):97–149.
3. Wassef M, Blei F, Adams D, Alomari A, Baselga E, Berenstein A, Burrows P, Frieden IJ, Garzon MC, Lopez-Gutierrez JC, Lord DJ, Mitchel S, Powell J, Prendiville J, Vikkula M, ISSVA Board and Scientific Committee. Vascular anomalies classification: recommendations from the International society for the study of vascular anomalies. Pediatrics. 2015;136(1): e203–14.
4. Patan S. Vasculogenesis and angiogenesis. Cancer Treat Res. 2004;117:3–32.
5. Berlien HP, Poetke M, Philipp C. Phakomatosen. In: Transitionsmedizin. Stuttgart: Oldhafer Schattauer; 2016. p. 169–80.
6. Poetke M. Laser treatment in haemangiomas and vascular malformations. In: Berlien H-P, Müller G, editors. Applied laser medicine. Berlin/New York: Springer; 2003.
7. Burns AJ, Kaplan LC, Mulliken JB. Is there an association between hemangioma and syndromes with dysmorphic features? Pediatrics. 1991;88:1257–67.
8. Mulliken JB. Capillary malformations, hyperceratotic stains, teleangiectasias and miscellaneous vascular blots. In: Mulliken JB, Burrows PE, Fishman SJ, editors. Mulliken and youngs vascular anomalies: hemangiomas and malformations. 2nd ed. New York: Oxford University Press; 2013. doi:10.1093/med/9780195145052.003.0013.
9. Urban P, Philipp CM, Poetke M, Berlien HP. Value of colour coded duplex sonography in the assessment of haemangiomas and vascular malformations. Med Laser App. 2005;20(4):267–78.
10. Urban P, Berlien H-P, Tinschert S. Vascular malformations in particular syndromes with regional overgrowth. Eur J Vasc Med. 2013;42:35–26.
11. Happle R. Phacomatosis pigmentovascularis revisited and reclassified. Arch Dermatol. 2005;141(3):385–8. doi:10.1001/archpedi.161.4.356.
12. Mandal RK. Sturge-Weber syndrome in association with Klippel-Trenaunay syndrome and phakomatosis pigmentovascularis type IIb. Indian J Dermatol Venerol Leprol. 2014;80:51–3.
13. Sürücü O, Sure U, Stahl S, et al. Neue CCM1-Mutation bei einem 2-jährigen. Monatsschr Kinderheilkunde. 2007;155:1161–5.

Part V

**Contemporary Diagnosis
of CVM: Imaging Modalities**

Jovan N. Markovic and Cynthia K. Shortell

Congenital vascular malformations (CVMs) represent complex group of vascular lesions caused by embryologic dysmorphogenesis with normal rate of endothelial proliferation that can lead to anomalies of the vascular system characterized by wide range of presenting symptoms and often unpredictable clinical course [1–5]. Clinical evaluation often underestimates the involvement of deep structures such as muscles, bones, joints, or abdominal viscera and is not sufficient to differentiate high-flow from low-flow lesions and malformations from tumors in some of the more complex cases [6–9]. Limitations in diagnosis and treatment resulted from inadequate classification schema and diagnostic algorithms that traditionally characterized management of these vascular lesions [10, 11]. A relatively recent advancement in the diagnostic and treatment modalities have resulted in a better understanding of the pathophysiology and natural history of CVMs and improved management of these lesions.

Diagnostic techniques that were traditionally the most frequently used for the evaluation of CVMs include plain radiography, duplex ultrasonography, computed tomography (CT), magnetic resonance imaging (MRI), and angiography [12–15]. Nuclear medicine tests, such as transarterial

lung perfusion scintigraphy (TLPS), radionuclide lymphoscintigraphy (LSG), and whole-body blood pool scintigraphy (WBBPS), have also been utilized for the diagnostic work-up of these lesions [16, 17].

The role of plain films is limited because of low soft tissue contrast resolution. Plain films are most useful to demonstrate soft tissue and bony hypertrophy, limb length discrepancy, and phleboliths in the patients with localized intravascular coagulopathy. Duplex ultrasonography is a portable, non-invasive imaging technique that provides real-time arterial and venous flow velocities as well as real-time visualization during intervention for vascular access [18]. It yields both functional and anatomic data in the evaluation of CVMs. It is particularly helpful in defining the flow characteristics within the anomaly, thus aiding in differentiating among venous, arterial, and mixed malformations. On duplex ultrasonography, venous malformations demonstrate monophasic, biphasic, and no detectable flow in 78%, 6%, and 16% of cases, respectively, while HFVMs duplex ultrasonography is characterized by multidirectional blood flow, rapid arteriovenous shunting and high-amplitude arterial waveform with spectral broadening [18]. On grayscale ultrasonography venous malformations appear as hypoechoic or heterogeneous lesions with anechoic structures visible in <50% of cases [18]. In approximately 16% of cases will demonstrate no detectable flow [18]. In these cases flow in venous malformations is only detectible on ultrasonography with

J.N. Markovic, MD (✉) • C.K. Shortell, MD, FACS (✉)
Duke University Medical Center, Durham, NC, USA
e-mail: jovan.markovic@duke.edu;
Cynthia.shortell@dm.duke.edu

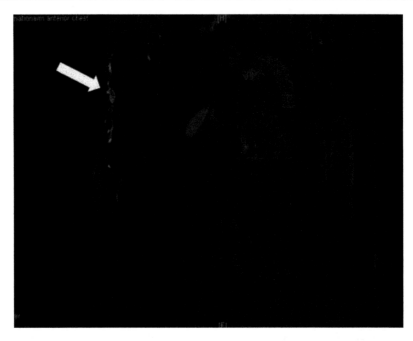

Fig. 21.1 Coronal T2-weighted MRI demonstrates hyperintense signal in the venous malformation involving the anterolateral aspect of the right upper extremity

provoking maneuver (i.e., compression and release of the malformation). Ultrasound can be also used for identification of phleboliths which are visualized as pathognomonic echogenic acoustical shadowing. Although duplex ultrasonography is usually the first examination to be considered in CVMs by a large number of practitioners, in part due to relative low cost compared to other techniques, ultrasonography is frequently inadequate to demonstrate the extent of the lesion, relationship with surround anatomic structures, and communication with deep venous system. In addition ultrasound is characterized by low spatial resolution and a narrow field of view that is frequently not sufficient to include the entire lesion. A high-frequency linear array transducer of 5–10 MHz or even 15 MHz should be used for optimal imaging [18].

CT use in the evaluation of CVMs is limited as even with contrast administration, CT usually provides poor lesion conspicuity relative to adjacent structures and does not always provide assessment of internal vascular architecture within the malformation. These two characteristics are critical for preoperative planning and treatment selection. On CT without contrast, venous malformations appear as low attenuation and are homogeneous. This radiologic characteristic is used to differentiate them from high-flow lesions. However, if there is coexisting adipose infiltration, low-flow malformations can appear heterogeneous which can lead to an inconclusive or erroneous CT results. Contrast-enhanced CT can identify the location of the malformation, vessel ectasia, and/or aneurysm formation. Compared to MRI, CT may better define alterations in bony architecture as well as phleboliths or other dystrophic calcifications. True extent of the lesion into soft tissue however is often underestimated on CT scans as only contrast-enhanced vessels opacity within the lesion.

MRI has been the imaging modality of choice in the evaluation of CVMs as it gives a bright T2-weighted spin-echo sequences hypersignal that delineates the extent of the malformation throughout the involved tissues [19]. In T2-weighted sequence, low-flow malformations are characterized by high signal intensity (an imaging propriety used to differentiate them from high-flow lesions) (Fig. 21.1). In addition, MRI shows the lesion's flow characteristics in relation to normal circulation and provides good soft tissue definition [20]. An equivocal MRI usually prompted catheter-directed

Fig. 21.2 dceMRI demonstrates a lesion during the arterial phase what confirms a large HFVM involving the lateral aspect of the proximal upper extremity. dceMRI information is used for differential diagnosis and treatment planning

angiography to rule out a high-flow arterial component. This is of critical value in the management of CVM as treatment options for high-flow and low-flow lesions are different, and the presence of arterial component represents absolute contraindication for transcutaneous sclerotherapy (due to increased risk of distal embolic events and extensive tissue necrosis) which can be effectively used in the treatment of LFVM.

Whole-body blood pool scintigraphy can be used in patients with diffuse CVMs as an optional test to evaluate the lesions scattered throughout the body and also for the evaluation of the lymphatic malformations by their negative blood pool findings. TLPS is not indicated for the initial evaluation of the CVMs. Its major role is to rule out the presence of combined arteriovenous lesions as TLPS can detect a micro-shunting within the lesion which can be occasionally missed even with conventional arteriography. LSG can be useful for the evaluation of the combined CVMs when it is important to rule out lymphatic component. It is worth emphasizing that these nuclear tests were utilized only in highly specialized vascular clinics in the past and that currently their role has more didactic rather than clinically applicable purpose.

Although widely accepted in the past, above-mentioned (nonnuclear medicine) diagnostic techniques are frequently inconclusive in complex cases, and consequently a significant number of patients have required evaluation with more invasive catheter-based angiography. Relatively recently introduced technique of dynamic contrast-enhanced MRI (dceMRI), which is based on time-resolved imaging of contrast kinetics and time-resolved echo-shared angiographic techniques, is very useful in this regard and has been validated as clinically applicable to definitively distinguish HFVM from LFVM with accuracy rate of approximately 84%, leaving relatively small number of inconclusive cases that require confirmatory angiography [21, 22]. In addition to flow characteristics, dceMRI yields more information regarding extent of the malformation, soft tissue involvement, and the relationship to normal anatomy, all of which becomes important in treatment planning. Pretreatment imaging with dceMRI provides valuable information prior to intervention and provides both high spatial and temporal resolution allowing for precise lesion characterization and treatment planning (Fig. 21.2). At our institution dceMRI serves as the mainstay of diagnostic evaluation for patients with clinically suspected

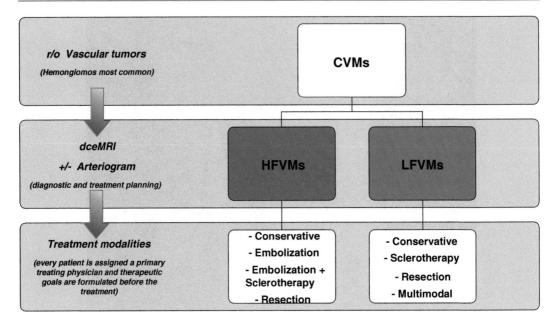

Fig. 21.3 Diagnostic and therapeutic algorithm used for multidisciplinary treatment of congenital vascular malformations (CVMs). *dceMRI* dynamic contrast-enhanced magnetic resonance imaging, *HFVMs* high-flow vascular malformations, *LFVM* low-flow vascular malformations

CVM [23]. Information obtained from such imaging allows the patient to be stratified into a high-flow or low-flow vascular malformation group based on a simplified diagnostic stratification scheme, such that an appropriate therapeutic plan can be formulated and unnecessary invasive testing can be avoided in most patients (Fig. 21.3).

In summary, management of CVMs requires an accurate diagnosis before intervening. Above-described diagnostic algorithm with novel imaging techniques avoids noncontributory imaging and has been validated as clinically applicable for making an accurate anatomical and hemodynamic assessment of CVMs and for treatment planning in majority of patients. The hemodynamic and anatomic characteristics determined by dceMRI allow for implementation of catheter-based embolization for high-flow lesions, or transcutaneous sclerotherapy for low-flow lesions, as well as the use of surgical resection, depending on the extent of the lesion, its intrinsic morphology, and involvement of vital anatomic structures. The utility of a dceMRI-focused diagnostic algorithm to fully evaluate lesion characteristics is of upmost importance as once

hemodynamic physiology is discerned, focused, and individualized treatment strategies can be applied, and a significant majority of the patients with both LFVM and HFVM can be managed to attain treatment goals set by both the patient and provider in a comprehensive and streamlined fashion. This ultimately allows for more efficient treatment of CVMs and thus improved patient outcomes and patient satisfaction.

References

1. Cohen Jr MM. Vasculogenesis, angiogenesis, hemangiomas, and vascular malformations. Am J Med Genet. 2002;108(4):265–74.
2. Diehl S et al. Altered expression patterns of EphrinB2 and EphB2 in human umbilical vessels and congenital venous malformations. Pediatr Res. 2005;57(4):537–44.
3. Boon LM, Mulliken JB, Vikkula M, et al. Assignment of a locus for dominantly inherited venous malformations to chromosome 9p. Hum Mol Genet. 1994;3:1583–7.
4. Calvert JT et al. Allelic and locus heterogeneity in inherited venous malformations. Hum Mol Genet. 1999;8(7):1279–89.
5. Irrthum A, Brouillard P, Boon LM, Warman ML, Olsen BR, Mulliken JB, Enjolras O, Vikkula M. Linkage

disequilibrium narrows locus for venous malformations with glomus cells (VMGLOM) to a single 1.48-Mbp YAC. Eur J Hum Genet. 2001;9:34–8.

6. Belov S. Anatomopathological classification of congenital vascular defects. Semin Vasc Surg. 1993;6:219–24.

7. Lee BB, Laredo J. Classification of congenital vascular malformations: the last challenge for congenital vascular malformations. Phlebology. 2012;27(6):267–9.

8. Lee BB, Laredo J, Lee TS, Huh S, Neville R. Terminology and classification of congenital vascular malformations. Phlebology. 2007;22(6):249–52.

9. Marler JJ, Mulliken JB. Vascular anomalies: classification, diagnosis, and natural history. Facial Plast Surg Clin North Am. 2001;9(4):495–504.

10. Lee BB, Laredo J, Seo JM, Neville R. Chapter 29. Treatment of lymphatic malformations. In: Mattassi, Loose, Vaghi, editors. Hemangiomas and vascular malformations. Milan, Italy: Springer-Verlag Italia; 2009. p. 231–50.

11. Lee BB. Advanced management of congenital vascular malformation (CVM). Int Angiol. 2002;21(3):209–13.

12. Lee BB, Mattassi R, Choe YH, Vaghi M, Ahn JM, Kim DI, Huh SH, Lee CH, Kim DY. Critical role of duplex ultrasonography for the advanced management of a venous malformation (VM). Phlebology. 2005;20:28–37.

13. Gold L, Nazarian LN, Johar AS, Rao VM. Characterization of maxillofacial soft tissue vascular anomalies by ultrasound and color Doppler imaging: an adjuvant to computed tomography and magnetic resonance imaging. J Oral Maxillofac Surg. 2003;61(1):19–31.

14. Rauch RF, Silverman PM, Korobkin M, et al. Computed tomography of benign angiomatous lesions of the extremities. J Comput Assist Tomogr. 1984;8: 1143–6.

15. Burrows PE, Mulliken JB, Fellows KE, Strand RD. Childhood hemangiomas and vascular malformations: angiographic differentiation. AJR Am J Roentgenol. 1983;141(3):483–8.

16. Lee BB, Mattassi R, Kim BT, Park JM. Advanced management of arteriovenous shunting malformation with transarterial Lung Perfusion Scintigraphy (TLPS) for follow up assessment. Int Angiol. 2005;24(2):173–84.

17. Lee BB, Mattassi R, Kim BT, Kim DI, Ahn JM, Choi JY. Contemporary diagnosis and management of venous and AV shunting malformation by whole body blood pool scintigraphy (WBBPS). Int Angiol. 2004;23:355–67.

18. Lee BB, Bergan J, Gloviczki P, Laredo J, Loose DA, Mattassi R, Parsi K, Villavicencio JL, Zamboni P. Diagnosis and treatment of venous malformations – Consensus Document of the International Union of Phlebology (IUP)-2009. Int Angiol. 2009;28(6):434–51.

19. Moukaddam H, Pollak J, Haims AH. MRI characteristics and classification of peripheral vascular malformations and tumors. Skeletal Radiol. 2009;38(6):535–47.

20. Konez O, Burrows PE. Magnetic resonance of vascular anomalies. Magn Reson Imaging Clin N Am. 2002;10(2):363–88.

21. Van Rijswijk CS, van der Linden E, van der Woude HJ, van Baalen JM, Bloem JL. Value of dynamic contrast-enhanced MR imaging in diagnosing and classifying peripheral vascular malformations. AJR Am J Roentgenol. 2002;178(5):1181–7.

22. Lidsky M, Spritzer C, Shortell C. The role of dynamic contrast-enhanced magnetic resonance imaging in the diagnosis and management of patients with vascular malformations. J Vasc Surg. 2011;53(1):131–7.

23. Markovic JN, Shortell CK. Multidisciplinary treatment of the extremity vascular malformations. J Vasc Surg-Venous Lymphat Disord. 2015;3:209–18.

Jovan N. Markovic and Cynthia K. Shortell

Introduction

Historically, the diagnosis and treatment of congenital vascular malformations (CVMs) have been hampered by the complex nature of these vascular lesions, the persistence of outdated and often inconsistent terminology, as well as the absence of defined imaging protocols and therapeutic algorithms [1–5]. As vascular malformations range in severity from trivial to life-threatening, from focal to diffuse and extensive, and vary significantly with regard to composition, the ability to use a single imaging modality to distinguish between high-flow and low-flow lesions is essential when the goal is to avoid noncontributory and/or invasive imaging modalities, select proper treatment modality, avoid unnecessary invasive catheter-based procedures, and avoid potentially life-threatening side effects [6–9].

Multiple diagnostic modalities are used (alone or combined) to evaluate vascular malformations and to confirm the initial clinical diagnosis including US imaging, CT scan, catheter-based angiography, and MRI [10–15]. Although still frequently used US and CT scan provide variable degrees of diagnostic accuracy or frequently insufficient information with regard to pre-procedural planning. Consequently a significant number of patients was left undiagnosed or required evaluation with a catheter-based angiography.

Magnetic Resonance Imaging

Given the abovementioned limitations, MRI become the imaging modality of choice in the confirmation, characterization, and differentiation between vascular malformations and their subtypes. MRI gives a bright signal on T2-weighted spin-echo sequences for the parenchymal portions of vascular lesions which is not only useful to delineate the extent of the malformation throughout the involved tissues, but it also allows for treatment planning and can be used for objective assessment of the treatment efficacy [15]. The full extent of tissue involvement is readily depicted when T1 and T2 or short-tau inversion recovery (STIR) images are acquired [16, 17].

Low-flow malformations have characteristically augmented intraluminal signal on T2-weighted images [17]. There is frequently an intraluminal signal on the T1-weighted images as well. Low-flow lesions enhance with contrast and normally do not contain flow voids. A low signal on T2-weighted images in low-flow malformations is concerning for thrombosis, and a very focal area of low signal can represent a phlebolith [15]. Venous malformations commonly present as solitary or multiple lobulated, cavitary, or infiltrative masses that are usually isointense or

J.N. Markovic, MD (✉) • C.K. Shortell, MD, FACS (✉)
Duke University Medical Center, Durham, NC, USA
e-mail: jovan.markovic@duke.edu;
Cynthia.shortell@dm.duke.edu

© Springer-Verlag Berlin Heidelberg 2017
Y.-W. Kim et al. (eds.), *Congenital Vascular Malformations*, DOI 10.1007/978-3-662-46709-1_22

hypointense on T1-weighted and hyperintense on T2-weighted or STIR images. As mentioned above, signal voids are indicative of thrombosis in the vessels or phleboliths. Macrocystic lymphatic malformations are often differentiated from venous malformations by their predominantly cavitary, lobulated, and septated appearance that is characterized by hypointense signal on T1-weighted and hyperintense signal on T2-weighted and STIR images. Distinct from venous malformations, macrocystic lesions do not enhance with an exception of "rings and arcs" appearance within cyst wall or septa [15]. Macrocystic lesions are more likely to demonstrate fluid-fluid levels. Microcystic lesions are differentiated from macrocystic lesions by the absence of dominant cystic spaces and lack of contrast enhancement, and this is used as criteria to differentiate them from venous malformations [17].

High-flow vascular malformations typically do contain flow voids that can be identified on T1- and T2-weighted images (Fig. 22.1). This radiologic characteristic is used for distinguishing them from low-flow lesions. High-flow lesions are also frequently visualized as dilated feeding arteries and draining veins with a paucity of venous lakes [17].

Conventional MRI was not used only for evaluation of a lesion but for the evaluation of deep venous system. This is very important as the prevalence of deep venous system anomalies is high in CVM patients and the status of deep

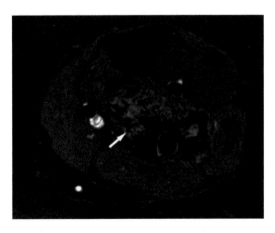

Fig. 22.1 Conventional MRI: T1-weighted fat-saturated gadolinium-enhanced imaging of arteriovenous malformation reveals multiple flow voids (*arrow*)

venous system and its relation to CVMs is used for treatment planning. In a study of 392 patients with CVM, Eifert et al. documented that in 8% of CVM patients (with venous predominance) aplasia or hypoplasia of deep venous trunks was present [18]. In these patients venous blood flow from the affected limbs depends on superficial and abnormal vessels. Obliteration of these vascular structures would jeopardize the venous circulation of the affected limb. Therefore evaluation of patency and anatomic variations of the entire venous system (deep and superficial) is vital in these patients. It has been reported that prevalence of deep venous anomalies is even higher (18%) in patients with KTS [19].

Dynamic Contrast-Enhanced MRI

Although conventional MRI shows the lesion's flow characteristics in relation to normal circulation and provides good soft tissue definition, it is frequently not adequate to differentiate between different types of CVMs in more complex cases as it does not provide hemodynamic data. In addition, many particulars can mitigate conventional MRI findings, for example, a blood vessel that courses within an imaging plane may produce an intraluminal signal despite fairly fast flow, falsely suggesting a low-flow malformation which can potentially lead to catastrophic side effects if the lesion is treated as low-flow malformation.

To avoid this, dceMRI can be used to more accurately assess flow within the lesion since it yields more information with regard to hemodynamic characteristics of CVM by utilizing time-resolved imaging of contrast kinetics (TRICKS) and time-resolved echo-shared angiographic techniques (TREAT) where images are acquired sequentially (Fig. 22.2) [20]. This dynamic image acquisition produces multiple image volume sets, each at a different time points that are subsequently converted to a maximum-intensity projection, which are displayed in a way that vessel and lesion enhancement are the only structures visualized. This technique generates the appearance of dceMRI images that are analogous

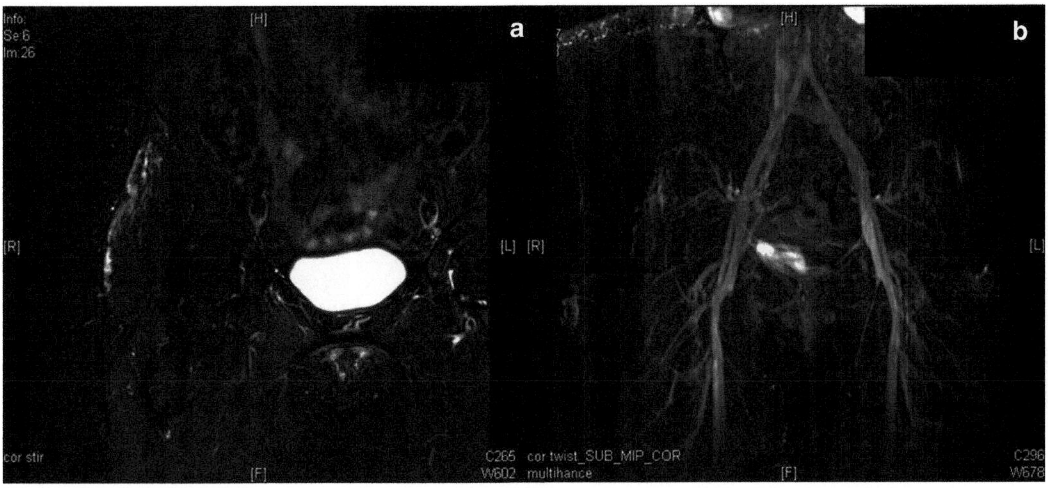

Fig. 22.2 A low-flow vascular malformation is seen in conventional and dynamic contrast-enhanced magnetic resonance imaging. (**a**) A short-tau inversion recovery (STIR) image of a low-flow vascular malformation. (**b**) Low-flow vascular malformation is seen in late venous phase of dynamic contrast-enhanced magnetic resonance imaging

to a display of a conventional digital arteriogram with background subtraction [21]. In this way, main vascular components of the lesion are enhanced, which provides better definition and more accurate differentiation between high-flow and low-flow lesions than conventional MRI. In addition, dceMRI has the advantage of being able to detect dominant or multiple feeding vessels in CVMs, what is critical for treatment planning [20, 22–24].

dceMRI has characteristic imaging properties that can be obtained either on 1.5T scanners or 3T scanners: Avanto [Siemens Medical Systems, Malvern, Pa] or Signa hdx [General Electric Healthcare, Piscataway, NJ]. First, multiplanar T1-weighted spin echo and T2-weighted fast spin echo or fast STIR images are initially obtained. Slice thickness, spatial resolution, matrix, and coil selection are dependent on the area to be imaged and the scanner used. Following this a power injector is used to intravenously administer 5–20 mL of contrast (gadolinium diethylenetriamine pentaacetate or gadolinium benzyloxypropionictetraacetate). Image acquisition extends from the arterial to the late venous phase using time-resolved imaging of contrast kinetics, time-resolved echo-shared angiographic technique, or time-resolved angiography with stochastic trajectories dynamic sequences. Effective image temporal resolution is usually 3–8 s. Finally, post-contrast T1-weighted spin-echo images are acquired. After acquisition, images are reviewed on a picture archiving platform and communication system workstation.

Individual studies and volume sets can be interrogated on a Vitrea three-dimensional workstation (Vital Images, Minnetonka, Minn) if needed. Besides defining the extent of the abnormality, dceMRI result interpretations include information with regard to the type of vascular malformation as well as the flow velocity within the lesion. If the dynamic gadolinium-enhanced sequences identified flow within the lesion at or preceding the visualization of arterial flow within normal vessels, the lesion is considered to be a high-flow lesion. The presence or absence of early venous return from veins draining the lesion or true immediate arterial venous shunting (i.e., an arterial venous malformation) through the lesion is used to describe the flow characteristics. If the lesion is not apparent on the dynamic gadolinium-enhanced images until the capillary phase, or more typically the venous phase, as determined by a comparison with visualization of normal vessels, the lesion is considered to be a low flow (Fig. 22.3). In contrast high-flow malformations visualized from early arterial to late venous phase (Fig. 22.4).

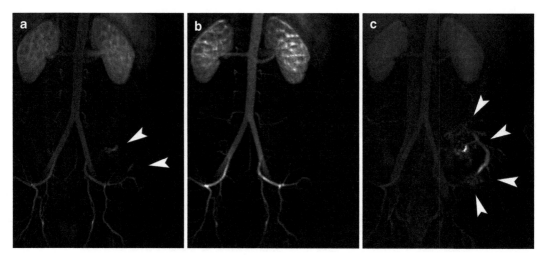

Fig. 22.3 dceMRI coronal MIP time-resolved images: (**a**) early venous phase demonstrates initial opacification of part of the malformation (*arrowheads*). (**b**) Arterial phase image demonstrates no vascular abnormality. (**c**) Late venous phase image demonstrates full opacification of the venous malformation (*arrowheads*)

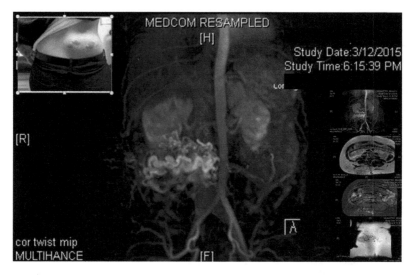

Fig. 22.4 On dceMRI imaging sequences a high-flow vascular malformation is visualized in early arterial through late venous phase

Dynamic Contrast-Enhanced MRI: Clinical Evaluation

In 2002, Rijswijk et al. published data from a prospective study resulted from blinding two independent observers as they reviewed conventional MRI and dceMRI imaging performed on 27 patients with clinically suspected high-flow vascular malformations [25]. All patients underwent dceMRI as well as diagnostic angiography. The sensitivity of conventional MRI in differentiating venous and non-venous lesions was 100%. However, data from this study showed an increase in the specificity of MRI from 24–33 to 95% with the addition of dynamic contrast-enhanced sequences [25].

At our institution we reviewed our experience with CVM evaluation by above-described technical protocol for dceMRI [26]. Data from our study showed that this imaging modality can be used to definitively distinguish HFVM from LFVM in as high as approximately 84% of CVM patients [26]. The patients with equivocal dceMRI underwent evaluation by arteriogram. This represents a significant diagnostic work-up improvement as historically, a significantly larger subgroup of patients would be reevaluated with catheter-based angiography.

Our data based on the evaluation of 122 patients showed that clinically relevant high-flow malformations were never missed on dceMRI: none of the dceMRI-diagnosed low-flow vascular malformations treated invasively had a high-flow component, and flow quality of indeterminately diagnosed low-flow vascular malformations was confirmed with secondary studies. As mentioned earlier, dceMRI alone was sufficient to diagnose flow characteristics in at least 83.8% of patients. The location of the lesion did not correlate with a resulting indeterminate dceMRI, and there were no obvious patient-specific or lesion-specific characteristics that predicted indeterminate imaging studies. Furthermore, our data demonstrated the dceMRI sensitivity and specificity for diagnosing HFVMs of 78.6% and 85.2%, respectively. Respective rates for LFVMs were 85.2% and 78.6% [26].

CAPRT Time-Resolved Imaging

Cartesian acquisition with projection reconstruction-like sampling (CAPR time-resolved imaging) has been reported as an advanced imaging technique to be able to provide high temporospatial resolution imaging that allows for highly accurate characterization of the CVMs and treatment planning.

In a small series of patients with VMs authors demonstrated excellent correlation between CAPR time-resolved technique imaging results and conventional angiography (which was performed at the time of treatment) [16]. Data of this study also suggested that delayed imaging should be utilized to capture complete filling of very slow CVMs. Although initial results associated with CAPR time-resolved imagining are promis-

ing, larger clinical trials are needed before this imaging modality can be accurately evaluated in the management of VMs.

Angiography

When dceMRI is not definitive in assessing flow status, arteriography is performed not only to confirm the diagnosis but also to identify the communication pattern with the draining venous system and to provide an opportunity for treatment planning and/or intervention (Fig. 22.5). Angiography also allows the classification of the VM based on its anatomy in regard to the communication pattern with the draining venous system. Based on the appearance of the VMs and the draining venous system during phlebography, all VMs can be classified into four distinct groups: Type I (isolated VMs without phlebographically appreciable venous drainage), Type II and Type III VMs (demonstrate normal-sized and enlarged venous drainage, respectively), and Type IV VMs (characterized by essentially ectatic dysplastic veins). Although abovementioned phlebographic classification does not provide information regarding the location of the VMs or the involvement of surrounding anatomical structures, it provides useful data for treatment planning, especially when the sclerotherapy is considered as a treatment option. Puig et al. [3] demonstrated that sclerotherapy can be safely performed in low-risk patients with Type I and Type II lesions, while patients with Type III and Type IV VMs were at the increased risk of perioperative complications due to efflux of sclerosant from the VM during sclerotherapy and potentially lethal distal embolic events [3].

Although highly specific, arteriography is limited in its ability to delineate a lesion relative to its adjacent anatomic structures. This is an important limitation as CVMs frequently infiltrate muscle, encircle nerves, and can invade adjacent vital tissues. In addition arteriography is considered an invasive technique as it carries significant risk for complications including groin hematoma, pseudoaneurysm, arteriovenous fistula, acute arterial

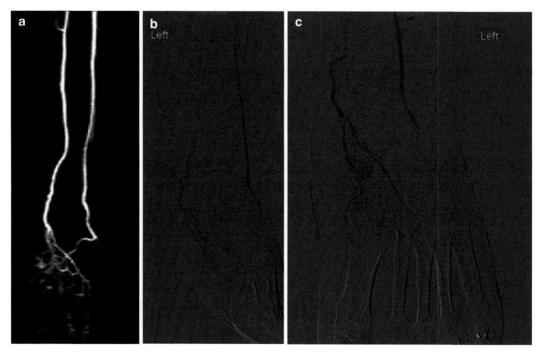

Fig. 22.5 dceMRI shows questionable early filling suggestive of arterial flow (**a**). Subsequent confirmatory arteriography demonstrates the absence of arterial shunting (**b, c**)

thromboembolic events, and infection. These complications have been reported in approximately 1.5–9% of patients [27, 28].

Conclusion

Although multiple imaging modalities are available for the management of CVMs, dceMRI provides the most critical information, especially regarding CVMs that will be treated. Above described diagnostic algorithm with novel imaging techniques avoids noncontributory imaging and has been validated as clinically applicable for making an accurate anatomical and hemodynamic diagnosis of CVMs and for treatment planning in majority of patients. In addition, it avoids unnecessary diagnostic arteriograms, in most of the cases, allowing a significant number of CVM patients to be spared the expense, risk, and inconvenience of a catheter-based diagnostic study, as well as delayed or erroneous diagnosis.

References

1. Degni M, Gerson L, Ishikava K, et al. Classification of the vascular diseases of the limbs. J Cardiovasc Surg (Torino). 1973;14:109–16.
2. Belov S. Anatomopathological classification of congenital vascular defects. Semin Vasc Surg. 1993;6:219–24.
3. Puig S, Aref H, Chigot V, Bonin B, Brunelle F. Classification of venous malformations in children and implications for sclerotherapy. Pediatr Radiol. 2003;33:99–103.
4. Marler JJ, Mulliken JB. Vascular anomalies: classification, diagnosis, and natural history. Facial Plast Surg Clin North Am. 2001;9(4):495–504.
5. Bartels C, Horsch S. Classification of congenital arterial and venous vascular malformations. Angiology. 1995;46(3):191–200.
6. Lee BB. Critical issues in management of congenital vascular malformation. Ann Vasc Surg. 2004;18(3):380–92.
7. Lee BB et al. Congenital vascular malformations: general diagnostic principles. Phlebology. 2007;22(6):253–7.
8. Erin FDM et al. Clinical characteristics and management of vascular anomalies: findings of a

multidisciplinary vascular anomalies clinic. Arch Dermatol. 2004;140(8):979.

9. Lee BB, Bergan JJ. Advanced management of congenital vascular malformations: a multidisciplinary approach. Cardiovasc Surg. 2002;10(6):523–33.

10. Burrows PE, Laor T, Paltiel H, Robertson RL. Diagnostic imaging in the evaluation of vascular birthmarks. Dermatol Clin. 1998;16(3):455–88.

11. Trop I, Dubois J, Guibaud L, et al. Soft-tissue venous malformations in pediatric and young adult patients: diagnosis with Doppler US. Radiology. 1999;212:841–5.

12. Paltiel HJ, Burrows PE, Kozakewich HP, Zurakowski D, Mulliken JB. Soft-tissue vascular anomalies: utility of US for diagnosis. Radiology. 2000;214:747–54.

13. Legiehn GM, Heran MK. Venous malformations: classification, development, diagnosis, and interventional radiologic management. Radiol Clin North Am. 2008;46:545–97.

14. Lee BB, Antignani PL, Baraldini V, Baumgartner I, Berlien, P, Blei F, Carrafiello GP, Grantzow R, Rabe E, Ianniello A, Laredo J, Loose D, Lopez Gutierrez JC, Markovic JN, Mattassi R, Parsi K, Shortell C, Tamburini M, Vaghi M. ISVI-IUA consensus document diagnostic guidelines of vascular anomalies: vascular malformations and hemangiomas. Int Angiol. 2015;34(4):333–74.

15. Fayad LM, Hazirolan T, Bluemke D, Mitchell S. Vascular malformations in the extremities: emphasis on MR imaging features that guide treatment options. Skeletal Radiol. 2006;35:127–37.

16. Mostardi PM, Young PM, McKusick MA, Riederer SJ. High temporal and spatial resolution imaging of peripheral vascular malformations. J Magn Reson Imaging. 2012;36(4):933–42.

17. Moukaddam H, Pollak J, Haims AH. MRI characteristics and classification of peripheral vascular malformations and tumors. Skeletal Radiol. 2009;38:535–47.

18. Eifert S, Villavicencio JL, Kao TC, Taute BM, Rich NM. Prevalence of deep venous anomalies in congenital vascular malformations of venous predominance. J Vasc Surg. 2000;31:462–71.

19. Browse NL, Burnand KG, Lea TM. The klippel trenaunay syndrome. In: Browse NL, Burnand KG, Thomas ML, editors. Diseases of the veins: pathology, diagnosis and treatment. London: Edward Arnold; 1988. p. 609–25.

20. Prince MR. Contrast-enhanced MR angiography: theory and optimization. Magn Reson Imaging Clin N Am. 1998;6(2):257–67.

21. Lidsky ME, Markovic JN, Miller Jr MJ, Shortell CK. Analysis of the treatment of congenital vascular malformations using a multidisciplinary approach. J Vasc Surg. 2012;56(5):1355–62.

22. Konez O, Burrows PE. Magnetic resonance of vascular anomalies. Magn Reson Imaging Clin N Am. 2002;10:363–88. vii

23. Hovius SE, Borg DH, Paans PR, Pieterman H. The diagnostic value of magnetic resonance imaging in combination with angiography in patients with vascular malformations: a prospective study. Ann Plast Surg. 1996;37:278–85.

24. Rinker B, Karp NS, Margiotta M, Blei F, Rosen R, Rofsky NM. The role of magnetic resonance imaging in the management of vascular malformations of the trunk and extremities. Plast Reconstr Surg. 2003;112:504–10.

25. van Rijswijk CS, van der Linden E, van der Woude HJ, van Baalen JM, Bloem JL. Value of dynamic contrast-enhanced MR imaging in diagnosing and classifying peripheral vascular malformations. AJR Am J Roentgenol. 2002;178:1181–7.

26. Lidsky ME, Spritzer CE, Shortell CK. The role of dynamic contrast-enhanced magnetic resonance imaging in the diagnosis and management of patients with vascular malformations. J Vasc Surg. 2012;56(3):757–64.

27. Nasser TK, Mohler 3rd ER, Wilensky RL, Hathaway DR. Peripheral vascular complications following coronary interventional procedures. Clin Cardiol. 1995;18(11):609–14.

28. Lumsden A, Peden E, Bush RL, Lin PH. Complications of endovascular procedures. In: Rutherford RB, editor. Vascular surgery. Philadelphia: Elsevier Saunders; 2005. p. 809–20.

Ultrasonography in the Diagnosis of Congenital Vascular Malformation

23

Massimo Vaghi

In the diagnostic workflow of the vascular malformations, duplex ultrasound represents the basic investigation. This role is related to the large availability of the equipment, the low cost of the investigation, and the absence of radiation exposure. Other interesting features are represented by the lack of invasiveness and the real-time investigation.

Duplex instruments can scan both the morphology and the hemodynamic features of vascular anomalies and tumors. We can collect numerical values for size of the vascular malformation. The limits of the investigation are related to the limited spatial resolution and investigation field. The temporal resolution is very high and allows real-time examinations and a precise hemodynamic evaluation.

It is important to underline that the procedure is operator dependent, and the results of the investigation are related not only to the technical skills of the operator but more to his knowledge of the pathology. There is some agreement for the necessity to standardize the examination and to perform it according to different depths [1].

In case of limb involvement, both limbs should be extensively investigated and morphological and hemodynamic parameters should be assessed.

The first step in the diagnosis of a vascular malformation is to recognize its presence. The differential diagnosis is represented by hemangiomas and malignant tumors.

The second step is to characterize the malformation according to the hemodynamic parameters (slow flow-high flow) and the vessels involved. It is mandatory to define the malformation according to the embryological development into truncular or extratruncular.

In truncular malformation the hemodynamic impairment is predominant while in extratruncular malformations the organ involvement is predominant [2–4].

The third step is the guide for therapy (percutaneous, endovascular, surgical) [5, 6, 9–11].

Regarding the examination's methodology, we have to stress that the B mode examination is fundamental and should be done before any flow examinations. B mode elicits to discover disorders of the main vessels like hypoplasia, aplasia, and diffuse dilation or aneurysmal dilatation [7, 8]. In the presence of dilated vessels or the presence of cysts, the compression of these structures will reveal if these are thrombosed (incompressible tubes) or, in case of dilated spaces, there are lymph cysts (not compressible).

The B mode evaluation allows to visualize the dynamic of involved muscles and the presence of major nervous trunks around the malformation (Fig. 23.1). It is very important to underline that ultrasound is a real-time examination and it can be performed in supine and

M. Vaghi, MD
Vascular Surgery Department, Hospital G. Salvini, Garbagnate Milanese, Italy
e-mail: vaghim@yahoo.it

© Springer-Verlag Berlin Heidelberg 2017
Y.-W. Kim et al. (eds.), *Congenital Vascular Malformations*, DOI 10.1007/978-3-662-46709-1_23

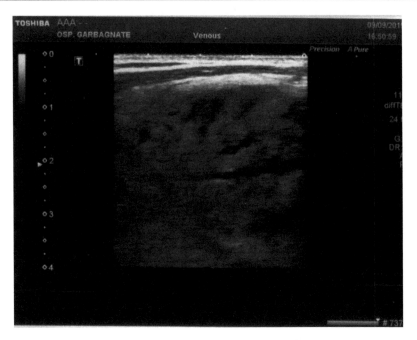

Fig. 23.1 Semimembranosus muscles infiltrated by venous and lymphatic malformation

upright position and during movement. Some venous and also lymphatic malformations may collapse in supine position and may be detectable only in orthostatism.

According to the hemodynamic features, the malformations may have the following flow profiles at Doppler examination: spontaneous high flow with normal resistance index, spontaneous high flow with low resistance index, spontaneous low flow, induced low flow, and no flow.

Doppler examination is based on color Doppler examination and spectral analysis. In both cases the pulse repetition frequency should be adjusted to the flow velocity of the investigated vessel. The Doppler visualization is important to detect the flow anomalies but also the morphological characteristics of A-V shunt or pattern of venous incompetence (Figs. 23.2 and 23.3).

The vessels should be followed in order to get an anatomic map of the malformation.

We should be aware that sometimes vascular malformations are like iceberg and that the deep and hidden part of the malformation may be the most important in terms of hemodynamic involvement, and we should sure to investigate all the vessels of the anatomic area. The setting of

the equipment is very important in order to detect the flow anomalies: it should be different for high- and low-flow malformations (Fig. 23.4).

In this case the color Doppler should be turned to real time (no delay and no overwriting by the software) in case of high-flow malformations and to power Doppler for low-flow malformations. Spectral analysis should include the velocity, the flow direction, and the characteristics of flow (e.g., the presence of pulsatile flow in veins). Derived parameters like acceleration blood flow volume, resistance index should be included in order to gain a data set which is very important in controlling the evolution of the pathology. This evolution may be spontaneous or conditioned by a therapeutic approach.

A-V shunts usually have a honeycomb appearance on B mode examination and are not compressible. It is important to detect the morphology of the shunt in order to have an idea of the shunt's morphology and how many arterial and venous vessels are involved. The classification of Park-Do [11] is very important in this case.

Intraosseous A-V shunt may be detected by setting the equipment for transcranial investigations.

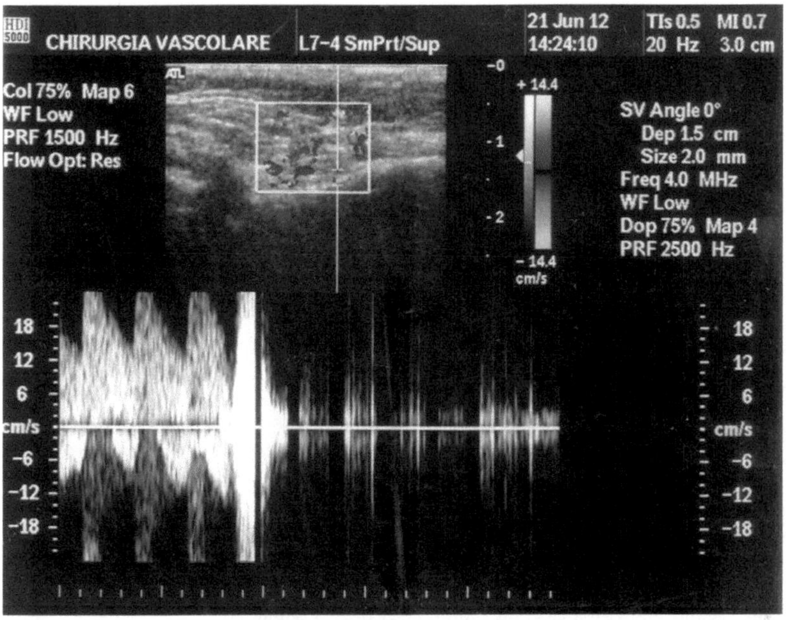

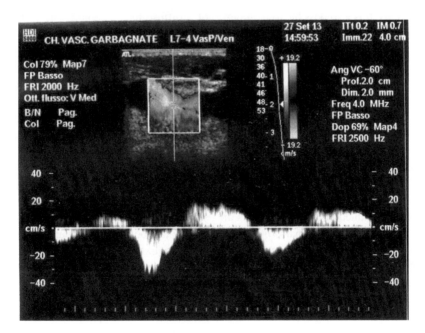

Fig. 23.2 High-flow malformation: the presence of diastolic high-velocity flow in an extratruncular malformation

Fig. 23.3 Pattern of venous reflux at duplex examination

Low-resistance flow is a peculiar characteristic of A-V malformation, but it is also possible after muscular exercise, in the presence of infantile or congenital hemangiomas and malignant tumors. The differential diagnosis is based on clinical examination in cases of hemangiomas and on the B mode picture in case of nonvascular tumors.

Venous malformations are the most frequent vascular malformations. It is possible to detect hypoplasia, aplasia, and aneurysmal dilatation [12]

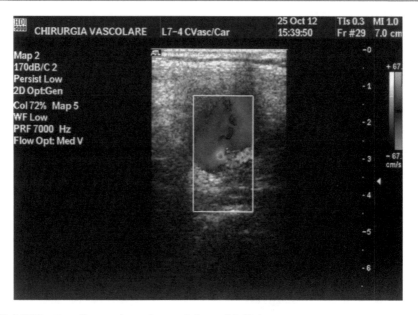

Fig. 23.4 High PRF setting allows to detect the morphology of A-V shunt

of the truncal veins. It is also possible to highlight the presence of accessory vessels which should involve after birth like the marginal vein persistence.

Extratruncular malformations usually infiltrate neighboring tissues. They are prone to develop thrombosis. Thrombosed vessels should be described as the flow pattern which may be spontaneous, present after augmentation or absent. The presence of soft tissues calcifications called phlebolith is typical of venous malformations and is the result of multiple episodes of thrombosis. The hemodynamic evaluation of all the vessels of the anatomic area involved by the malformation is crucial to plan a therapeutic intervention.

In case of lymphatic malformation, it is possible to detect some blood flow in the cystic walls or near the lymphatic structures. It is not possible to detect the lymph flow and it elicits that for lymphatic malformation only morphological data are measurable. Functional data can be collected only with lymphatic scintigraphy. In this case the presence of edema and its extension and the presence of cysts and their dimensions should be investigated. Microcystic lesion gives the image of a diffuse hyperechoic tissue in reason of the multiple reflecting areas [15].

Lymphatic malformations may infiltrate neighboring tissues and this should be described.

Duplex scanning is also useful in the exploration of visceral vessels in order to detect [14] congenital aneurysm of the splanchnic arteries, A-V shunts in the renal arteries, and hepatic circulation. This latter is frequent in Rendu-Osler syndrome. Duplex scanning is also useful in the detection of venous compression like May-Thurner syndrome and the nutcracker syndrome.

The hemodynamic evaluation of venous compression like nutcracker syndrome is possible using duplex scanning. In these cases the hemodynamic data collected by duplex scanning should be confirmed by the invasive measurement of the venous pressure gradient across the stenosis like in the case of nutcracker syndrome [16, 17].

Impaired venous flow and the presence of reflux in the jugulars and azygos veins may be detected with duplex scanning although this type of diagnosis is very operator dependent [13].

References

1. Laroche JP, Becker F, Khau-Van-Kien A, Baudoin P, Brisot D, Buffler A, Coupé M, Jurus C, Mestre S, Miserey G, Soulier-Sotto V, Tissot A, Viard A, Vignes S, Quéré I. Quality standards for ultrasonographic assessment of peripheral vascular malformations and vascular tumors. Report of the French Society for vascular medicine. J Mal Vasc. 2013;38(1):29–45.
2. Lee BB, Antignani PL, Baraldini V, Baumgartner I, Berlien P, Blei F, Carrafiello GP, Grantzow R, Ianniello A, Laredo J, Loose D, Lopez Gutierrez JC, Markovic J, Mattassi R, Parsi K, Rabe E, Roztocil K, Shortell C, Vaghi M. ISVI-IUA consensus document diagnostic guidelines of vascular anomalies: vascular malformations and hemangiomas. Int Angiol. 2015;34(4):333–74. Epub 2014 Oct 6. PubMed PMID: 25284469
3. Lee BB, Baumgartner I, Berlien P, Bianchini G, Burrows P, Gloviczki P, Huang Y, Laredo J, Loose DA, Markovic J, Mattassi R, Parsi K, Rabe E, Rosenblatt M, Shortell C, Stillo F, Vaghi M, Villavicencio L, Zamboni P. Guideline. Diagnosis and treatment of venous malformations. Consensus document of the international union of phlebology (iup): updated-2013. Int Angiol. 2014. [Epub ahead of print] PubMed PMID: 24961611.
4. Stillo F, Baraldini V, Dalmonte P, El Hachem M, Mattassi R, Vercellio G, Amato B, Bellini C, Bergui M, Bianchini G, Diociaiuti A, Campisi C, Gandolfo C, Gelmetti C, Moneghini L, Monti L, Magri C, Neri I, Paoloantonio G, Patrizi A, Rollo M, Santecchia L, Vaghi M, Vercellino N; Italian Society for the study of Vascular Anomalies (SISAV). Vascular Anomalies Guidelines by the Italian Society for the study of Vascular Anomalies (SISAV). Int Angiol. 2015;34(2 Suppl 1):1–45. PubMed PMID: 26159424.
5. Lee BB, Mattassi R, Choe YH, Vaghi M, Ahn JM, Kim DI, Huh SH, Lee CH, Kim DY. Critical role of duplex ultrasonography for the advanced management of a venous malformation (VM). Phlebology. 2005;20:28–37.
6. Trop I, Dubois J, Guibaud L, Grignon A, Patriquin H, McCuaig C, Garel LA. Soft-tissue venous malformations in pediatric and young adult patients: diagnosis with Doppler US. Radiology. 1999;212(3):841–5.
7. Maleti O, Lugli M, Collura M. Anévrysmes veineux poplités: expérience personnelle. Phlebologie. 1997;50: 53–9.
8. Katz ML, Comerota AJ. Diagnosis of a popliteal venous aneurysm by venous duplex imaging. J Ultrasound Med. 1991;10:171.
9. Offergeld C, Schellong SM, Daniel WG, Huttenbrink KB. Value of color-coded duplex ultrasound in interstitial laser therapy of hemangiomas and vascular malformations. Laryngorhinootologie. 1998;77(6):342–6.
10. Puig S, Casati B, Staudenherz A, Paya K. Vascular low-flow malformations in children: current concepts for classification, diagnosis and therapy. Eur J Radiol. 2005;53(1):35–45.
11. Park KB, Do YS, Lee BB, Kim DI, Wook Kim Y, Shin BS, et al. Predictive factors for response of peripheral arteriovenous malformations to embolization therapy: analysis of clinical data and imaging findings. J Vasc Interv Radiol. 2012;23(11):1478–86.
12. Bush S, Khan R, Stringer M. Anterior jugular venous aneurysm. Eur J Pediatr Surg. 1999;9(1):47–8.
13. Menegatti E, Zamboni P. Doppler haemodynamics of cerebral venous return. Curr Neurovasc Res. 2008;5(4):260–5.
14. Matter D, Grosshans E, Muller J, et al. Apport de l'échographie à l'imagerie des vaisseaux lymphatiques par rapport aux autres méthodes. J Radiol. 2002;83:599–60.
15. Paltiel HJ, Burrows PE, Kozakewich HP, Zurakowski D, Mulliken JB. Soft-tissue vascular anomalies: utility of US for diagnosis. Radiology. 2000;214:747–54.
16. Villavicencio JL. The desperate plea of women with the nutcracker syndrome. Phlebologie. 2010;39:1–8.
17. Takebayashi S, Ueki T, Ikeda N. Diagnosis of the nutcracker syndrome with color Doppler sonography: correlation with flow patterns on retrograde left renal venography. Am J Roentgenol. 1999;172:29–43.

CT and CT Angiogram in the Diagnosis of Congenital Vascular Malformations

Massimo Vaghi and Andrea Ianniello

In the setting of pediatric vascular anomalies, multiple imaging modalities can be used to evaluate characteristic of the lesions, such as size, flow velocity, flow direction in relation to the surrounding structures (vessels, muscle, nerve, bone, skin), and lesion content [1].

Compared to magnetic resonance (MR, the imaging modality of choice for diagnosing and characterizing vascular anomalies), contrast enhancement computed tomography (CT) has some advantages particularly in vascular malformation of the bowel and lung, due to its better spatial resolution than MR that, on the other hand, present a higher-contrast resolution which means a better definition of the vascular malformation [2, 3].

The use of CT is mandatory in all patients with contraindications to MR. Due to its low execution study time, CT is preferable to MR in patients with unstable cardiovascular status or respiratory time: with the introductions of multislice CT scanners, large vascular territories can now be imaged in few seconds, minimizing the detrimental effect of motion on image quality [3].

Image processing workstations facilitate rapid creations of multiplanar and three-dimensional images thereby improving scan interpretation and treatment planning, particularly useful in case of complex vascular anomalies; they are also useful to document aneurysm formations in high-flow vascular malformation [2].

CT, even with contrast enhancement, usually provides poor lesion conspicuity relative to adjacent potentially critical structures and does not usually provide assessment of internal malformation vascular architecture [1].

Of course the main disadvantage of CT is the radiation exposure, with doses that are particularly high when multiphasic scans are performed to resolve arterial and venous phase of enhancement: this aspect is of particular importance considering the young ages of patients usually affected by vascular malformation. For this reason CT scan, when feasible, should be replaced by other diagnostic modalities that do not use ionizing radiations, such as ultrasound or MR [3].

Lymphatic malformations (LM) consist of masses of endothelial-lined, thin-walled channels that contains lymphatic fluids. It usually appear in early childhood, although some may appear in adulthood. LM are classified as diffused or focal and microcystic or macrocystic [3, 4]. LM most commonly occur in the cervicofacial region (approximately 75%), but they can involve any structure except the brain [3].

Macrocystic LM, composed of large, multiple clearly defined cysts and septa, usually appear as

M. Vaghi (✉)
Department of Vascular Surgery, AO. G. Salvini Hospital, Garbagnate Milanese, Italy
e-mail: vaghim@yahoo.it

A. Ianniello (✉)
Department of Radiology, AO. G. Salvini Hospital, Garbagnate Milanese, Italy
e-mail: ianand@libero.it

© Springer-Verlag Berlin Heidelberg 2017
Y.-W. Kim et al. (eds.), *Congenital Vascular Malformations*, DOI 10.1007/978-3-662-46709-1_24

hypodense lesions occasionally with fluid-fluid levels within the cyst because of protein or blood content. The septations and wall of the cysts may enhance after intravenous contrast administration while the cystic spaces do not enhance, which is an important feature in differentiating LM from venous malformations (VM) [4].

Microcystic LM are characterized with multiple, no visible, small cystic lesion; on CT scan appears as low attenuation masses; they may have no enhancement or may show a mild diffuse enhancement pattern due to the small septations, similar to that seen in more solid masses [4].

Enhancement of the cysts may occasionally be seen after treatment or in mixed lymphaticovenous malformations [4, 5].

VM, the most common type of VM, usually present at birth, may not become symptomatic until later life; they may involve only the skin, but they can also extant to the muscles, joint, and bone [4].

On non-contrast CT, VM are usually of low attenuation and appear homogeneous or, as is commonly the case, heterogeneous if infiltrated with adipose tissue. The margins of the lesion are often lobulated [6, 7].

Because VM contain dilated slow-flow vascular spaces, enhancement of the channels is typically seen after intravenous contrast administration, with a similar pattern of gradual peripheral to central enhancement as is seen in hepatic hemangiomas [4, 7].

However, contrast CT can still underestimate lesion extent [7, 8].

CT scan is particularly helpful to identify both dystrophic calcifications and phleboliths when present and to provide detailed anatomic information regarding adjacent bony pathology: intraosseous involvement may be apparent as focal areas of cortical thinning with increased trabeculae [4].

In Klippel-Trenaunay patients, it is possible to evaluate large body segments and, with subsequent multiplanar reconstructions, their largely macroscopic "truncular" nature. Recently described techniques of multidetector CT venography for this subgroup of patients have allowed detection of abnormalities of the superficial and deep venous systems: the use of this diagnostic technique, which involve the use of ionizing radiation, has had little spread preferring other imaging modalities for the evaluation of deep or superficial venous system such as Doppler ultrasound or indirect MR venography [9, 10].

High-flow arteriovenous malformation (AVM) is characterized by an abnormal network of connections interposed between feeding arteries and draining veins, resulting in a complex vascular anomaly [4]. In these types of vascular malformation, normal arterioles or capillary bed are absent: the central confluence of vessels form the *nidus* of the AVM [4].

On CT scan, an AVM appear as a highly enhancing lesion with multiple feeding arteries associated with dilated draining veins, usually without soft tissue component or identifiable mass [2]. There are some exceptions to this latter point: first, an AVM may take on a mass like appearance if compact or "confined" as within a fascial space or muscle sheath; second, skin thickening and fatty hypertrophy associated with AVM may create the appearance of a mass in some lesions; and third, edema or contrast enhancement in the periphery of the "nidus" of an AVM can give the lesion a mass-like appearance of a mass in some lesion [4, 5].

In some cases, it may be difficult to distinguish an AVM from a malignant vascular tumors such as rhabdomyosarcoma, soft tissue sarcoma, angiosarcoma, and hemangiopericytoma. Helpful signs of an AVM include the presence of fat within the lesion, muscle atrophy, and the absence of surrounding edema; however, aggressive, enlarging lesions may require surgical biopsy. Lesions which appear to be vascular at the periphery but solid at the center require particular caution [11].

Contrast-enhanced CT scan, with angiography phase, in AVMs is significantly more informative than in other vascular malformations because it provides a distinct three-dimensional data set for accurate mapping and measurement of arterial, nidal, and venous structures and assessment of flow patterns for interventional radiologic or surgical planning [6].

AVM can involve cutis and sub-cutis, muscle and also bone-producing lytic bone expansion, lacy or hyperostotic changes, or cortical thinning. CT scan in particular is helpful to identify direct bone involvement showing not only high-flow intraosseous channels but also lytic and sclerotic changes [3] (Figs. 24.1, 24.2 and 24.3).

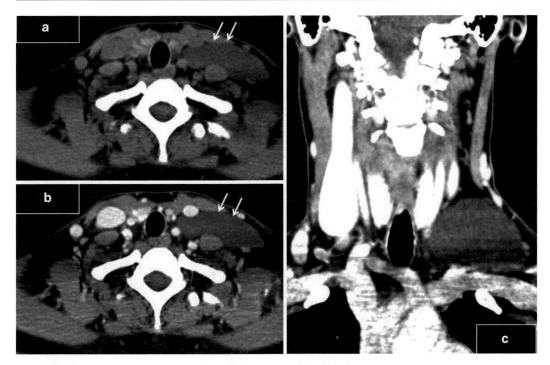

Fig. 24.1 Neck lymphatic malformation. CT scan without contrast (**a**) shows a homogeneous ipodense cystic lesion without septation and without fluid–fluid levels (*arrows*). After contrast media administration (**b** axial plane, **c** coronal plane) no enhancement is recognizable peripherally and inside the lesion (*arrows*)

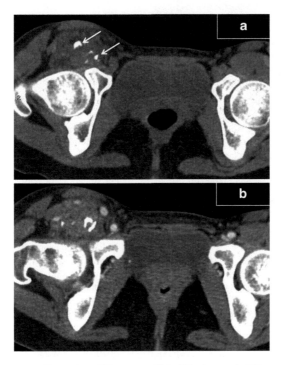

Fig. 24.2 Psoas muscle venous malformation. CT scan without contrast (**a**) show a soft ipo-isodense sort tissue mass infiltrating the psoas muscle containing several phleboliths (*arrows*). CT scan after contrast media administration (**a**) shows a mild enhancement of the mass and better identify the relationship with other structures

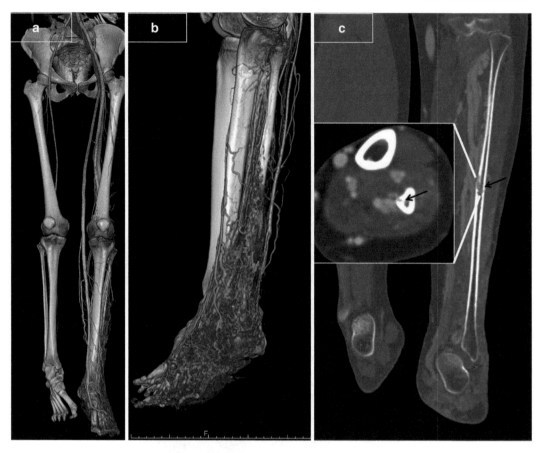

Fig. 24.3 Lower left limb arteriovenous malformation (Fig. 24.1a, b: *VR* volume-rendering reconstructions; Fig. 24.1c: *MIP* maximum intensity projection reconstruction) shows a poor identifiable mass composed of multiple enlarged feeding arteries and dilated draining veins infiltrating muscles (especially the posterior tibialis muscle) and bone causing a small area of cortical osteolysis (*arrows*) to the middle third of the fibular shaft

References

1. Hyodoh H, Hori M, Akiba H, Tamakawa M, Hyodoh K, Hareyama M. Peripheral vascular malformations: imaging, treatment approaches, and therapeutic issues. Radiographics. 2005;25(Suppl 1):S159–71.
2. Dubois J, Soulez G. Role of MR and CT in diagnostics. In: Hemangiomas and vascular malformations: an atlas of diagnosis and treatment. 2nd ed. Milano/Heidelberg: Springer; 2015.
3. Konez O, Hopkins KL, Burrows PE. Pediatric techniques and vascular anomalies. In: Rubin GD, Rofosky NM, editors. CT and MR angiography. Lippincott, Philadelphia. 2009. p. 1118–87.
4. Konez O, Burrows PE. Magnetic resonance of vascular anomalies. Magn Reson Imaging Clin N Am. 2002;10(2):363–88.
5. Legiehn GM, Heran MK. Classification, diagnosis, and interventional radiologic management of vascular malformations. Orthop Clin North Am. 2006;37(3):435–74.
6. Dubois J, Soulez G, Oliva VL, et al. Soft-tissue venous malformations in adult patients: imaging and therapeutic issues. Radiographics. 2001;21(6):1519–31.
7. Legiehn GM, Heran MK. Venous malformations: classification, development, diagnosis, and interventional radiologic management. Radiol Clin North Am. 2008;46(3):545–97.
8. Dubois J, Garel L. Imaging and therapeutic approach of hemangiomas and vascular malformations in the pediatric age group. Pediatr Radiol. 1999;29:879–93.
9. Mavili E, Ozturk M, Akcali Y, et al. Direct CT venography for evaluation of the lower extremity venous anomalies of Klippel-Trénaunay syndrome. AJR Am J Roentgenol. 2009;192:W311–6.
10. Bastarrika G, Redondo P. Indirect MR venography for evaluation and therapy planning of patients with Klippel-Trenaunay syndrome. AJR Am J Roentgenol. 2010;194(2):W244–5.
11. Abernethy LJ. Classification and imaging of vascular malformations in children. Eur Radiol. 2003;13(11):2483–97.

Radionuclide Scintigraphy for Congenital Vascular Malformations

Joon Young Choi

Introduction

Radionuclide scintigraphy is a kind of diagnostic imaging modalities which utilizes radiopharmaceuticals or radiotracer and a gamma camera. Radiopharmaceutical or radiotracer consists of a radionuclide which emits radiation and a tracer which has a specific property such as drug, ligand, metabolites or flow tracer. When a radiopharmaceutical is administered into patients, it distributes through the body according to its property and emits specific radiation, usually gamma ray. A gamma camera accepts that kind of radiation, transforms it into an electrical signal and generates images which reflect the distribution of that radiopharmaceutical at the time of image acquisition. In pathological condition, the biodistribution of radiopharmaceutical is different from that of normal or physiological condition, which results in the different images from that of normal or physiological condition. There are several kinds of image acquisition methods in radionuclide scintigraphy. In terms of extent, it divides into regional imaging and whole-body imaging. Two-dimensional acquisition is called as planar imaging, and three-dimensional acquisition generates single-photon emission

computed tomography (SPECT) images. In terms of time and acquisition number, radionuclide scintigraphy includes static and dynamic/serial acquisition. The advantages of radionuclide scintigraphy include high sensitivity, capability of whole-body imaging, serial imaging and/or tomography, presentation of functional/metabolic diagnostic information and relatively low costs compared to CT/MRI.

For evaluating congenital vascular malformations (CVMs), there are several kinds of radionuclide scintigraphy to be clinically used: whole-body blood pool scan (WBBPS) and SPECT, transarterial lung perfusion scintigraphy (TLPS) and lymphoscintigraphy. In this chapter, the imaging principles, methods and clinical applications of those radionuclide scintigraphies are described.

Imaging Principles and Methods

WBBPS and SPECT

The most commonly used radiopharmaceutical for whole-body blood pool scan is Tc-99m-labelled autologous red blood cells (RBCs), which means that the RBCs derived from a patient are attached with Tc-99m, a radioisotope. The radiopharmaceutical is intravenously administered into the patient, and it distributed in the blood-pooling spaces such as the heart and blood vessels. Image acquisition is possible 5–10 min after the injection of the radiotracer. Whole-body

J.Y. Choi, MD, PhD
Department of Nuclear Medicine, Samsung Medical Center, Sungkyunkwan University School of Medicine, Seoul, South Korea
e-mail: gyrus@skku.edu

© Springer-Verlag Berlin Heidelberg 2017
Y.-W. Kim et al. (eds.), *Congenital Vascular Malformations*, DOI 10.1007/978-3-662-46709-1_25

imaging including both anterior and posterior images is recommended to characterize and screen CVMs. If necessary, dynamic acquisition for the specific interesting part is performed immediately after the injection of radiotracer. After whole-body imaging, optional SPECT acquisition can be done to characterize further. For example, for CVMs located in the head and neck and body, SPECT is helpful to localize and to characterize the CVMs due to their deep-seated location and complex anatomy [14].

Although there are no specific preparations of patients for this scan, several drugs such as heparin, methyldopa, digoxin, propranolol and iodinated contrast media can interfere with the labelling of Tc-99m and RBCs, which potentially may affect the image quality [5]. Figure 25.1 demonstrates the normal biodistribution of

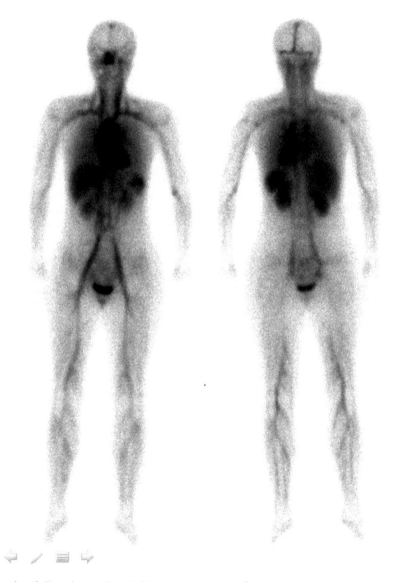

Fig. 25.1 Anterior (*left*) and posterior (*right*) whole-body blood pool scan images of a 45-year-old female. Physiologically, there are significant high uptakes in the heart, blood vessels, liver, spleen, kidney and nasal mucosa. Sometimes, mild physiological uptake can be observed in the uterus, testicles and muscles. Significant uptakes in the ureter and urinary bladder result from excreted radiotracer via urine

Tc-99m RBCs. If there are significant uptakes except those normal blood-pooling organs and excretory organs related to radiotracer or asymmetric/focal uptakes in those normal blood-pooling organs, they can be considered pathological blood-pooling lesions including CVMs. To quantify the severity and extent of abnormal blood-pooling lesions, a lesion-to-whole-body count ratio can be measured, which also can be used for evaluating therapeutic response [12]. In CVMs of the lower extremities, the count ratio between iliac vessels can be used to differentiate arteriovenous shunting from non-arteriovenous shunting malformations [3].

TLPS

The radiopharmaceutical for TLPS is Tc-99m-labelled macroaggregated albumin (MAA), which is commonly used in the lung perfusion scan. The particle size of Tc-99m MAA is usually between 10 and 90 μm. Therefore, when it is intravenously injected, most Tc-99m MAA is trapped in the lung capillary, where the size is mostly between 5 and 10 μm. For TLPS, this radiotracer is injected into the artery proximal to the CVM lesion. If there is no significant arteriovenous shunting in the lesion, most radiotracer is trapped in the capillaries distal to the injected artery. If there is significant arteriovenous shunting, a part of radiotracer is trapped in the capillaries distal to the injected artery. On the contrary, the remaining radiotracer enters venous circulation via arteriovenous shunting and is trapped in the lung capillary. Using this principle, in TLPS Tc-99m MAA is injected twice, intravenously at first and intraarterially later. The dynamic images in the lung are continuously acquired before and after the two-time injection of the radiotracer. In case of arteriovenous shunting, significant increased uptake is found in the lungs after the second injection into the artery. To measure shunt fraction, the time-activity curve of the lungs is used. Figure 25.2 demonstrated the measurement of shunt fraction from the time-activity curve of the lungs [4, 13, 16]. After the lung imaging, additional whole-body images are acquired to verify the right intraarterial injection.

Although there are no specific preparations of patients for this scan, in case of significant right-to-left cardiac/extracardiac shunt or paediatric patients, the decrease of MAA particle number is necessary to prevent systemic embolism by MAA particles entered into arteries [15]. If the lesion locates in the head and neck, chest or abdomen, it is difficult to perform TLPS, because the intraarterial injection proximal to the lesion is not possible in a gamma camera room. Therefore, TLPS is used to evaluate CVMs in the extremities.

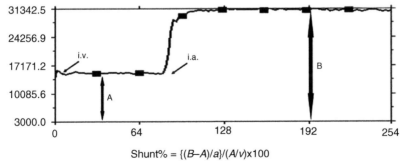

Shunt% = {(B–A)/a}/(A/v)x100

A: average count of lung after intravenous injection
B: average count of lung after intraarterial injection
v: net dose for venous injection
a: net dose for arterial injection

Fig. 25.2 The measurement of arteriovenous shunting fraction from the time-activity curve of the lungs (Reproduction from Chung et al. [4] permitted by *Nuclear Medicine and Molecular Imaging journal*)

Extremity Lymphoscintigraphy

The radiopharmaceutical for lymphoscintigraphy is a radiolabelled colloid such as Tc-99m antimony colloid, Tc-99m tin colloid, Tc-99m phytate or Tc-99m nanocolloid. When this kind of radiolabelled colloid is subcutaneously injected into interdigital space of the hands or feet, it enters into the lymphatic system and moves according to the lymphatic flow. To enhance the lymphatic transport, exercises such as walking, bicycling and hand grip are encouraged immediately after the injection. For imaging, whole-body acquisition usually 1–2 h after the injection is performed to evaluate CVMs, especially lymphatic malformation in the extremities, chest wall and pelvis. If necessary, dynamic or delayed images can be obtained, along with semiquantitative measurements. Therefore, lymphoscintigraphy shows the functional lymphatic flow and lymph nodes in vivo, which is helpful to diagnose chronic lymphedema and to evaluate the severity and therapeutic response in chronic lymphedema [1, 2, 6–8, 17, 18].

Lymphoscintigraphy can be used to evaluate significant lymphedema or lymphatic malformation which results in lymphatic functional derangement. However, it is difficult to perform lymphoscintigraphy for evaluating lymphatic malformation in the head and neck, lungs and abdomen, because of difficult injection of the radiotracer into the relevant site. Representative image findings suggesting significant lymphatic functional impairment include decreased lymph node/lymphatic vessel uptake, visualization of collateral lymphatic vessels and the presence of dermal backflow.

Clinical Applications

Diagnosis and Characterization of Vascular Malformations

It is clinically important to diagnose and to determine the type of CVMs, because the treatment plan and prognosis are different. Radionuclide scintigraphy is helpful to diagnose and to characterize CVMs. In case of pure venous malformation, there are abnormal blood-pooling lesions on WBBPS, no significant abnormal findings on lymphoscintigraphy and/or no significant shunt on TLPS. In pure lymphatic malformations, there are no significant blood-pooling lesions on WBBPS. On lymphoscintigraphy, if the lymphatic malformation communicates with major lymphatic vessels or induces functional impairment, abnormal findings are observed. However, if the lymphatic malformation is isolated from major lymphatic vessels, there may be no significant abnormal findings on lymphoscintigraphy. In pure arteriovenous malformations, there are abnormal blood-pooling lesions on WBBPS with asymmetric increased uptake in the draining vessels proximal to the lesion, normal lymphoscintigraphy and/or increased shunt fraction on TLPS.

WBBPS showed a good sensitivity of more than 90% to diagnose blood-pooling CVMs such as venous malformation and arteriovenous malformation [9–12, 14]. The overall characterizing accuracy of extremity CVMs by WBBPS and/or lymphoscintigraphy was more than 90% [9, 10]. In head and neck CVMs, blood pool SPECT showed a good result of 83% accuracy to characterize the lesions [14]. To diagnose arteriovenous malformation specifically, TLPS presented a good sensitivity of 94% and specificity of 100% with a cutoff shunt fraction of 20% [4]. False-negative findings in TLPS could be observed in the small micro-arteriovenous malformations [4, 13]. However, TLPS is relatively invasive and technically difficult due to intraarterial injection than WBBPS. WBBPS may be also used to diagnose arteriovenous malformation. In CVMs of the lower extremities, the count ratio between iliac vessels in WBBPS can be used to differentiate arteriovenous shunting from non-arteriovenous shunting malformations, which was well correlated with the shunt fraction measured by TLPS [3].

Figure 25.3 demonstrates the representative images of radionuclide scintigraphy according to the type of CVMs.

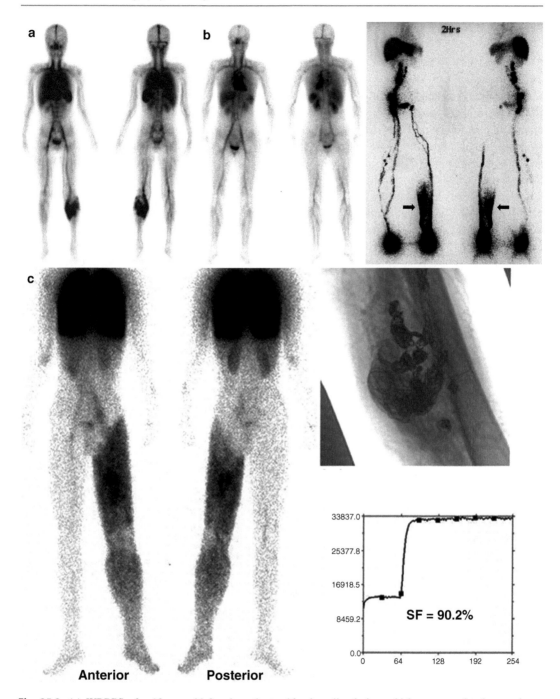

Anterior **Posterior**

Fig. 25.3 (**a**) WBBPS of a 10-year-old female patient shows a focal abnormal blood-pooling lesion in the left calf, which was proved to be pure venous malformation (Reproduction from Kim et al. [10] permitted by Elsevier Limited). (**b**) WBBPS (*left*) and lower extremity lymphoscintigraphy (*right*) of a 45-year-old female patient show abnormal dermal backflow (*arrow*) and collateral lymphatic vessel in the left lower extremity without abnormal blood-pooling lesion, which was proved to be pure lymphatic malformation (Reproduction from Kim et al. [10] permitted by Elsevier Limited). (**c**) TLPS (*left*), angiography (*right upper*) and time-activity curve (*right lower*) of a 30-year-old male patient show increased shunt fraction of 90.2%, which was proved to be arteriovenous malformation (Reproduction from Chung et al. [4] permitted by *Nuclear Medicine and Molecular Imaging journal*)

Extent of Vascular Malformations

CVMs are a kind of systemic disease, which means that malformation can occur in any vessels of the whole body. Screening clinically unsuspected CVM lesions is also important, because they can progress during follow-up. Early detection of those lesions is helpful to determine the follow-up plan and early intervention. WBBPS is useful to screen blood-pooling CVMs due to its whole-body coverage, high sensitivity and relatively low costs compared to CT/MRI. A recent study reported that WBBPS could detect 41 additional abnormal vascular lesions that were not found during initial clinical evaluation in 17% of the patients with venous malformations [10]. Figure 25.4 demonstrates the representative image of WBBPS which detected clinically unsuspected lesions.

Therapy Response Evaluation and Follow-Up

In blood-pooling CVMs such as venous malformation and arteriovenous malformation, multis-ession sclerotherapy or embolization therapy can be performed. WBBPS is helpful to evaluate the response to those treatment and disease progression, because of whole-body coverage, easy interpretation, capability of quantitation, convenient repetitive exam, non-invasiveness and relatively low costs compared to CT/MRI [11, 12]. A lesion-to-whole-body count ratio may be used as a quantitative index representing the disease severity and therapeutic response. Figure 25.5 demonstrates the representative image of WBBPS which shows a good response to multisession sclerotherapy in venous malformation. In extremity arteriovenous malformations, the shunt fraction measured by TLPS is good to evaluate the response to sclerotherapy or embolization therapy, which is well correlated with clinical and angiographic response [4, 13]. However, TLPS is relatively invasive than WBBPS due to intraarterial injection and cannot be applied for arteriovenous malformations except those in extremities. In lymphatic malformation combined with significant lymphedema, lymphoscintigraphy may be used to assess the extent and severity of

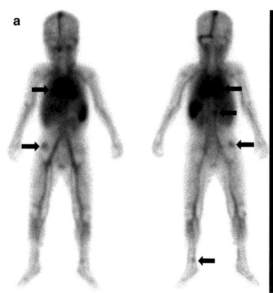
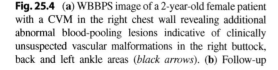
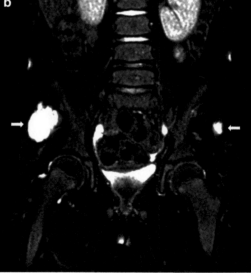

Fig. 25.4 (a) WBBPS image of a 2-year-old female patient with a CVM in the right chest wall revealing additional abnormal blood-pooling lesions indicative of clinically unsuspected vascular malformations in the right buttock, back and left ankle areas (*black arrows*). (b) Follow-up coronal T2 fat-suppressed magnetic resonance imaging scan revealing a high-signal intensity lobulating mass involving both gluteus medius muscles suggesting low-flow type of vascular malformations (*white arrows*) (Reproduction from Kim et al. [10] permitted by Elsevier Limited)

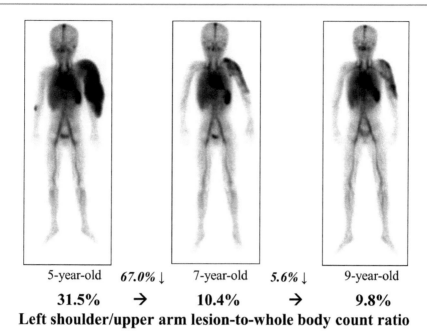

5-year-old   *67.0%* ↓   7-year-old   *5.6%* ↓   9-year-old

31.5%   →   10.4%   →   9.8%

Left shoulder/upper arm lesion-to-whole body count ratio

Fig. 25.5 Serial WBBPS images of a female patient with venous malformation in the left shoulder and upper arm demonstrate a good response to multisession sclerother-apy by a significant decrease in the lesion-to-whole-body count ratio

lymphedema, to evaluate the response to therapy and to predict the prognosis [2, 6–8, 18].

Conclusions

In CVMs, several kinds of radionuclide scintigraphy are useful to diagnose, to characterize, to screen and to evaluate the response to therapy. High sensitivity, whole-body coverage, non-invasiveness and relative low costs are the main advantages of radionuclide scintigraphy for evaluating CVMs. However, the number of published studies is relatively small. Further validation studies are necessary.

References

1. Cambria RA, Gloviczki P, Naessens JM, Wahner HW. Noninvasive evaluation of the lymphatic system with lymphoscintigraphy: a prospective, semi-quatitative analysis in 386 extremities. J Vasc Surg. 1993;18:773–82.
2. Choi JY, Hwang JH, Park JM, Lee KH, Kim SE, Kim DI, et al. Risk assessment of dermatolymphan-gioadenitis by lymphoscintigraphy in patients with lower extremity lymphedema. Korean J Nucl Med. 1999;33:143–51. [Korean]
3. Chung HW, Choi JY, Lee SJ, Lee EJ, Kim YH, Choi Y, et al. Differential diagnosis between arteriovenous and non-arteriovenous malformations of the lower extremities using whole-body blood pool scintigraphy. J Nucl Med. 2005;46 Suppl:276P. [Abstract].
4. Chung JW, Choi JY, Kim YW, Kim DI, Do YS, Lee EJ, et al. Diagnosis and post-therapeutic evaluation of arteriovenous malformations in extremities using transarterial lung perfusion scintigraphy. Nucl Med Mol Imaging. 2006;40:316–21. [Korean].
5. Hesslewood S, Leung E. Drug interactions with radio-pharmaceuticals. Eur J Nucl Med. 1994;21:348–56.
6. Hwang JH, Kwon JY, Lee KW, Choi JY, Kim B-T, Lee BB, et al. Changes in lymphatic function after complex physical therapy for lymphedema. Lymphology. 1999;32:15–21.
7. Hwang JH, Choi JY, Lee JY, Hyun SH, Choi Y, Choe YS, et al. Lymphoscintigraphy predicts response to complex physical therapy in patients with early stage extremity lymphedema. Lymphology. 2007;40:172–6.
8. Jung JY, Hwang JH, Kim DH, Kim HS, Jung SH, Lee KW, et al. Predicting the effect of complex physical therapy: utility of manual lymph drainage performed on lymphoscintigraphy. J Korean Acad Rehab Med. 2004;28:78–82. [Korean]
9. Kim YH, Choi JY, Kim YW, Kim DI, Do YS, Hwang JH, et al. Characterization of congenital vascular malformation in extremities using whole body blood pool

scintigraphy and lymphoscintigraphy. Lymphology. 2009;42:77–84.

10. Kim YH, Choi JY, Kim YW, Kim DI, Do YS, Choe YS, et al. Diagnosis and whole body screening using blood pool scintigraphy for evaluating congenital vascular malformation. Ann Vasc Surg. 2014;28: 673–8.

11. Lee BB, Kim B-T, Choi JY, Cazaubon M. Management of congenital vascular malformation in 2003: role of whole body scintigraphy in evolutive survey. Angeiologie. 2003;55:17–26. [French].

12. Lee BB, Mattassi R, Kim BT, Kim YW, Ahn JM, Choi JY. Contemporary diagnosis and management of venous and arterio-venous shunting malformation by whole body blood pool scintigraphy. Int Angiol. 2004;23:355–67.

13. Lee BB, Mattassi R, Kim YW, Kim BT, Park JM, Choi JY. Advanced management of arteriovenous shunting malformation with transarterial lung perfusion scintigraphy for follow-up assessment. Int Angiol. 2005;24:173–84.

14. Lee JY, Choi JY, Kim YH, Kim DI, Kim YW, Kim KH, et al. Characterization of congenital lymphatic and blood vascular malformations in the head and neck using blood pool scintigraphy and SPECT. Lymphology. 2010;43:149–57.

15. Parker JA, Coleman RE, Grady E, Royal HD, Siegel BA, Stabin MG, et al. SNM practice guideline for lung scintigraphy 4.0. J Nucl Med Technol. 2012;40:57–65.

16. Partsch H. Non-invasive investigations, measurement of shunting volume in vascular malformation of the limbs. In: Belov ST, Loose DA, Weber J, editors. Vascular malformations. Reinbek: Einhorn-presse Verlag GmbH; 1989. p. 99–103.

17. Szuba A, Shin WS, Strauss HW, Rockson S. The third circulation: radionuclide lymphoscintigraphy in the evaluation of lymphedema. J Nucl Med. 2003;44:43–57.

18. Yoo J, Choi JY, Hwang JH, Kim DI, Kim YW, Choe YS, et al. Prognostic value of lymphoscintigraphy in patients with gynecological cancer-related lymphedema. J Surg Oncol. 2014;109:760–3.

Indocyanine Green (ICG) Lymphography

26

Takumi Yamamoto

Introduction

Primary lymphedema is considered one of clinical aspects of lymphatic malformation, and lymph flow evaluation is important for its management. There are several imaging modalities to visualize lymph flows for lymphedema evaluation. Near-infrared fluorescent lymphography using indocyanine green (ICG) is becoming popular, because ICG lymphography allows clear visualization of superficial lymph flows in real time without risk of radiation exposure unlike lymphoscintigraphy [1–5]. Although deep lymph flows (>2 cm in depth) cannot be directly visualized, ICG lymphography provides much clearer images compared with lymphoscintigraphy and allows real-time navigation during interventions such as manual lymph drainage and lymphatic surgery. Dynamic ICG lymphography allows evaluation of lymph pump function and circulation conditions with one ICG injection [6, 7].

Protocol of Dynamic ICG Lymphography

Dynamic ICG lymphography consists of two-phase observations: early transient phase for evaluation of lymph pump function and late plateau phase for evaluation of lymph circulation [6, 7].

Dynamic ICG lymphography is performed as follows: an examinee is kept still for 15 min,, and 0.05–0.20 ml of 0.25% ICG is injected; 0.2 ml ICG is intradermally injected at the second web space of the foot and at a point lateral to the Achilles' tendon for leg and genital lymphedema evaluation, 0.1 ml at the second web space of the hand and at a point ulnar to the palmaris longus tendon for arm lymphedema evaluation, and 0.05 ml at the glabella and at the philtrum for head and neck lymphedema evaluation [1–7]. Fluorescent images are obtained using an infrared camera system immediately after ICG injection. An examinee is kept still in a supine position during 5 min of lymph pump function measurement; lymph pump function is measured using ICG velocity (distance of ICG movement divided by time). ICG velocity represents lymph transportation capacity and is useful for evaluation of intervention's efficacy by comparing ICG velocity before and after intervention.

After measurement of ICG velocity at early transient phase, an examinee is instructed to move her/his extremity rigorously to facilitate ICG diffusion. Two to 72 h after ICG injection, ICG movement reaches a plateau. Lymph circulation

T. Yamamoto, MD
Department of Plastic and Reconstructive Surgery,
The University of Tokyo, Hongo 7-3-1, Bunkyo-ku,
Tokyo 113-8655, Japan
e-mail: tyamamoto-tky@umin.ac.jp

© Springer-Verlag Berlin Heidelberg 2017
Y.-W. Kim et al. (eds.), *Congenital Vascular Malformations*, DOI 10.1007/978-3-662-46709-1_26

is evaluated based on ICG lymphographic find-ings, which allows pathophysiological classifi-cation of lymphedema [6–8]. When lymphatic surgery is planned, ICG is injected the day before surgery; ICG velocity is measured at the day before surgery, lymph circulation is evaluated at the operation day, and lymph flow navigation is performed during lymphatic surgery [6, 7, 9–13].

ICG Lymphography Findings

Findings of ICG lymphography are largely clas-sified into normal linear pattern and abnormal dermal backflow (DB) pattern. DB pattern is sub-divided into three patterns: splash pattern (mild DB pattern), stardust pattern (moderate DB pat-tern), and diffuse pattern (severe DB pattern) [1–5, 8]. Linear pattern is linear fluorescent image, splash pattern tortuous fluorescent lines, stardust pattern many fluorescent spots without line, and diffuse pattern diffusely fluorescent image with-out spot or line (Fig. 26.1).

Lymph flows in lymphatic collectors in a nor-mal condition, which is shown as linear pattern on ICG lymphography. When lymph flows are obstructed in proximal region(s) by lymphatic malformation, lymphatic collectors become dilated and lymphatic valvular insufficiency and lymph backflow occur distal to the obstruction [9, 11, 14–16]. Precollecting lymphatic vessels and lymphatic capillaries become dilated to compensate lymph overload (collateral lymph pathways), which is shown as splash pattern on ICG lymphography. When collateral lymph pathways are not enough to compensate lymph overload, lymph extravasation takes place, and extravasation points are shown as spots on ICG lymphography (stardust pattern). As lymph extravasation and lymphosclerosis become severe, extravasation points are not differenti-ated from each other, which is shown as diffuse pattern on ICG lymphography. With progression of lymph flow obstruction, ICG lymphography patterns change from linear to splash, to star-dust, and finally to diffuse pattern (Fig. 26.2). For primary lymphedema with proximal lymph flow obstruction (obstruction proximal to the

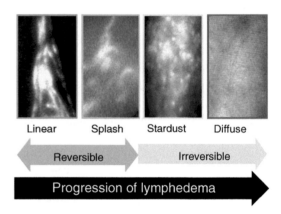

Fig. 26.2 Indocyanine green lymphography pattern change with progression of lymphedema

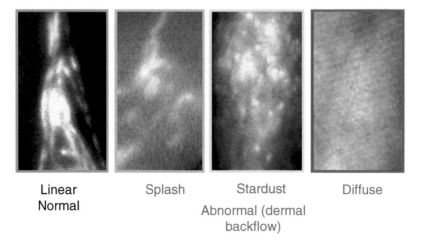

Fig. 26.1 Characteristic indocyanine green lymphography patterns. Linear (*left*), splash, (*center left*), stardust (*center right*), and diffuse (*right*) pattern

DB stage	ICG pattern	ICG distribution
Stage 0	DB(-)	Only Linear pattern seen
Stage I	Splash(+)	Splash around axilla/groin
Stage II	Stardust(+)	Stardust limited to elbow/knee
Stage III	Stardust(++)	Stardust exceeding elbow/knee
Stage IV	Stardust(+++)	Stardust in whole limb
Stage V	Diffuse(+)	Diffuse with Stardust

Fig. 26.3 Dermal backflow (DB) stages for pathophysiological severity evaluation of obstructive lymphedema

inguinal/axillary lymph nodes), DB stages are useful for pathophysiological severity staging system (Fig. 26.3) [2, 3].

Differentiation of DB patterns is clinically important, because each DB pattern indicates different prognosis [17, 18]. Splash pattern represents a reversible lymph circulatory change, and a patient with splash pattern can be improved to normal lymph circulatory condition (linear pattern) without any intervention; some patients suffer from progressive lymphedema. Stardust/diffuse pattern represents an irreversible lymph circulatory change, and a patient with stardust/diffuse pattern can never be improved to normal condition even with conservative treatments; all patients suffer from progressive lymphedema. Although clinically progressive, lymphedema with stardust pattern can be improved by lymphovenous shunt operations, because lymphatic vessels are not severely sclerotic. On the other hand, lymphedema with diffuse pattern can hardly be improved by lymphovenous shunt operations, because lymphatic vessels are severely sclerotic with no lymph flow [9, 11, 14].

ICG lymphography has higher sensitivity and specificity to detect abnormal lymph circulation in extremities compared with lymphoscintigraphy [2, 3, 5]. Using DB stage, International Society of Lymphology stage 0 can be further classified into DB stage 0/I/II. As mentioned above, it is important to diagnose patients based on DB stage, because different DB stage indicates different prognosis [17].

In conditions other than proximal lymph flow obstruction such as lymphatic hypoplasia/aplasia or dysfunction, uptake of ICG is decreased or even none. In such cases, ICG lymphography shows less enhanced areas with linear pattern or no fluorescent image.

Primary Lymphedema Classification

Primary lymphedema can be classified into four patterns using ICG lymphography: proximal DB (PDB) pattern, distal DB (DDB) pattern, less enhancement (LE) pattern, and no enhancement (NE) pattern (Fig. 26.4) [19].

In PDB pattern, ICG lymphography shows distally extending DB patterns similar to findings of cancer-related obstructive lymphedema; DB patterns extend distally from the axilla/groin as in breast/pelvic cancer-related arm/leg lymphedema [2, 3]. Malignancy should be ruled out first, when ICG lymphography shows PDB pattern on a patient without past history of malignancy. Primary localized (axillary/inguinal or more proximal) lymphatic abnormalities (lymphatic vessels and/or lymph nodes) are considered a cause of lymphedema.

ICG lymphography classification

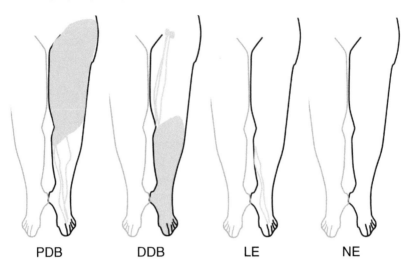

PDB   DDB   LE   NE

Fig. 26.4 Indocyanine green lymphography classification for primary lymphedema

DB pattern is also shown in DDB pattern, indicating obstructive mechanism as a cause of lymphedema. Distribution of DB pattern is different between PDB and DDB pattern; DB pattern is seen only in the distal region of limbs in DDB pattern, and no DB pattern is detected in the proximal (axillary/inguinal) region. Patients with DDB pattern are usually associated with past history of cellulitis. Distal localized lymphatic vessels' abnormalities are considered a cause of lymphedema, and lymphatic inflammation due to cellulitis aggravates the disease's course.

In LE pattern, no DB pattern is detected, and linear pattern is shown only in a part of limbs; Linear pattern is seen only in the distal region (forearm/leg), and no enhanced image is obtained in more proximal region. This indicates there is no obstructive mechanism such as localized lymphatic aplasia as a cause of lymphedema. Superficial lymphatic dysfunction or dysplasia can be a cause of lymphedema. Congenital or severe case is very rare in patients with LE pattern, and clinical symptoms become worse gradually with aging. Since lymph transportation capacity decreases with aging, aging in the setting of subclinical lymphatic dysfunction would be one of the causes [6, 7].

In NE pattern, no enhanced lymphatics is detected other than ICG injection sites. Severe lymphatic abnormality is considered as a cause of lymphedema, such as whole limb lymphatic aplasia and severe malabsorption of lymph. Most patients with NE pattern suffer from congenital unilateral lymphedema and have no past history of cellulitis. Primary lymphedema with NE pattern is likely to be more severe than those with other ICG patterns.

ICG Lymphography Classification for Lymphedema Management

The ICG lymphography classification of primary lymphedema, categorized according to abnormal lymph circulation, has a potential to be a useful tool not only for understanding pathophysiology of the disease but also for lymphedema management (Fig. 26.5) [19]. Basically, conservative treatments should be commenced first when diagnosis of lymphedema is made. However, lymphedema with moderate–severe DB (stardust or diffuse pattern) is progressive and refractory to conservative treatments, and further surgical treatment is required to improve the disease's condition [12, 13].

In PDB pattern and DDB pattern, DB patterns are observed as in obstructive lymphedema secondary to cancer treatments. Since obstructive

ICG	Suspected pathophysiology	Recommended management
PDB	Lymph flow obstruction proximal to axilla/groin	Lymphatic bypass
DDB	Lymph flow obstruction distal to axilla/groin	Lymphatic bypass
LE	Pump dysfunction Superficial lymphatic system hypoplasia	Strict compression
NE	Whole limb aplasia Lymph mal – absorption	Lymph node transfer Liposuction

Fig. 26.5 Management of primary lymphedema based on indocyanine green lymphography classification

mechanism is suspected, lymph flow bypass, bypassing the obstruction site, is considered a useful therapeutic option [12, 13, 20]. When extensive diffuse pattern is observed, lymphatic bypass can hardly be effective, because lymphatic vessels are too sclerotic to expect bypass effect [9, 11, 17]. For patients with diffuse pattern or with severely sclerotic lymphatic vessels, vascularized lymph node transfer is indicated. When lymphedematous limb is associated with extensive fat deposition, debulking surgery such as liposuction is useful to improve the limb's shape.

For patients with LE pattern, no DB pattern is shown, indicating no or incomplete obstructive mechanism. Lymphatic bypass operation may be ineffective for this non-obstructive lymphedema, and vascularized lymph node transfer seems too invasive because lymphedema with LE pattern is usually mild. Strict compression therapy is recommended with or without manual lymph drainage.

In NE pattern, no lymphatic image is visualized on ICG lymphography, indicating no collecting lymphatic vessels or severe dysfunction of lymph absorption. Since lymphedema with NE pattern is usually severe refractory to conservative treatments, surgical treatments are required to improve the disease's condition. Lymphatic bypass surgery is impossible for lymphatic aplasia cases and is of no clinical effect for cases of lymph malabsorption [20]. Vascularized lymph node transfer is effective

by creating a new lymph drainage system in an affected limb to improve lymph circulation, and liposuction is helpful to reduce lymphedematous volume with fat deposition.

References

1. Yamamoto T, Narushima M, Doi K, Oshima A, Ogata F, Mihara M, Koshima I, Mundinger GS. Characteristic indocyanine green lymphography findings in lower extremity lymphedema: the generation of a novel lymphedema severity staging system using dermal backflow patterns. Plast Reconstr Surg. 2011;127(5):1979–86.
2. Yamamoto T, Matsuda N, Doi K, Oshima A, Yoshimatsu H, Todokoro T, Ogata F, Mihara M, Narushima M, Iida T, Koshima I. The earliest finding of indocyanine green (ICG) lymphography in asymptomatic limbs of lower extremity lymphedema patients secondary to cancer treatment: the modified dermal backflow (DB) stage and concept of subclinical lymphedema. Plast Reconstr Surg. 2011;128(4):314e–21e.
3. Yamamoto T, Yamamoto N, Doi K, Oshima A, Yoshimatsu H, Todokoro T, Ogata F, Mihara M, Narushima M, Iida T, Koshima I. Indocyanine green (ICG)-enhanced lymphography for upper extremity lymphedema: a novel severity staging system using dermal backflow (DB) patterns. Plast Reconstr Surg. 2011;128(4):941–7.
4. Yamamoto T, Iida T, Matsuda N, Kikuchi K, Yoshimatsu H, Mihara M, Narushima M, Koshima I. Indocyanine green (ICG)-enhanced lymphography for evaluation of facial lymphoedema. J Plast Reconstr Aesthet Surg. 2011;64(11):1541–4.

5. Yamamoto T, Yamamoto N, Yoshimatsu H, Hayami S, Narushima M, Koshima I. Indocyanine green lymphography for evaluation of genital lymphedema in secondary lower extremity lymphedema patients. J Vasc Surg Venous Lymphat Disord. 2013;1(4):400–5.
6. Yamamoto T, Narushima M, Yoshimatsu H, Yamamoto N, Oka A, Seki Y, Todokoro T, Iida T, Koshima I. Indocyanine green velocity: lymph transportation capacity deterioration with progression of lymphedema. Ann Plast Surg. 2013;71(5):59–594.
7. Yamamoto T, Narushima M, Yoshimatsu H, Yamamoto N, Kikuchi K, Todokoro T, Iida T, Koshima I. Dynamic indocyanine green lymphography for breast cancer-related arm lymphedema. Ann Plast Surg. 2014;73(6):706–9. 2013 Jul 25 [Epub ahead of print].
8. Yamamoto T, Koshima I. Splash, stardust, or diffuse pattern: differentiation of dermal backflow pattern is important in indocyanine green lymphography. Plast Reconstr Surg. 2014;133(6):e887–8.
9. Yamamoto T, Yamamoto N, Azuma S, Yoshimatsu H, Seki Y, Narushima M, Koshima I. Near-infrared illumination system-integrated microscope for supermicrosurgical lymphaticovenular anastomosis. Microsurgery. 2014;34(1):23–7.
10. Yamamoto T, Yoshimatsu H, Koshima I. Navigation lymphatic supermicrosurgery for iatrogenic lymphorrhea: supermicrosurgical lymphaticolymphatic anastomosis and lymphaticovenular anastomosis under indocyanine green lymphography navigation. J Plast Reconstr Aesthet Surg. 2014;67(11):1573–9.
11. Yamamoto T, Yamamoto N, Numahata T, Yokoyama A, Tashiro K, Yoshimatsu H, Narushima M, Kohima I. Navigation lymphatic supermicrosurgery for the treatment of cancer-related peripheral lymphedema. Vasc Endovascular Surg. 2014;48(2):139–43.
12. Yamamoto T, Narushima M, Kikuchi K, Yoshimatsu H, Todokoro T, Mihara M, Koshima I. Lambda-shaped anastomosis with intravascular stenting method for safe and effective lymphaticovenular anastomosis. Plast Reconstr Surg. 2011;127(5):1987–92.
13. Yamamoto T, Narushima M, Yoshimatsu H, Seki Y, Yamamoto N, Oka A, Hara H, Koshima I. Minimally invasive lymphatic supermicrosurgery (MILS): indocyanine green lymphography-guided simultaneous multi-site lymphaticovenular anastomoses via millimeter skin incisions. Ann Plast Surg. 2014;72(1): 67–70.
14. Yamamoto T, Yamamoto N, Narushima M, et al. Lymphaticovenular anastomosis with guidance of ICG lymphography. J Jpn Coll Angiol. 2012;52:327–31.
15. Yamamoto T, Matsuda N, Todokoro T, Yoshimatsu H, Narushima M, Mihara M, Uchida G, Koshima I. Lower extremity lymphedema index: a simple method for severity evaluation of lower extremity lymphedema. Ann Plast Surg. 2011;67(6):637–40.
16. Yamamoto T, Yamamoto N, Hara H, Mihara M, Narushima M, Koshima I. Upper extremity lymphedema (UEL) index: a simple method for severity evaluation of upper extremity lymphedema. Ann Plast Surg. 2013;70(1):47–9.
17. Yamamoto T, Koshima I. Subclinical lymphedema: understanding is the clue to decision making. Plast Reconstr Surg. 2013;132(3):472e–3e.
18. Yamamoto T, Yamamoto N, Yamashita M, Furuya M, Hayashi A, Koshima I. Efferent lymphatic vessel anastomosis (ELVA): supermicrosurgical efferent lymphatic vessel-to-venous anastomosis for the prophylactic treatment of subclinical lymphedema. Ann Plast Surg. 2016;76(4):424–7.
19. Yamamoto T, Yoshimatsu H, Narushima M, Yamamoto N, Hayashi A, Koshima I. Indocyanine green lymphography findings in primary leg lymphedema. Eur J Vasc Endovasc Surg. 2015;49:95–102.
20. Yamamoto T, Koshima I, Yoshimatsu H, Narushima M, Mihara M, Iida T. Simultaneous multi-site lymphaticovenular anastomoses for primary lower extremity and genital lymphoedema complicated with severe lymphorrhea. J Plast Reconstr Aesthet Surg. 2011;64(6):812–5.

Microscopic Lymphangiography

Claudio Allegra, Michelangelo Bartolo,
and Anita Carlizza

Like the blood capillaries, the lymphatic microvessels are formed by a thin layer of endothelial cells resting on a delicate basal membrane. This structure, particularly at the initial segment, is widely fenestrated. The cells are anchored to filaments which, as interstitial pressure increases, are believed to open the fenestrations and allow the lymph to enter the lymphatic microvessel [1, 2]. The cutaneous microlymphatic circulation is formed by two superficial networks joined by small perpendicular vessels through which the lymph drains from the superficial into the deep network. This deep network is connected by channels that run in a perpendicular direction from the skin downward to the lymphatic precollectors [1–3]. The lymphatic system is currently conceptualized as an integral component of a drainage network originating from the venous end of microcirculation. Together with the venous portion of the capillary circulation and the interstitium, it constitutes a single system that may be defined as a functional microcirculatory unit [2–6]. The venous and the lymphatic systems work together (Fig. 27.1); they are connected by tiny lymphovenous anastomoses that activate when the pressure in the lymphatic system rises [7–9]. Persistent venous stasis will lead to functional overload in the lymphatic system that may result in dynamic insufficiency because the fluid overload exceeds the transport capacity of the lymphatics.

In these conditions, lymphangiopathy develops and, in turn, exacerbates edema, which is no longer only of venous but also of lymphatic origin [3, 10–15].

With today's technologies, the initial lymphatics in any body compartment can be visualized to study microlymphatic vessel by microlymphography technique.

Microlymphography is performed using a moving arm with a fluorescence video microscope (Wild Leitz). Using magnification (1×), the microlymphatic network is visualized after a subepidermal injection of 0.01 mc dextran 150,000 (25%) 5 cm above the medial malleolus under microscopic control. Photomicrographs are filmed using video camera (Ikegami ITC-410) and transformed into video signals to a digital video recorder (Sony SLV-415) and simultaneously depicted on two or more monitors. Recordings lasted for at least 15 min.

From these images, we analyze:

(a) Morphology of the lymphatic network [1, 16–18]
(b) Mean diameter of the microlymphatics using morphometric computerized elaboration and

C. Allegra (✉)
San Giovanni Hospital, Rome, Italy
e-mail: allegra@mclink.it

M. Bartolo • A. Carlizza
Department of Angiology, S. Giovanni Hospital, Rome, Italy

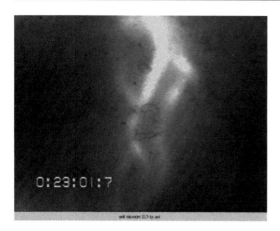

Fig. 27.1 Anastomosis between microlymphatic system fluorescent and blood capillaries

estimated (in μ) choosing among ten of the best stained meshes [1, 16–18]

(c) Velocity of fluorescence staining or the time needed to visualize (i.e., stain) the microlymphatic network from the time of intradermal inoculation [1, 16–18]

(d) "Permanency" or the amount of time that the microlymphatic remains stained

(e) "Extension" or the distance from the inoculation area to depiction of the microlymphatic network

(f) Diffusion or the loss of fluorescent dye into perilymphatic tissues (transudation or dissolution of the microlymphatic)

The above parameters (from C to F) are directly correlated with the opening of lymphatic collectors, degree of lymphatic hypoplasia, and the integrity of the lymphatic vessel in response to increased cutaneous pressure.

The servo-nulling system apparatus (Mod 5A) consists of a pressure transducer (Mod 915), a video signal control (515), and a micromanipulator. With 3.2× magnification, we measure [24–26]:

(a) Intraluminal lymphatic pressure by introducing a 7–9 μ microneedle probe on the micromanipulator into the most densely stained lymphatic and connected it to the Mod 5A to yield an intraluminal pressure for at least 1 min. Computer analysis thereafter provides the range and mean of the intraluminal lymphatic pressure recorded.

(b) By manipulating the microneedles into the adjacent tissue, interstitial pressure is determined and used as a reference for intralymphatic pressure readings including initial lymphatics highlighted by following the diffusion of fluorescent dextran.

Studies by Allegra et al. using the system have improved our knowledge of the pathophysiology of the lymphatic circulation in healthy subjects and in patients with chronic venous disease, lymphedema, and other vascular conditions [19, 20, 22, 23].

Besides intramicrolymphatic pressure, this method can be used to measure interstitial pressure in healthy individuals and in those with chronic venous disease and lymphedema.

Lymphatic Vasomotion and Lymphatic Flow Motion

Several important findings were discovered by chance. After having recorded thousands of microlymphographs and fast-forwarded several images, we noticed that it was sometimes possible to recognize, even with the naked eye, the flow movement inside the microlymphatics.

We digitized several microlymphographs and observed and measured lymphatic flow. For the first time, the velocity of lymphatic flow was visualized and measured in vivo in a human. We noted two different types of intramicrolymphatic flow: a very slow granular flow, which we termed "lymphatic flow motion" (about 10 ± 4 m/s), and a pulsating "stop-and-go" flow pattern, faster than the former (about 91 ± 58 m/s), with periodic accelerations, which we termed "lymphatic vasomotion."

The periodicity of the flow accelerations was about 1 min $\pm$ 25 s.

We were unable to visualize either type of flow pattern in healthy subjects; however, in patients with CVD (CEAP 2,3), we sometimes found a pulsating flow (lymphatic vasomotion) in the proximity of the precollectors, but never granular flow (lymphatic flow motion). In patients with soft edema, we more often found a granular flow pattern, but rarely a periodic flow pattern in the proximity of the precollectors [19, 20, 22, 23].

That granular flow pattern is visible only in a setting of soft lymphedema, but not in patients with CVD or healthy subjects; it may be linked to an increase in the superficial flow that compensates for obstruction of normal deep flow.

In the setting of lymphedema, the presence of a pulsating flow (lymphatic vasomotion) is related to deep drainage because of the opening of the precollectors, probably resulting from critical pressure levels. As regards CVD, the pulsating flow pattern is related to similar dynamics, even if the underlying pathophysiological mechanism is failure of the microlymphatic system and increased interstitial pressure due to capillary stasis [19, 20, 22, 23]. In healthy subjects, neither flow pattern is detected since the lymph flows not in the superficial but, rather, in the deep network through the collectors and therefore cannot be visualized. Recent developments in monitoring and studying lymphatic flow have provided insights into the pathophysiology of lymphatic circulation (Table 27.1).

Microlymphography in Healthy Individuals, in Chronic Venous Disease, and in Lymphedema

Because microlymphography permits the visualization and study of microlymphatic vessels, it can be employed to study lymphatic pathophysiology in common micro- and macrocirculatory diseases [13]. In healthy individuals, few microlymphatics are ordinarily visualized because there is good drainage of contrast material into the deep lymphatic circulation [16] (Fig. 27.2). Involvement of the microlymphatics in chronic venous disease (CVD) offers a characteristic microlymphatic pattern, displaying an increased number of loops and typical fragmentation [1, 19, 20] (Fig. 27.3).

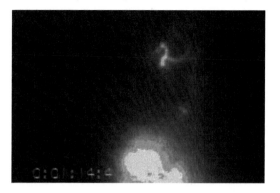

Fig. 27.2 Microlymphography in healthy subject

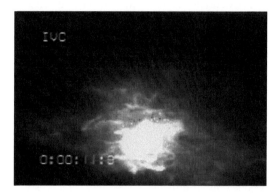

Fig. 27.3 Microlymphography in chronic venous disease, CEAP 2,3

Table 27.1 Microlymphatic network changes in primary lymphedema using fluorescent microlymphography

Parameters	Compressible	Moderately compressible	Noncompressible	Control
No(???) of initial lymphatics	32 ± 5	30.6 ± 8.23	10.6 ± 7.2	7 ± 5.03
Diameter (μm)	121 ± 48	166 ± 51	142 ± 47	54 ± 1
Velocity (sec)	1.5 ± 0.6	120 ± 42	250 ± 39	1 ± 0.3
Diffusion (μm)	13.83 ± 7	21 ± 11	32 ± 16	3.07 ± 1.1
Extension (μm)	40 ± 8.7	30 ± 2.5	18 ± 1	6 ± 2
Permanence (min)	8 ± 3.5	20 ± 4.8	17 ± 5.9	0.48 ± 1.7

Measured values were expressed as x(???) ±SD

Compressible Primary Lymphedema

Compared with healthy subjects, initial lymphatics are greater in number and enlarged and organized into a more extensive network. Moreover, after injection of fluorescent dextran, the microlymphatic network is rapidly depicted similar to controls, but diffusion into the surrounding tissue is slower and persistence of microlymphatic staining is prolonged [1–14]. Endolymphatic pressure also increases as interstitial pressure [23].

Moderately Compressible Primary Lymphedema

Compared with healthy subjects, the microlymphatic network is again greater, more enlarged, but with slower diffusion, reduced velocity of microlymphatic staining, and greater permanence of staining. Although the microlymphatic network is more extensive than in controls, it is less extensive than in compressible primary lymphedema. Both endolymphatic and interstitial pressure is higher than in controls and higher than in compressible primary lymphedema [23].

Noncompressible Primary Lymphedema

At this more advanced stage, microlymphography becomes more difficult. Fewer lymphatic vessels are depicted. Moreover, they appear tortuous, sometimes damaged or obstructed albeit dilated, but, nonetheless, still more extensive than in healthy subjects, yet less than compressible and moderate compressible lymphedema and quite irregular. Staining is much slower and more retarded than in

compressible and moderate compressible lymphedema. Diffusion is slower and permanence greater and similar or worse. Endolymphatic and interstitial pressures are both significantly increased andgreater [23] (Table 27.2).

In early-stage lymphedema, the number of microlymphatic loops is particularly high, and the microlymphatic pressure is much higher than the normal range. This finding can be interpreted as a mechanism of initial insufficiency (Fig. 27.4) [1, 21, 22].

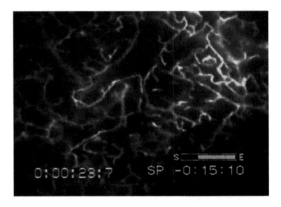

Fig. 27.4 Microlymphography in lymphedema

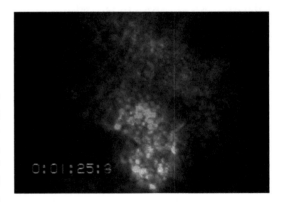

Fig. 27.5 Microlymphography in fibrosis

Table 27.2 Microdynamic pressures in primary lymphedema

Pressure (mmHg)	Compressible	Moderately compressible	Noncompressible	Control
EP	8.2 ± 1.7	10.03 ± 2.1	11 ± 1.5	4.19 ± 1.9
IP	4.31 ± 1.98	5.18 ± 1.48	7.2 ± 1.9	0.65 ± 1

EP endolymphatic pressure, *IP* interstitial pressure

In long-standing lymphedema, the microlymphatics cannot be seen because of the presence of fibrosis [1, 23] (Fig. 27.5).

When the data from dynamic capillaroscopy and capillary blood velocity (CBV) are combined with microlymphography, a more complete picture can be obtained for understanding the pathophysiology of a microcirculatory unit [1–3, 5, 8, 16, 17, 27].

References

1. Bollinger A, Fagrell B. Clinical capillaroscopy. Toronto: Hogrefe & Huber Publishers; 1990.
2. Pratesi F. Sistema microvasculotessutale: morfologia funzionale. In: Microcircolazione e microangiologia. Torino: Ed.Min. Med; 1990. p. 17–30.
3. Allegra C, Carlizza A. Oedema in chronic venous insufficiency: physiopathology and investigation. Phlebology. 2000;15:122–5.
4. Allegra C. Endotelio come organo. Pragma Ed: Milano; 1991.
5. Allegra C, Carioti B. Diffusione endoteliale capillare in vivo. Minerva Angiol. 1993;18(1 Suppl 1):245–51.
6. Allegra C, Carlizza A. Rheopletysmography and laser-Doppler velocimetry in the study of microcirculatory flow variability. In: Allegra C, Intaglietta M, Messmer K, editors. Vasomotion and flowmotion. Progress in applied microcirculation, vol. 20. Basel: Karger; 1991.
7. Allegra C. *Appunti di Flebologia*. Arti Grafiche Istaco Ed. 1991:15–9.
8. Allegra C, Carlizza A. Constitutional functional venopathy. Adv Vasc Pathol. Int Congress Series 1150. 1997;123–9.
9. Spiegel M, Vesti B, Shore A, Franzeck UK, Bollinger A. Pressure of lymphatic capillaries in human skin. Am J Physiol. 1992;262:H1208–10.
10. Speicer DE, Bollinger A. Microangiopathy in mild chronic venous incompetence: morphological alterations and increased transcapillary diffusion detected by fluorescence videomicroscopy. Int J Microcirc Clin Exp. 1991;10:55–66.
11. Allegra C. The role of the microcirculation in venous ulcers. Phlebolymphology. 1994;2:3.
12. Husmann MJ, Barton M, Vesti BR, Franzeck UK. Postural effects on interstitial fluid pressure in humans. J Vasc Res. 2006;43(4):321–6.
13. Agus GB, Allegra C. Guidelines for diagnosis and therapy of diseases of the veins and lymphatic vessels. Int Angiol. 2013;32(Suppl 1):71–3.
14. Gretener SB, Lauchli S, Franzeck UK. Effect of venous and lymphatic congestion on lymph capillary pressure of the skin in healthy volunteers and patients with lymphedema. J Vasc Res. 2000;37(1):61–7.
15. Guyton AC. Interstitial fluid pressure. Physiol Rev. 1971;51:527–32.
16. Bartolo Jr M, Allegra C. Image: can we see lymphatics? Int J Microcirc Clin Exp. 1994;14(Suppl 1):191.
17. Allegra C. Microcirculatory techniques and assessment of chronic venous insufficiency. Medicographia. 1996;18:30.
18. Lauchli S, Haldimann L, Leu AJ, Franzeck UK. Fluorescence microlymphography of the upper extremities. Evaluation with a new computer programme. Int Angiol. 1999;18(2):145–8.
19. Bartolo Jr M, Carioti B, Cassiani D, Allegra C. Lymphatic capillary pressure in human skin of patients with chronic venous insufficiency. Int J Microcirc Clin Exp. 1994;14(Suppl 1):191.
20. Allegra C, Bartolo Jr M. Haemodynamic modifications induced by elastic compression therapy in CVI evaluated. by microlymphography. Phlebology '95. 1995;1:9–17.
21. Fischer M, Costanzo U, Hoffmann U, Bollinger A, Franzeck UK. Flow velocity of cutaneous lymphatic capillaries in patients with primary lymphedema. Int J MicrocircClin Exp. 1997;17(3):143–9.
22. Allegra C. Lymphatics of the skin in primary lymphoedemas. Int J Microcirc Clin Exp. 1996;16(Suppl 1):114.
23. Allegra C, Bartolo Jr M, Sarcinella R. Morphologic and functional changes of the microlymphatic network in patients with advanced stages of primary lymphedema. Lymphology. 2002;35:114–20.
24. Wunderlich P, Scherman J. Continuous recording of hydrostatic pressure in renal tubules and blood capillaries by use of a new pressure transducer. Pflugers Arch. 1969;313:89–94.
25. Intaglietta M. Pressure measurements in the microcirculation with active and passive transducers. Microvasc Res. 1973;5:317–23.
26. Intaglietta M, Tompkins WR. Simplified micropressure measurements via bridge current feedback. Microvasc Res. 1990;39:386–9.
27. Byung-Boong L, Bergan J, Rockson Stanley G. Lymphedema : a concise compendium of theory and practice. Springer- Verlag London Limited Ed.; 2011. p. 191–7.

MR Lymphangiography

28

Ningfei Liu

The imaging of lymphatic system is much diffi-cult than that of blood circulation due to several reasons. Firstly, lymphatic vessels are slender, fragile, and transparent. Thus, to approach lym-phatic vessel and deliver contrast directly is not easy. Secondly, the diameters of lymphatic vessel are small and the wall has less smooth muscle cell that leads to a weak contraction at a low rhythm. Lymph flow at a lower speed is a non-constant stream under normal condition. Therefore, lymphatic pathway may not always be visualized during imaging. Thirdly, the composi-tion of lymphatic system network is more com-plex than the blood system. There are around 600 of lymph nodes in human body, which distribute between every two or more efferent and afferent lymphatic vessels [1]. The commonly used lym-phoscintigraphy with isotopic contrast agent has insufficient resolution to accurately outline the internal anatomy of lymph node and lymphatic vessels. Lymphangiography using iodine oil agent, which is capable of visualizing the lym-phatics, is no longer routinely performed because it is highly invasive and difficult to perform and also can lead to life-threatening complications.

As a new diagnostic test, 3D high-resolution MR lymphangiography (MRL) has been proven to be useful in the diagnosis of peripheral lymphatic system disorders in recent years [2–5]. Around 2000 patients have been examined in the author's clinic since 2007. MR lymphangiography with gadobenate dimeglumine quickly and sufficiently visualizes the lymphatic pathway and lymph nodes draining from the intracutaneously injec-tion sites in lymphedematous limbs and gives both morphological and functional assessments of tested lymphatic system.

Contrast Agent and Material Administration

The specificity of absorption and transportation of the contrast agent by lymphatic system made it possible to visualize the finely detailed morpho-logical changes of lymphatic as well as regional lymph node under high-resolution MR imaging. Paramagnetic contrast agent gadobenate dimeglu-mine (Gd-BOPTA) (MultiHance, Bracco, Milano, Italy) is an extracellular, water-soluble, small molecular (molecular weight 1 kDa) para-magnetic contrast agent with a gadolinium (Gd) concentration of 0.5 mol/L. This contrast agent is not subject to metabolization and is excreted unchanged by passive glomerular filtration. Experimental animal models have demonstrated merely minor tissue damage after nonintravenous injection or extravasation [6]. Therefore, the

N. Liu, MD, PhD
Lymphology Center of Department of Plastic and Reconstructive Surgery, Shanghai Ninth People's Hospital, Shanghai Jiao Tong University School of Medicine, 639 Zhi Zao Ju Road, Shanghai, China, 200011
e-mail: liuningfei@126.com

agent offers an acceptable safety profile for intra-cutaneous administration. For injection of Gd-BOPTA, a thin needle (24 gauge) is used. A total amount of 8 mL contrast material and 1 mL mepivacainhydrochloride 1% are subdivided into eight portions and injected intradermally into the dorsal aspect of each foot or hand in the region of the four interdigital webs. Mepivacainhydrochloride 1% is administered with the contrast material to alleviate the pain for the patients at the time of injection.

MRL Examination

Patient is in the prone position for lower limb and pelvic cavity inspection and in the supine position for the examination of arm lymphedema. MR examinations are performed with a clinical 3.0 T MR unit (Achiva, software release 2.1; Philips Medical Systems, Best, the Netherlands) with a maximum gradient strength of 80 mT/m and a slew rate of 200 mT/(mms). Patient is placed in the supine position with feet first. Four stations are examined: the lower leg inferior segment and foot region, the lower leg superior segment and upper leg inferior segment including knee region, middle upper leg, and the inguinal region and the proximal upper leg. In these stations, a dedicated six-element phased-array sensitivity encoding (SENSE) cardiac reception coil is used (Philips Medical Systems, Best, the Netherlands). Before interstitial MRL, a 3D heavily T2-weighted MRI with an optimized protocol is performed for imaging stationary fluid to obtain high signal intensity. The serial turbo sequences included fat saturation and half-scan acquisition single-shot fast spin-echo sequence (SSFSE). The fast spin echo is a strong T2-weighted multi-echo sequence with a repetition time (TR) of 2820 ms and an echo time (TE) of 740 ms. The scan field of view (FOV) is 360 × 285. Fifty five to 85 slices with 2-mm thickness and a 240 × 190 matrix are selected in SSFSE. Maximum intensity projection (MIP) and source images are used to reconstruct images of the lymphatic system.

For MRL, 3D fast-spoiled gradient-recalled echo T1-weighted images with a fat saturation

technique (T1 high-resolution isotropic volume excitation, THRIVE) are initially acquired prior to the administration of gadopentetate dimeglumine. The MR imaging parameters are as follows: TR/TE, 3.5/1.7; flip angle, 25; FOV, 360 cm×320 cm; matrix, 300 × 256; slices, 55–95; voxel size, 1.5 mm × 1.2 mm × 1.2 mm; the number of signal average, 2; and acquisition time, 0 min 40 s. The first station is repeated at 5, 10, 15, 20, 25, and 30 min after intracutaneous application of the contrast material. The remained three stations are subsequently examined once after first station completion. To outline lymphatic vessels, MIP reconstruction images are calculated as well.

Image Interpretation

After data acquisition, image post-processing and subsequent analysis is performed. The MR images are evaluated on a workstation connected to the MR unit (ViewForum, Version 2.5, Philips, the Netherlands). Each data set is given a unique code, and all annotations are removed from each original image before image analysis. For the 3D data sets, both source and MIP images are reviewed. Lymphatic vessels are evaluated regarding their visibility with a beaded appearance, size, and collaterals. According to these features, the visualized dilated lymphatic vessels are counted and compared in MIP. The contrast enhancement of the lymphatic vessels and lymph nodes of lower extremity and inguinal region can be qualitatively and quantitatively evaluated. The appearance and distribution pattern of lymphatic pathway in the diseased extremities and the morphological characteristics of inguinal nodes on pre- and post-contrast MR images are analyzed. In the meantime, the existence and location of edema in the affected limbs are also evaluated.

Quantitative analysis, including:

1. The rapid transportation of contrast agent by draining lymphatic and regional lymph node ensures a consecutive and real-time inspection of transporting function of lymphatic and lymph node within a reasonable length of

time. Tracing the movement of enhanced flow within lymphatic vessel allowed quantitative assessment of abnormal lymph flow kinetics. Assessment of the time course of enhancement of lymph flow in vessels directly draining from the injection sites. After contrast injection, the measurement of contrast movement in a contrast-enhanced lymphatic is started from the ankle region along its course toward proximal part in a series of 5–6 successive images along the enhanced lymphatic vessel with clear outline. The length of the enhanced vessel on the final image is recorded, and the speed of contrast movement is calculated with formula as speed (cm) = total length of visualized lymphatic vessel (cm)/ inspection time (minute).

The measurements of contrast-enhanced speed of lymph flow are made in a group of 25 cases. Among them 23 limbs in 20 cases are available for dynamic observation of the contrast-enhanced flow at a series time points. The speed of enhanced lymph flow in this study ranged from 0.301 to 1.48 cm/min (Fig. 28.1). It is notable that the speed of lymph transport might be largely individually dependent. For example, a patient with primary lymphedema on the left lower extremity over 20 years, the tested speed of flow is 1.25 cm/min, which is among the highest scores of those patients, while the diameter of the tested vessel is 6.1 mm, also in the highest range.

The appearance of enhanced lymphatic channel in post-contrast MR image reflected that the lymphatics remained spontaneous contraction and transportation capability in the examined primary and secondary lymphedema limbs.

2. The assessment of enhancement of inguinal lymph node directly draining from the injection sites. For evaluating the results of enhancement of these lymph nodes, the ratio of signal intensity (SI) of lymph node against signal intensity of adjacent muscle is estimated. The operator-defined regions of interest (ROIs) are drawn on the coronal post-contrast images. At least one pair of inguinal nodes is measured. The ROI on muscles is selected in the upper portion of the thigh near inguinal region with approximately equal size of lymph node. The ratio of node/muscle SI is compared between lymphedema and contralateral limbs on post-contrast MR images. In patients the dynamic enhancement of contrast in bilateral nodes is estimated, the wash-in and wash-out curves are derived from designated ROI, and the peak enhancement time and lymph node/muscle SI ratio at peak time are directly compared.

The inspection of the enhancement of contrast in inguinal nodes started 30–40 min after intracutaneously contrast agent injection. At this time, the inguinal nodes of the healthy volunteers

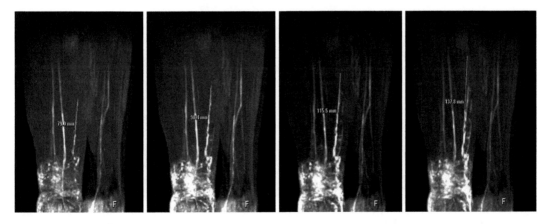

Fig. 28.1 Real-time observation of the velocity of lymph flow by measuring the enhanced lymphatic vessel after intradermal injection of contrast

and the clinical non-edema limbs are markedly enhanced. The comparison of lymph node versus muscle signal intensity ratio between nodes of edema limbs and contralateral nodes showed remarkable asymmetrical accumulation of contrast between the nodes of edematous limbs and contralateral limbs of patients with unilateral lymphedema (Fig. 28.2) as well as in patients with bilateral lymphedema in whom edema is serious in one limb and mild in the other. Therefore, comparison of dynamic nodal enhancement between edema and contralateral limbs and analysis of the time-signal intensity curves could clarify the delayed or declined transport of lymph in individual node and allow quantitative assessment of abnormal nodal lymph flow kinetics.

Qualitatively and morphological observation:

1. Lymphatic drainage patterns

The enhancement of these lymphatic pathways persisted throughout the examination time around 40 min. On the initial images, the enhancement of lymphatic channels may be light and discontinued. But the signal intensity increased and the channels gradually become

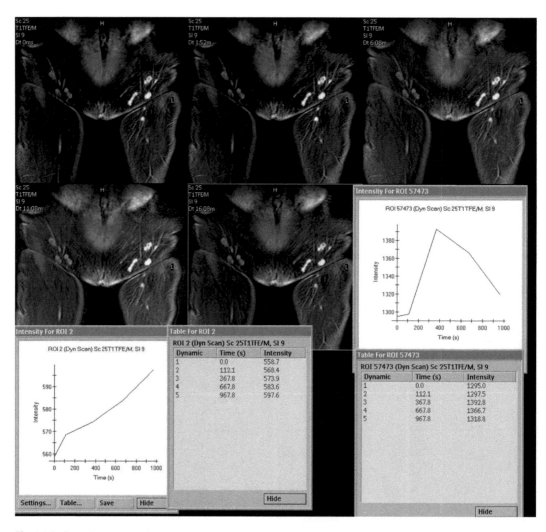

Fig. 28.2 Real-time observation of contrast flow in and flow out through the inguinal lymph nodes of lymphedema patient. The filling of contrast in the lymph nodes was slower in *right side* (lymphedema limb) and was significantly delayed than that in lymph nodes of *left* (no lymphedema limb)

totally opacified with time. The lymphatic vessels in the edematous limbs are irregular in shape or uneven in diameter and twisted; the characters made it easily being distinguished from venous. The number of contrast-enhanced lymphatics in lymphedematous limbs varied from single to numerous. The diameters of visualized lymphatics ranged from 1.2 to 8 mm. The identical patterns of lymphatic pathway in the primary lymphedema limb are diverse [(7)]: radiating arranged enhanced vessels in the lower leg assemble to the medial portion of the knee and went up to the thigh, discontinued, and lightly enhanced but dilated the vessels in the medial portion of the lower limb; bunches of extremely dilated and significantly highlighted lymph are located mainly in the media and less in the lateral portion of the thigh; remarkably dilated and opacified lymph went from the lower

leg directly to the inguinal node with few branches (Fig. 28.3a–c). In secondary lymphedema limb after tumor surgery, there are numerous opacified collateral lymphatic vessels with relatively even diameter indicative of lymphatic neovascularization [8] (Fig. 28.4). Leakage of contrast from the lymphatic vessels may see in lymphedematous limbs of secondary etiology at a relatively early stage [9].

The visualization of contrast-enhanced lymphatic channel in the affected limb is coexistent with accumulation of edema fluid in the tissue in almost all tested cases. Therefore, lymphatic circulation disorder should highly be suspected when contrast-enhanced lymphatics are visualized with this test. Generally no or single contrast-enhanced lymphatic vessel is visualized in limbs of healthy individuals, neither in limbs with lipedema [2].

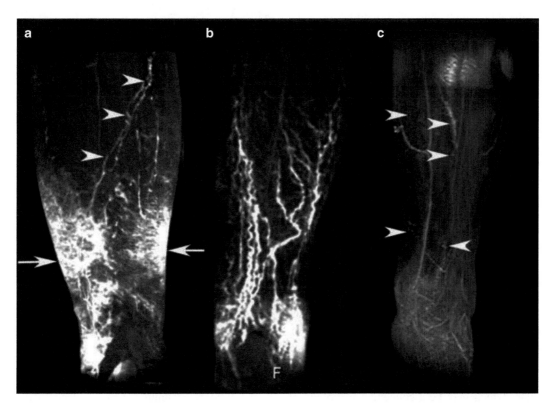

Fig. 28.3 Dynamic three-dimensional MR angiography showed a variety of malformations of lymphatic vessels in the lower extremities of primary lymphedema. (**a**) A fewer dilated lymphatic vessels (*arrowheads*) and dermal back-

flow (*arrows*); (**b**) radiating arranged dilated vessels in the lower leg of primary lymphedema; (**c**) enhanced lymphatic vessels (*arrowheads*) distributed as slender network over the lower extremity

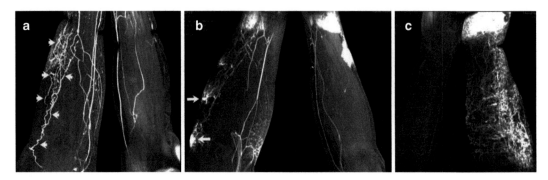

Fig. 28.4 MR lymphangiography of secondary arm lymphedema. (**a**). Tortuous and significantly dilated collecting lymphatics (*arrows*). (**b**) Lymphatic collector disruption and lymphorrhea (*arrows*) in the forearm. (**c**) Significantly dilated lymphatic collectors with extensive opening of numerous communication branches

2. Morphologic characteristics of inguinal lymph nodes

Lymphatic circulation disorders may be caused solely by lymph node abnormal or a lymphatic vessel problem, or a combination of lymphatic and lymph node abnormalities [7]. The morphological changes including nodal size, internal lymph node architecture, and lymph node borders are evaluated. The shape of inguinal lymph node in contralateral side and healthy volunteers is spherical or oval, numbered from 2–3 to 7–8 with a diameter around 1.0 cm. Compared with contralateral limbs, the morphological abnormalities of inguinal nodes in edema limbs observed in present study are absent of node, single large or multi-small fibrotic nodes, small nodules, node with irregular border and hemogeneous structure, irregular nodal outline with homogeneous architecture, and markedly enlarged nodes with increased number (Fig. 28.5). Dynamic MR demonstrated abnormal patterns of contrast filling in the draining inguinal nodes. Post-contrast MR lymphangiographic images however displayed more structural abnormalities as no contrast enhancement in the nodes which may indicate a total fibrosis of the nodes, uneven nodal enhancement which indicates structural anomalies, and partial enhancement within the nodes which may be a congenital pathology of the nodes. Moreover enhanced MR lymphangiography has been proved a promising imaging modality in diagnosing and staging of malignant lymph nodes [10].

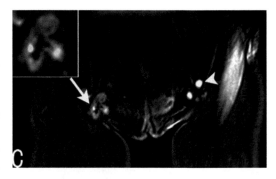

Fig. 28.5 MR lymphangiography shows inguinal lymph nodes (*arrow*) with irregular shape and partial contrast filling on the right limb of primary lymphedema and homogeneous filling of contrast in the lymph nodes (*arrowhead*) of no edema limb post-contrast injection

The combination of the lymphatic and lymph node images may then outline the integral picture of the affected lymphatic system.

3. Lymphedema confirmation

The morphological and structural characteristics of lymphedematous limbs are evaluated for confirmation of clinic diagnosis during MR inspection [2]. The pre- and post-contrast MR image not only provided detailed information of the lymphatic system but also extralymphatic involvement such as (1) the location and extent of edema fluid (in general the fluid is accumulated above deep facial membrane or diffused in subcutaneous in the late stage of the disease edema within muscles and intramuscular space resulting from venous backflow disorder) (Fig. 28.6); (2) fat

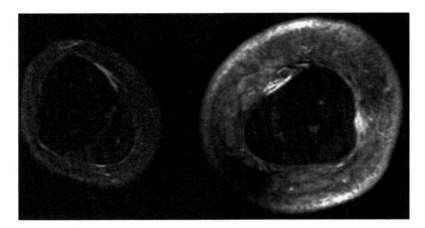

Fig. 28.6 MRI shows lymphedema at an early stage with small amount of water in the subcutaneous layer of the limb (*left*) and a significant thickening and fat tissue deposition in the subcutaneous (*right*).

tissue deposition, which is prominent in very thick subcutaneous tissue (Fig. 28.6); and (3) blood vascular abnormalities as hemangioma and varicose vein. Based on the information by MR imaging, it is easy to stage a lymphedematous limb and differentiate lymphedema from venous edema or lipedema. In the meantime, "dermal backflow," that is, the contrast-enhanced stagnant lymph fluid flow back into the dermal tissue, is a common phenomenon in chronic lymphedematous tissue

Contrast MR lymphangiography with gadobenate dimeglumine is able to visualize the precise morphological status of lymphatic vessels and lymph nodes in lymphedematous limb. In the meantime, it provided comprehensive information concerning the function status of lymph flow transportation in lymphatic and the nodes. This method is minimally invasive, easy, and safe and combines morphological and functional examination in a single acquisition, and the enriched data suffice to characterize lymphatic and lymph nodes in the limb with lymphatic circulation disorders. The comprehensive information provided by contrast MR lymphangiography may also be useful in staging and classification of primary lymphostatic diseases and assessment of the response of treatment. It is also helpful in seeking more direct and effective treatment, avoiding damage of lymphatic and lymph nodes still working during surgical procedure.

References

1. Kubik S. Anatomy of the lymphatic system. In: Foldi M, Foldi E, Kubik S, editors. Textbook of lymphology. München: Elsevier GmbH; 2003. p. 34–5.
2. Liu NF, Lu Q, Jiang ZH. Anatomic and functional evaluation of lymphatics and lymph nodes in diagnosis of lymphatic circulation disorders with contrast magnetic resonance lymphangiography. J Vasc Surg. 2009;49:980–7.
3. Liu NF, Lu Q, Wu XF. Comparison of radionuclide lymphoscintigraphy and dynamic magnetic resonance lymphangiography for investigating extremity lymphoedema. Br J Surg. 2010;97:359–65.
4. Lohrmann C, Foeldi E, Bartholome JP. Godoteridol for MR imaging of lymphatic vessels in lymphoedematous patients:initial experience after intracutaneous injection. Br J Radiol. 2007;80:569–73.
5. Lu Q, Xu J, Liu N. Chronic lower extremity lymphedema: a comparative study of high- resolution interstitial MR lymphangiography and heavily T2-weighted MRI. Eur J Radiol. 2010;73:365–73.
6. Ruehm SG, Corot C, Debatin JF. Interstitial MR lymphgraphy with a conventional extracellular gadolinium-based agent:assessment in rabbits. Radiology. 2001;218:664–9.
7. Liu NF, Yan ZX. Classification of lymphatic system malformations in primary lymphoedema based on MR lymphangiography. Eur J Vascu Endovasc Surg. 2012;44:345–9.
8. Liu NF, Wang BS. Functional lymphatic collectors in breast cancer-related lymphedema arm. Lymphat Res Biol. 2014;12:232–7.
9. Liu NF, Yan ZX, Wu XF, Luo Y. Spontaneous lymphatic disruption and regeneration in obstructive lymphoedema. Lymphology. 2013;46:56–63.
10. Liu NF, Yan ZX, Lu Q, Wang CG. Diagnosis of Inguinal lymph node metastases using contrast enhanced high resolution MR lymphangiography. Acad Radiol. 2013; 20:218–23.

Part VI

Contemporary Management of CVM

Management of Congenital Vascular Malformation: Overview

29

Young-Wook Kim, Young Soo Do, and Byung-Boong Lee

Approaches to patients with congenital vascular malformation (CVM) have been changed not only in the diagnosis but also in the management through the last two decades. Newly established classification and understanding on the anatomic and biologic characteristics of various types of CVM lesions took the leading role to formulate contemporary management principles.

Ultimate goals of the CVM treatment include reduction or extirpation of CVM lesion with minimal recurrence and treatment-related complication rates.

To achieve these goals, minimal invasive or multidisciplinary approach is more frequently adopted in current management of CVM patients.

Y.-W. Kim, MD (✉)
Vascular Surgery, Samsung Medical Center,
Sungkyunkwan University School of Medicine,
Seoul, South Korea
e-mail: young52.kim@samsung.com;
ywkim52@gmail.com

Y.S. Do
Department of Radiology, Samsung Medical Center,
Sungkyunkwan University School of Medicine,
Seoul, South Korea

B.-B. Lee, MD, PhD, FACS
Professor of Surgery and Director, Center for the
Lymphedema and Vascular Malformations,
George Washington University, Washington, DC, USA

Adjunct Professor of Surgery, Uniformed Services,
University of the Health Sciences,
Bethesda, MD, USA
e-mail: bblee38@gmail.com

In general, following points are usually considered before treatment of CVM patients.

- Treat or "wait and see" – require evaluating risk versus benefits of each side.
- What is an expected natural course of the CVM lesion? – consider expected complications or sequelae when leave it untreated.
- If decided to treat, when is an optimal timing for the treatment?
- What are important structures around the CVM lesion?
- If decided to treat, how can we approach to the CVM lesion without or with minimal damage to the normal tissue or organs around the CVM lesion?
- If decided to treat, how can we reduce rates of recurrence and treatment-related complication?

Not all the CVMs would need the treatment or equally treated because they take different natural course with different prognosis. As described in previous chapters, CVM shows various clinical features and different clinical significance according to the type, anatomic site and extent of the CVM lesion, and age of the patients. For example, arteriovenous malformation (AVM) is considered as a potentially life- or limb-threatening condition in general, while venous malformation (VM) is not.

Head and neck CVMs usually present with cosmetic reasons, and CVM lesion close to the upper airway may cause breathing difficulty.

Patients with CVM lesions in the extremity often present with pain, swelling, and/or bleeding or lymphatic discharge from skin, while some patients present with serious limb length or size discrepancy, joint contracture, or foot ischemia.

Depth of CVM involvement and anatomic location of the CVM lesion are also important to determine an optimal treatment strategy.

When sclerotherapy is considered for treatment of CVM, chemical skin burn is worrisome in CVM lesion confined to facial skin, while functional defect due to nerve damage is more worrisome for patients with CVM lesion close to the major nerve in the extremity. According to the anatomic location of the CVM lesion, treatment plan can be different considering cosmetic or functional complications related with the treatment.

Age of patient is another important factor in determining treatment strategy for patients with CVM. CVM lesions may present at late days in the life though it is congenital abnormality of blood or lymphatic vessels. Regarding to an optimal timing for the treatment of CVM lesion, early extirpation of CVM lesion is theoretically reasonable. However, endovascular or surgical treatment in pediatric patients is challenging due to small size of blood vessels, limited safety margin of sclerosing agent, and radiation hazard by the endovascular sclerotherapy. Therefore, risk versus benefit analysis should be done before attempting surgical or endovascular treatment of CVM. On an analysis to predict response to the percutaneous ethanol sclerotherapy in patients with venous malformation (VM), we found that no or delayed visualization of drainage vein on an initial direct puncture venogram, well-defined VM margin on MR image, and female gender were predictors of "better response" to the sclerotherapy [1].

Lymphatic malformation showing macrocystic lesion is an exception to the delayed treatment. It can be treated with local percutaneous injection with sclerosing agents.

Sometimes, CVM may be detected at late in life by development of complications of hidden CVM lesion. For example, lower extremity lymphatic malformation (LM) may present with repeated episodes of cellulitis, and pelvic AVM lesion may present with polymenorrhea and chronic anemia. To detect the clinically unapparent CVM lesion, it is required high index of suspicion of CVM. For an optimal management CVM lesion, knowledge in clinical and biologic features of various types of CVM and precise anatomic information are required.

Regarding the optimal treatment method, endovascular embolo-sclerotherapy is most frequently adopted therapy and particularly for patients with surgically inaccessible CVM lesion such as *diffuse infiltrating* type of extratruncular CVM lesions involving extensive regions of tissues. Surgical excision of *limited and localized* CVM lesion can be adopted as long as complete excision of the lesion is available with acceptable risk of complication. Sometimes both treatment methods can be attempted concomitantly or as staged procedures.

However, incomplete or inadvertent surgical excision of CVM lesion can make it worse due to recurrence or even aggravation of the CVM lesion and interruption of endovascular access route.

In this part VI (contemporary management of CVM), authors described various types of treatment modalities for CVM patients according to the types and anatomic location of CVM lesions.

Reference

1. Yun WS, Kim YW, Lee KB, Kim DI, Park KB, Kim KH, Do YS, Lee BB. Predictors of response to percutaneous ethanol sclerotherapy in patients with venous malformations: Analysis of patient self-assessment and imaging. J Vasc Surg. 2009;50:581–9.

Endovascular Treatment of Vascular Malformation: An Overview

30

Wayne F. Yakes, Alexis M. Yakes,
Robert L. Vogelzang, and Krasnodar Ivancev

Vascular anomalies constitute some of the most difficult diagnostic and therapeutic enigmas that can be encountered in the practice of medicine. The clinical presentations are extremely protean and can range from an asymptomatic birthmark to fulminant, life-threatening congestive heart failure. Attributing any of these extremely varied symptoms that a patient may present with to a vascular malformation can be challenging to the most experienced clinician. Compounding this problem is the extreme rarity of these vascular lesions. If a clinician sees one patient every few years, it is extremely difficult to gain a learning curve to diagnose and optimally treat them. Typically, these patients bounce from clinician to clinician only to experience disappointing outcomes, complications, and recurrence or worsening of their presenting symptoms. Vascular malformations are truly an "orphan" disease in the medical world.

Vascular anomalies were first treated by surgeons. The early rationale of proximal arterial ligation of arteriovenous malformations (AVMs)

W.F. Yakes, MD (✉) • A.M. Yakes, BM
The Yakes Vascular Malformation Center,
Englewood, CO 80113, USA
e-mail: Wayne.yakes@vascularmalformationcenter.com

R.L. Vogelzang, MD
Northwestern Medical Center, Chicago, IL, USA

K. Ivancev, MD, PhD
Division of Vascular Surgery,
University of Hamburg Medical Center,
Hamburg, Germany

proved totally futile as the phenomenon of neovascular recruitment stimulated and reconstituted arterial inflow to the AVM nidus. Microfistulous connections became macrofistulous feeders over time. Complete surgical extirpation of an AVM nidus proved very difficult and extremely hazardous, necessitating suboptimal partial resections. Partial resections could cause an initial good clinical response, but with time the patient's presenting symptoms recurred or worsened at follow-up [1–3]. Because of the significant blood loss that frequently accompanied surgery, the skills of interventional radiologists were eventually employed to embolize and devascularize these vascular lesions preoperatively. This allowed for more complete resections; however, complete extirpation of an AVM was still extremely difficult and rarely possible. As catheter delivery systems improved and embolic agents more varied, embolotherapy has since emerged as a primary mode of therapy in the management of vascular anomalies. Anatomically, vascular malformations are often in surgically difficult or inaccessible areas, which has led to increased reliance on the sophisticated endosurgical skills of the interventional radiologist and interventional neuroradiologist in the management of these problematic patients.

Because the clinical and angiographic manifestations can be extremely varied, hemangiomas and vascular malformations have always been difficult to classify. Moreover, numerous descriptive terms have been applied to impressive clinical

© Springer-Verlag Berlin Heidelberg 2017
Y.-W. Kim et al. (eds.), *Congenital Vascular Malformations*, DOI 10.1007/978-3-662-46709-1_30

examples in the hopes of distinguishing them as distinct syndromes. This has resulted in significant confusion in the categorization and treatment of these complex vascular lesions. Some of the confusing terms include congenital arteriovenous aneurysm, interosseous arteriovenous malformation, cirsoid aneurysm, serpentine aneurysm, capillary telangiectasia, angioma telangiectaticum, angioma arteriole racemosum, angioma simplex, angioma serpiginosum, nevus angiectoides, hemangioma simplex, lymphangioma, hemangiolymphangioma, nevus flammeus, verrucous hemangioma, capillary hemangioma, cavernous hemangioma, and capillary-venous angiomata. Based on the landmark research of Mulliken et al. [4–9], a rational classification of hemangioma and vascular malformations has evolved that should be incorporated into modern clinical practice. This classification system, based on endothelial cell characteristics, has removed much of the confusion in terminology that is present in the literature today. Once all clinicians understand and utilize this important classification system, ambiguity and confusion will be removed, and all clinicians can speak a common language. The International Society for the Study of Vascular Anomalies (ISSVA) has adopted this classification system just for these reasons.

Endovascular Occlusive Agents

Endosurgical vascular ablation (embolotherapy) has evolved as one of the cornerstones of modern Interventional Radiology. The extensive array of catheters, guide wires, endovascular ablative agents (embolic materials), and imaging systems are a tribute to the hard work, insight, and imagination of the many dedicated investigators in this area. Because of significant laboratory research, clinical research, and extensive clinical experience, the judicious use of endosurgical vascular ablative therapy is common in modern clinical practice. Now that it is firmly established as an essential therapeutic tool, its role will only continue to grow.

There are now many endovascular ablative agents that are used in various clinical scenarios.

The choice of agent depends upon several factors: the vascular territory to be treated, the type of abnormality being treated, the possibility of superselective delivery of an occlusive agent, the goal of the procedure, and the permanence of the occlusion required. The following are some occlusive agents that have been used to treat vascular anomalies.

Gelfoam (*Upjohn Co., Kalamazoo, MI*): Autologous clot was the first widely used particulate agent, but Gelfoam, a gelatin sponge, has become a much more popular transcatheter embolic agent. It is initially used for surgical hemostasis, readily available, inexpensive, and easy to use. It is packaged in sheets that can be cut into pledgets of any size required by the Interventional Radiologist. Gelfoam induces mild-to-moderate tissue reactivity, which enhances its thrombogenic effects. It is not a permanently occluding agent with regard to vascular malformations. Recanalizations usually occur within 7–30 days of the procedure.

Gelfoam powder (*Upjohn Co., Kalamazoo, MI*): Gelfoam is available as a powder with the individual particles measuring approximately 40–60 μm in size. Because of this small particle size, deep penetration can be expected. In high-flow vascular malformations, shunting to the pulmonary arterial bed will occur. Gelfoam powder has the same properties as the gelatin sponge sheets. Because of its small particle size, small-vessel occlusion is possible. Therefore, in the pelvis, head, and neck regions, and the paraspinal area, it should be used only with extreme caution, if ever, to prevent possible denervation of nerves by occluding the vasa nervorum [10]. Other more suitable, larger-particle agents could be used that will decrease the chance of neuropathy. The use of Gelfoam powder is very limited in the management of vascular malformations because recanalizations always occur 100%.

Avitene (*Alcon Laboratories, Fort Worth, TX*): Avitene (microfibrillar collagen hemostat) is similar to Gelfoam in that it is inexpensive, readily available, and easy to use. It also is a nonpermanent occluding agent. Because of the small particles (approximately 200 μm) that are present in the mixture, the potential complications that can occur with Gelfoam powder are also possible with Avitene. Avitene is prepared from denatured bovine collagen and is, therefore, potentially antigenic. Animal and human studies have shown no significant antigenic effects, however. A solution of Avitene with 33% ethanol has shown promise as a good embolic agent in a pig model. We prefer to use Avitene instead of Gelfoam to induce acute thrombosis. Avitene in our experience appears to be superior and much more thrombogenic than Gelfoam. It is similarly used as a topical hemostatic agent. Avitene is much simpler to use because it does not have to be cut in pieces. It can be mixed in a slurry with contrast added to it very quickly. Again, recanalizations in AVM embolizations with Avitene alone are universal.

Angiostat (*Regional Therapeutics, Santa Monica, CA*): Angiostat (GAX) is a collagen-based embolic agent that has characteristics similar to Gelfoam and Avitene in that it is not a permanently occluding agent. As opposed to a particle, Angiostat is a fiber measuring 5×75 μm.

Polyvinyl alcohol foam (*Contour, Interventional Therapeutics Corp., South San Francisco, CA; PVA, Biodyne Inc., El Cajon, CA; PVA, Ingenor Medical, Paris, France*): Polyvinyl alcohol particles (PVA, Ivalon) are formed by the reaction of polyvinyl alcohol foam with formaldehyde. It is biologically inert and provokes a mild inflammatory reaction. Initially thought to be a permanently occluding agent, PVA is now known to recanalize when used to treat vascular malformations. PVA is usually supplied in suspensions in sizes of 150–300, 300–500, 500–700, 700–1000, 1000–1500, 1500–2000, and 2000–2500 μm [11].

Coils (*Cook Inc., Bloomington, IN; Target Therapeutics, Los Angeles, CA*): Metallic coils with or without attached cotton or Dacron fibers have long been used to induce vascular occlusion, first introduced by Cesart Gianturcó. Many coils have been developed that will pass through standard 4, 5, and 6.5 French (Fr) catheters, as well as the new microcatheter systems. These occluding spring coil emboli function similarly to an arterial ligation in that they occlude the artery where the coil is released and do nothing to the capillary bed distally. The later development in coil technology is the Ruby Coil (Penumbra

Inc.; Alameda, CA) which is a platinum coil that is very soft and radiopaque on fluoroscopy. It is advanced through a specialized microcatheter developed by Penumbra Inc. This coil, and other similar ones, is unique in that it has a weld at the end of the coil length to a wire. The coils can come in various lengths with various sizes of circular diameter helixes. After the coil has been properly placed within an aneurysm or whatever vascular pathology is being treated, the coil can then be detached uneventfully and left in place. This is a distinct advantage in that perfect control can always be maintained in coil placement and detachment. If the operator does not like a particular coil positioning, it can be totally retracted. Further, once in position and then ready for detachment, it will detach without any pulling force. This is especially important when placing coils within an aneurysm that could be ruptured by any tugging force at the neck. The Nester fibered platinum coil (Cook Inc., Bloomington, IN) is also an excellent coil for vascular occlusion. Precise placement is possible, but it cannot be repositioned as there is no attachment to a coil pusher.

"Glues" (*Histoacryl Blau, B. Braun, Inc., Melsungen, Germany*): Isobutyl 2-cyanoacrylate (IBCA) and N-butyl cyanoacrylate (NBCA) belong to a class of tissue adhesives that are used for endosurgical vascular ablation. NBCA has replaced IBCA and is used to treat AVMs and AVF. These "glues" remain in the liquid state until contact occurs with an ionic solution, such as contrast material, saline, or blood, whereby it polymerizes from its monomeric form to its polymeric form. In this polymerization process, the cyanoacrylates generate heat, which may contribute to some level of histotoxicity in the adjacent area and angioneurosis. Tantalum powder is used to opacify the embolic mixture, so it can be visualized fluoroscopically and on plain films. Pantopaque or acetic acid has been used to retard the polymerization time of the mixture so that it can effectively reach the embolization target and then solidify. The cyanoacrylates were initially thought to be permanent occluding agents; however, it is now well documented that recanalizations do occur [12, 13]. Once solidified intravascularly, the cyanoacrylates incite a mild inflammatory response. In the management of head and neck vascular malformations, the cyanoacrylates cause a rock-hard mass that is extremely undesirable cosmetically. Furthermore, white tantalum powder should be used in Caucasian patients, and black tantalum powder should be used in Black patients to minimize unwanted subcutaneous discoloration. Because of current restrictions by the FDA, no American company manufactures this agent.

Onyx (*Covidien Corp.; ev 3 Endovascular Inc.; Plymouth, MN*) is a liquid embolic agent developed for the presurgical embolization of brain AVMs. Onyx is comprised of ethylene vinyl alcohol (EVOH) copolymers dissolved in dimethyl sulfoxide (DMSO) and suspended micronized tantalum powder for visualization during fluoroscopy. The delivery microcatheter must be compatible for DMSO injection. Onyx is available as Onyx 18 (6% EVOH) and Onyx 34 (8% EVOH) with Onyx 34 having a higher viscosity. It was first developed for presurgical and preradiosurgical brain AVM embolizations. Onyx has been adapted for peripheral AVM embolization, but like the other polymerizing tissue adhesives (IBCA, NBCA) publications, it is not a curative embolic agent and is palliative at best. In the endovascular treatment of dural AVF, if properly deposited, it can be curative in dural AVF embolization. However, as in NBCA, previous Onyx "cures" of dural AVF documented to have recurred as well.

Ninety eight percent ethyl alcohol (*dehydrated alcohol injection USP, Abbott Laboratories, North Chicago, IL*): Ethanol is a well-known sclerosing agent that induces significant thrombosis from the capillary bed backward. This results in total tissue devitalization. Ethanol induces thrombosis by denaturing blood proteins, dehydrating vascular endothelial cells and precipitating their protoplasm, denuding the vascular wall of endothelial cells, and segmentally fracturing the denuded vessel wall to the level of the internal elastic lamina. In the treatment of vascular malformations, ethanol has demonstrated its curative potential, as opposed to the palliation seen with other embolic agents. As with Gelfoam powder, extreme caution and superselective catheter placement are requirements when using ethanol as an endovascular occlusive agent. Ethanol can induce significant pain due to pain caused in the vessel wall vasa nervorum when injected intravascularly. Proper anesthesia, such as deep IV sedation or general anesthesia, is required to minimize patient discomfort. Post-embolization edema always occurs with the use of ethanol. Extreme caution with superselective catheter/needle positioning must be taken with its use to minimize the possibility of nontarget embolization of normal tissues to prevent tissue necrosis and neuropathy. Technical intraprocedural requirements for the use of ethanol include the following: (1) superselective catheter placement or direct deposition of ethanol within the nidus of the vascular lesion; (2) avoidance of alcohol injection into normal vessels; (3) use of General Anesthesia with appropriate intraprocedural monitoring; (4) good immediate postoperative care, including the appropriate use of medications to reduce side effects; and (5) careful clinical follow-up with appropriate retreatment when necessary to produce the maximum benefit.

Sotradecol (*sodium tetradecyl sulfate, Elkins-Sinn Inc., Cherry Hills, NJ*): Sotradecol is another sclerosing agent available in a 1% or 3% aqueous solution. Its properties are similar to ethyl alcohol, and it contains 2% benzyl alcohol. The same caveats apply to the use of Sotradecol as to the use of ethyl alcohol and Gelfoam powder in neurologically sensitive areas.

Detachable balloons (*Becton Dickinson balloon, Franklin Lakes, NJ; Debrun balloon and Halt balloon, Ingenor Medical, Paris, France; Hieshima balloon, Interventional Therapeutics Corp., South San Francisco, CA*): Since first introduced by Serbinenko in 1974 [14], several detachable balloons have been developed, and they have been used to endovascularly treat carotid-cavernous fistulae, head and neck aneurysms, varicocele, and AVF. Amplatzer vascular plugs (St. Jude Medical, St. Paul, MN) is another detachable vascular occlusion device.

Endovascular Treatment of Arteriovenous Malformations

AVMs are congenital vascular anomalies typified by hypertrophied inflow arteries shunting through a primitive vascular nidus into tortuous dilated outflow veins. No intervening capillary bed is present. Symptoms are usually referable to the anatomic location of the AVM. The larger and the more central and anatomically close to the heart an AVM is, the greater the likelihood of high-output cardiac consequences. Other presenting symptoms can include pain, progressive nerve deterioration or palsy, disfiguring mass, tissue ulceration, hemorrhage, impairment of limb function, limiting claudication, and so on. Vascular malformations cause symptoms referable to the anatomic area they occupy.

The baseline imaging workup prior to any therapy includes extensive arteriography, color duplex image (CDI), CTA, and MR. Selective and superselective arteriography defines the AVM's angioarchitecture and identifies any dangerous arterial anastomoses to normal vascular structures, any aneurysms within the lesion, the venous drainage, and the potential routes of access for endosurgical vascular embolotherapy. Furthermore, these baseline studies are compared to follow-up studies to determine the efficacy of therapy.

Many endovascular occlusive agents have been used to treat AVMs. Most agents produce palliative results; however, follow-up procedures are required as recanalizations and neovascular recruitment stimulate renewed symptoms. With the use of ethanol, recanalizations and neovascular recruitment rarely if ever are observed. Furthermore, untreated inflow arterial feeders have decreased in size in response to the decreased AV shunt within the nidus being ablated. CDI provides physiologic data documenting decreased flow rates through arterial feeders at follow-up as well.

In treating AVMs, superselective catheter placement is absolutely essential. When this is not possible, then direct percutaneous puncture techniques should be used to circumvent catheterization obstacles. If superselective placement at the AVM nidus is not possible, then the use of ethanol must be avoided. Frequently, inflow occlusion is required to induce slower flow to maximize the thrombogenic sclerosant properties of ethanol. This can be achieved through the use of occlusion balloon catheters, blood pressure cuffs, tourniquets, and so on. We empirically use occlusive techniques for at least 10 min. The amount of ethanol used in each endosurgical vascular ablative procedure is tailored to the flow-volume characteristics of the individual lesion. No predetermined volume of ethanol is ever considered.

Endovascular ablation of AVMs with ethanol has ushered in a new era in the therapy of these problematic anomalies. Cures and permanent partial ablations have been documented in our patient series resulting in symptomatic improvement. Because neovascular recruitment and recanalizations have not been observed, permanent partial ablations have led to long-term symptomatic improvement, obviating the need for further treatment. Despite the success that is possible with ethanol, it must be remembered that it is an extremely dangerous intravascular sclerosant that can cause tissue necrosis and neuropathy used improperly. It is an unforgiving embolic agent totally dependent on the expertise of the embolotherapist. The occasional embolizer should refrain from treating AVMs, especially with ethanol. We have observed a 6% complication rate in our vascular malformation patient series.

In small AVMs, a single procedure may be sufficient to ablate the lesion. Treatment of large, complex lesions should be staged for several reasons. In a protracted procedure, contrast limits can be exceeded, and an interventionalist can become fatigued, thereby increasing the probability of a judgment error or technical mishap. Most importantly, serial treatments reduce the risks of too extensive individual ablation, thereby decreasing the risk of tissue injury or potential complications arising from post-thrombosis edema.

Endovascular Treatment of AVMs based on Yakes AVM Classification

Yakes Type I direct AV connections, as typically seen in pulmonary AVF and renal AVF, can be permanently ablated by occluding the AVF with mechanical devices. Coils, Amplatzer plugs, occluders, detachable balloons, and the like are universally successful to cure Yakes Type I AVMs. Ethanol can also be curative in Yakes Type I AVMs if the AVF is of a small caliber (Fig. 30.1). Yakes Type IIa and Type IIb AVMs with the "nidum" nest-like angioarchitecture can be permanently ablated with absolute ethanol

from a superselective transcatheter/transmicrocatheter arterial approach of the nidus (Fig. 30.2).

Also, a direct puncture into the artery(ies) supplying the AVM immediately proximal to the AVM "nidum" and distal to any parenchymal arterial branches, to then inject ethanol superselectively, can be employed to circumvent catheterization obstacles when a transcatheter/transmicrocatheter positioning to achieve the same position to deliver ethanol into the "nidum" is not possible. These two transarterial approaches allow ethanol to sclerose and permanently ablate the "nidum." Also the AVM "nidum" itself can be direct-punctured, and ethanol (undiluted) can be injected to sclerose it directly to effect cure in its

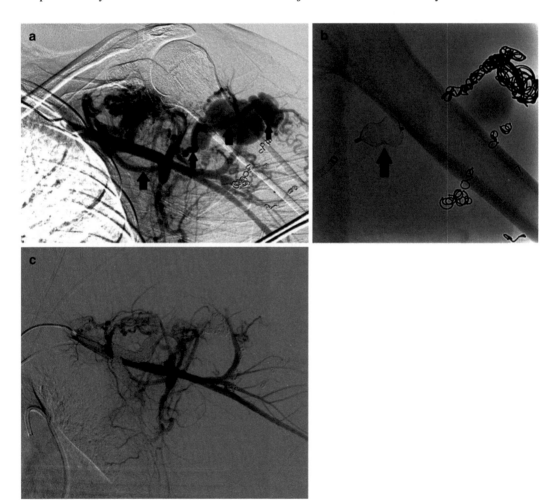

Fig. 30.1 (**a**) Yakes Type I AVM example. Left subclavian DSA demonstrating Yakes Type I AVM with direct AVF (*arrows*) of axillary artery branch into aneurysmal vein (**b**) Note deformity in occluding Amplatzer plug (*arrow*) (**c**) Left subclavian DSA demonstrating persistent cure of Yakes Type I AVF at 3-year follow-up

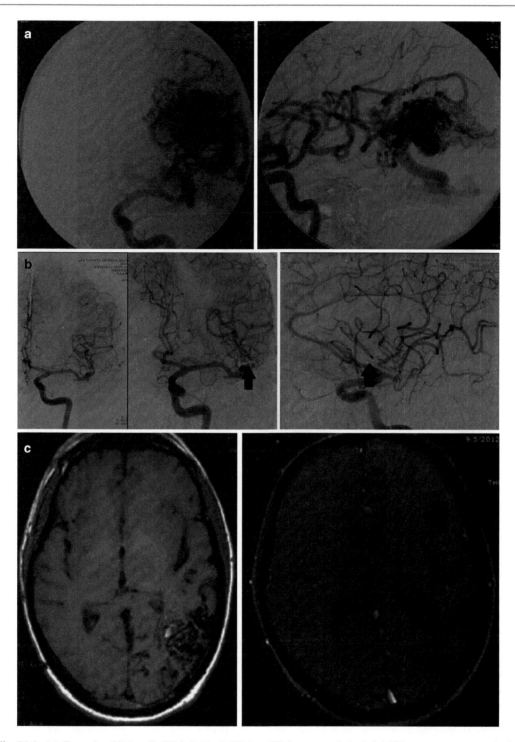

Fig. 30.2 (a) Example of Yakes II AVM, "nidus" AVM type. AP and lateral left internal carotid DSA demonstrating left brain Yakes Type IIa AVM supplied from left middle cerebral arterial branches. (b) AP and lateral left internal carotid artery DSA demonstrating cure of the left brain AVM at 16 year arteriographic follow-up. Once the AVM was cured, the left MCA aneurysm was surgically clipped (*arrows*). (c) Brain MR prior to ethanol embolotherapy (above) and 16-year follow-up demonstrating cure of AVM with brain volume loss resulting in ex vacuo enlargement of the left occipital horn of the lateral ventricle

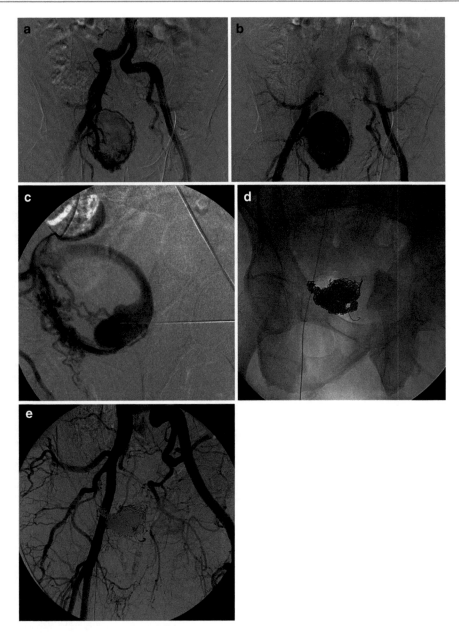

Fig. 30.3 (**a**) Example of Yakes Type IIIa AVM. AP pelvis DSA demonstrating right pelvic AVM with giant vein aneurysm. (**b**) AP pelvis DSA later phase. (**c**) Direct puncture DSA pre-coil embolization into giant vein aneurysm AVM "nidus" is in the vein wall itself. (**d**) Note tightly packed coil mass in vein aneurysm. (**e**) Oblique pelvis DSA demonstrating cure of right pelvic Yakes Type IIIa AVM at 3-year follow-up

multiple AVM compartments as well. In the Type IIb AVM, the vein aneurysm can be coil packed for curative treatment.

Yakes Type IIIa AVMs (multiple inflow arteries shunting into an aneurysmal vein with a single enlarged outflow vein) and Yakes Type IIIb AVMs (multiple inflow arteries into an aneurysmal vein with multiple enlarged outflow veins) can be curatively treated by several endovascular approaches (Figs. 30.3 and 30.4). The "nidum" in this type of angioarchitecture with an aneurysmal vein is within the vein wall itself. Superselective

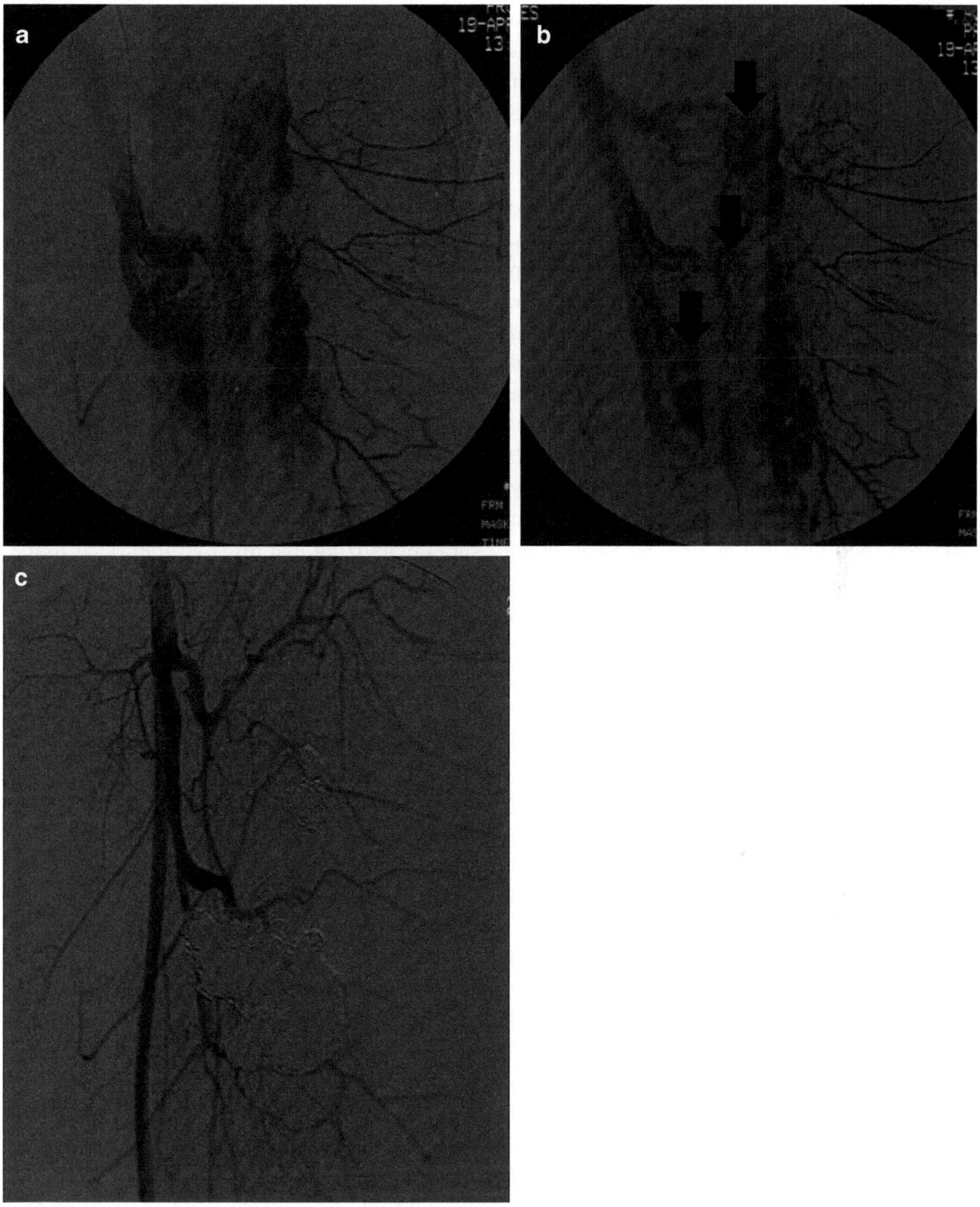

Fig. 30.4 (**a**) Example of Yakes Type IIIb AVM. AP left profunda femoris DSA demonstrating left femur intraosseous AVM, arterial phase. (**b**) Venous phase demonstrating multiple vein outflow from the intraosseous vein aneurysm (*arrows*). (**c**) AP left common femoral DSA demonstrating cure at 14-month follow-up. Note the coil placements into the various outflow vein aneurysmal segments

transarterial ethanol embolization distal to all parenchymal branches via transcatheter/transmicrocatheter and direct puncture endovascular approaches to the vein wall nidus can be curative but extremely difficult to treat all AVFs. A simpler additional curative endovascular approach for Type IIIa AVMs is to coil and embolize the aneurysmal vein cavity itself with, or without, concurrent ethanol injection into the coils within the aneurysmal vein. This is curative when the aneurysmal vein is totally and densely packed with coils. The aneurysmal vein can be accessed by direct 18 g needle puncture and by retrograde vein catheterization to achieve the same position within the aneurysmal vein sac to pack it with coils. The retrograde vein approach to curatively treat high-flow AVM vascular lesions was first published and illustrated in 1990 by Yakes et al. [15]. Yakes et al. described and illustrated cures of posttraumatic and congenital high-flow lesions from the vein approach. The second article articulating the vein approach to AVM treatment was subsequently published in 1996 by Jackson et al. [16]. Cures were documented in these published patient series. Jackson et al. described four cures of congenital AVMs by way of the retrograde vein approach in 1996. Cho and Do et al. also published the retrograde vein approach to curative Yakes Type IIIa/IIIb AVMs treatment in 2008 [17].

Yakes Type IIIb (aneurysmal vein with enlarged multiple outflow veins) can be cured by transarterial transcatheter ethanol embolization and can be cured by direct puncture and retrograde vein coiling techniques of the aneurysm sac and outflow veins. However, the aneurysmal vein portion and the immediate adjacent segments of each outflow vein must also be packed with coils completely to achieve cure. Yakes Type IIIb AVMs are more challenging to coil and cure than the Yakes Type IIIa AVMs due to the more complex multiple outflow veins morphology requiring coil treatment in these multiple aneurysmal vein compartments.

Yakes Type IV AVMs present a unique challenge to determine curative endovascular treatment strategies. AVMs, by definition, are direct AV connections without an intervening capillary bed (Yakes Types I–IV). Thus, superselective catheter and direct puncture needle positioning distal to *ALL* normal branches supplying parenchyma and immediately proximal to the AVM "nidum" itself will obviate tissue necrosis being that the capillary beds are not embolized and only the abnormal AV connections are sclerosed. However, Yakes Type IV AVMs infiltrate an entire tissue, thus termed as an "infiltrative" form of AVM. Being that the "infiltrated" tissue (e.g., auricular AVMs) is viable proves that capillary beds are undoubtedly interspersed along with the innumerable microfistulae throughout the involved tissue as well. Transarterial injection of ethanol by transcatheter/transmicrocatheter will sclerose the innumerable microfistulae but also would flood the capillary beds with ethanol devitalizing that diseased infiltrated tissue. Necrosis of that tissue would then ensue secondary to the concurrent occlusion of the capillary beds. Thus, Yakes Type IV AVMs posited a profound conundrum to treat by endovascular approaches (Fig. 30.5). Polymerizing agents would also occlude AVFs but also occlude the capillary beds as well causing massive tissue necrosis of that embolized tissue such as by glue and Onyx as well.

Thinking through this conundrum, one could rightly conclude that the only option is total surgical resection of that entire tissue as the only treatment option. After further reflection, an endovascular option for curative treatment, not palliative treatment, well considered was a strong possibility. Capillary beds have normal increased peripheral resistance which has a somewhat restrictive vascular flow pattern from artery to capillary to veins. AVMs/AVFs have abnormally lowered peripheral vascular resistance with rapid shunting into arterialized veins. The AVM outflow veins are then arterialized and hypertensive and have arterial pressures. The postcapillary outflow normotensive veins then compete with the higher arterialized pressure AVM outflow veins for outflow venous return. This vein hypertension then further restricts normal vein outflow, which in turn increases the systemic vascular resistance (SVR) of the normal arterioles immediately proximal to the capillary beds, now

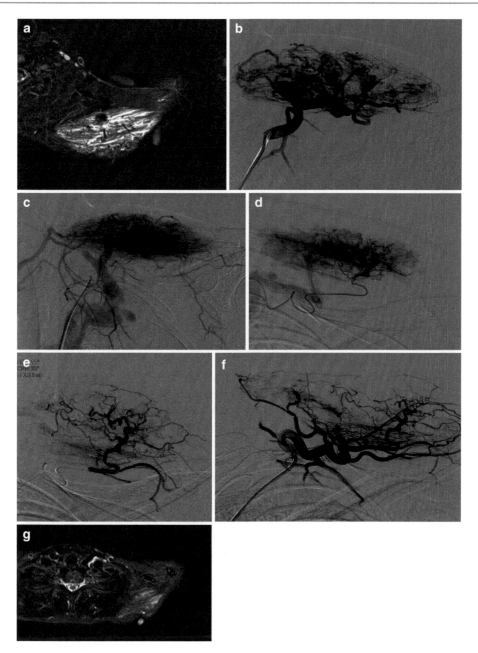

Fig. 30.5 (a) Axial left shoulder MR with STIR sequences demonstrating bright signal throughout left supraclavicular trapezius muscle. (b) Example of Yakes Type IV AVM. Selective DSA, early phase demonstrating total intramuscular infiltration of trapezius with AVM admixed with capillaries. (c) Selective DSA, venous phase demonstrating dense vascular stain with multiple outflow veins totally infiltrating the trapezius muscle. (d) Pre-embolization DSA with microcatheter superselectively placed to inject a 50% mixture of ethanol and non-ionic contrast. (e) Post-ethanol injection DSA. After embolization with 50% mixture of ethanol and non-ionic contrast, note that all arterial run-off branches are intact and there is no residual dense contrast tissue staining. Infiltrative Yakes Type IV AVM microfistulae have been occluded. The tissue capillary beds remain intact as evidenced by the excellent arterial run-off. (f) Global selective DSA demonstrating the absence of microfistula staining and normal arterial run-off supply. No tissue necrosis or injury occurred. (g) Axial MR STIR sequence demonstrating markedly decreased signal in left trapezius muscle. Compare to (a). Markedly decreased signal is consistent with significant ablation of Yakes Type IV AVM in the trapezius muscle. Compare to (a)

restricting arteriolar inflow to the capillary beds. The increased SVR into the capillaries coupled with abnormally low-resistance shunting into the admixed innumerable AVF allows for preferential vascular flow into the AVFs.

Mixing non-ionic contrast with absolute ethanol changes the viscosity and specific gravity of ethanol in this embolic mixture. Being "thickened" allows for preferential flow to the AVFs (lower-resistance vessels) and further restricts flow into the capillaries (higher-resistance vessels). Despite being 50% diluted with contrast, the ethanol can still effectively sclerose the innumerable microfistulae due to the small luminal diameters. This combination of preferential flow into the innumerable AVFs, the increased SVR into the capillaries restricting flow, the increased opacified ethanol viscosity, and changing the specific gravity with contrast of the ethanol 50% mixture all works to spare the capillaries and sclerose the innumerable AVF. Using pure ethanol would diminish this capillary sparing effect, and the AVFs and capillaries would both be sclerosed and occluded. This would cure the AVFs but would devitalize the tissue itself with occlusion of the capillaries. Use of various polymerizing embolic occlusive agents (NBCA; Onyx) would also cause the same devitalization of the tissues with occlusion of the capillaries. Particulate embolic agents (PVA, Contour Embolic, Embospheres, etc.) cannot permanently occlude the AVF and will make the capillaries ischemic with the proximal occlusion in the inflow arterioles but will not devitalize the tissues.

Summary

Yakes Type I: Can be permanently occluded, with mechanical devices such as coils, fibered coils, Amplatzer plugs, and other occluding devices. Ethanol alone can be curative in smaller diameter AVFs.

Yakes Type IIa: Can be permanently transarterially treated with undiluted absolute ethanol. At times, slowing the arterial inflow into the "nidum" with occlusion balloons, tourniquets, and blood pressure cuffs allows for less ethanol to be used to treat the AVM compartments. Direct puncture techniques into the inflow artery or AVM "nidum" allow ethanol to permeate and treat the AVM as well.

Yakes Type IIIa: Can be permanently occluded with transarterial, if possible, embolizations with ethanol of the vein wall "nidum" the same way as in the Yakes Type IIa AVM. They can also be permanently occluded by dense coil packing of the vein aneurysm sac itself with, or without, ethanol embolization. This can be accomplished via direct puncture of the vein aneurysm or by retrograde vein catheterization of the vein aneurysm cavity.

Yakes Type IIIb: Can be permanently occluded via transarterial approach as in Yakes Type II AVMs. They can be permanently occluded by treating the vein aneurysm itself and the multiple aneurysmal outflow veins also by coil embolization.

Yakes Type IV: Can be permanently occluded via transarterial superselective 50% mixture of non-ionic contrast and ethanol that treats the micro-AVFs and spares the higher-resistance capillaries. Direct puncture with 23 gauge needles into the microfistulous AV connections with 100% ethanol injections is also possible and curative.

References

1. Decker DG, Fish CR, Juergens JL. Arteriovenous fistulas of the female pelvis: a diagnostic problem. Obstet Gynecol. 1968;31:799–805.
2. Szilagyi DE, Smith RF, Elliott JP, Hageman JH. Congenital arteriovenous anomalies of the limbs. Arch Surg. 1976;111:423–9.
3. Flye MW, Jordan BP, Schwartz MZ. Management of congenital arteriovenous malformations. Surgery. 1983;94:740–7.
4. Mulliken JB, Glowacki J. Hemangiomas and vascular malformations in infants and children: a classification based on endothelial characteristics. Plast Reconstr Surg. 1982;69:412–20.
5. Mulliken JB, Zetter BR, Folkman J. In vitro characteristics of endothelium from hemangiomas and vascular malformations. Surgery. 1982;92:348–53.
6. Glowacki J, Mulliken JB. Mast cells in hemangiomas and vascular malformations. Pediatrics. 1982;70:48–51.

7. Finn MC, Glowacki J, Mulliken JB. Congenital vascular lesions: clinical application of a new classification. J Pediatr Surg. 1983;18:894–900.
8. Upton J, Mulliken JB, Murray JE. Classification and rationale for management of vascular anomalies in the upper extremity. J Hand Surg. 1985;6:970–5.
9. Mulliken JB, Young AE, editors. Vascular birthmarks: hemangiomas and malformations. Philadelphia: WB Saunders; 1988.
10. Lee DH, Wriest CH, Kaufman JCE, Pelz DM, Fox AJ, Vinuela F. Evaluation of three embolic agents in pig rete. AJNR. 1989;10:773–6.
11. Swarc TA, Carrasco CH, Wallace S, Richli W. Radiopaque suspension of polyvinyl alcohol foam for embolization. AJR. 1986;146:591–2.
12. Widlus DM, Murray RR, White Jr RI, et al. Congenital arteriovenous malformations: tailored embolotherapy. Radiology. 1988;169:511–6.
13. Rao VRK, Mandalam KR, Gupta AK, Kumar S, Joseph S. Dissolution of isobutyl 2-cyanoacrylate on long-term follow-up. AJNR. 1989;10:135–41.
14. Serbinenko FA. Balloon catheterization and occlusion of major cerebral vessels. J Neurosurg. 1975;41: 125–45.
15. Jackson JE, Mansfield AO, Allison DJ. Treatment of high-flow vascular malformations by venous embolization aided by flow occlusion techniques. Cardiovasc Intervent Radiol. 1996;19:323–8.
16. Cho SK, Do YS, Kim DI, Kim YW, Shin SW, Park KB, Ko JS, Lee AR, Choo SW, Choo IW. Peripheral arteriovenous malformations with a dominant outflow vein: results of ethanol embolization. Korean J Radiol. 2008;9:258–67.
17. Merland JJ, Riche MC, Chiras J. Intraspinal extramedullary arteriovenous fistula draining into medullary veins. J Neuroradiol. 1980;7:271–320.

Patricia E. Burrows

Introduction

Management of VMs varies for each patient depending on the extent and symptomatology of the lesion [1]. The usual indications for treatment include pain, swelling, disfigurement, bleeding, and consumption coagulopathy [2]. Focal VMs are typically treated with sclerotherapy (Fig. 31.1), while extensive diffuse VMs of the limbs are often managed primarily with compression garments. Diffuse VMs often contain painful focal venous expansions or varicosities that benefit from endovascular treatment (Fig. 31.2). Diffuse VM of the lower extremity typically has intra-articular involvement of the knee, which is known to cause progressive damage to the cartilage and degenerative arthritis. It is currently thought that early resection of the intra-articular VM may improve the prognosis for joint function [3, 4]. The most commonly used endovascular techniques for treating venous malformations are percutaneous injection of sclerosing medications, without and with permanent outflow occlusion, and endovenous laser treatment [5]. Except for very small lesions, patients should be evaluated with MRI and a coagulation profile. There are many indications for treatment, including pain, mass effect, and deformity. Endovascular treatment is usually performed in an angiography suite, although superficial lesions can be treated with ultrasound guidance in the clinic or operating room [6]. Resection can be effective for bulky lesions, especially when resection will not significantly affect function.

Techniques

Sclerotherapy or Percutaneous Embolization of Extra Truncal VM

Sclerotherapy is a technique in which a sclerosing drug is injected directly into the vascular malformation in order to achieve endothelial cell death and subsequent fibrosis. The most commonly used sclerosants are absolute ethanol, sodium tetradecyl sulfate (STS), polidocanol, and bleomycin. In general, the efficacy of the procedure depends upon the quality of contact of the concentrated sclerosant solution with all of the endothelial lining of the VM. STS and polidocanol are best administered as foam, as it has been shown that a foamed agent is more effective in displacing the blood and penetrating the VM. Foam can be created by mixing the agent with an equal amount of air across a three-way stopcock. Adding an epidural filter helps to produce a denser foam. The addition of oily contrast medium [Lipiodol] produces a foam that is more stable than that made with air alone. There is also

P.E. Burrows, MD
Medical College of Wisconsin, Children's Hospital of Wisconsin, Milwaukee, WI, USA
e-mail: PBurrows@chw.org

© Springer-Verlag Berlin Heidelberg 2017
Y.-W. Kim et al. (eds.), *Congenital Vascular Malformations*, DOI 10.1007/978-3-662-46709-1_31

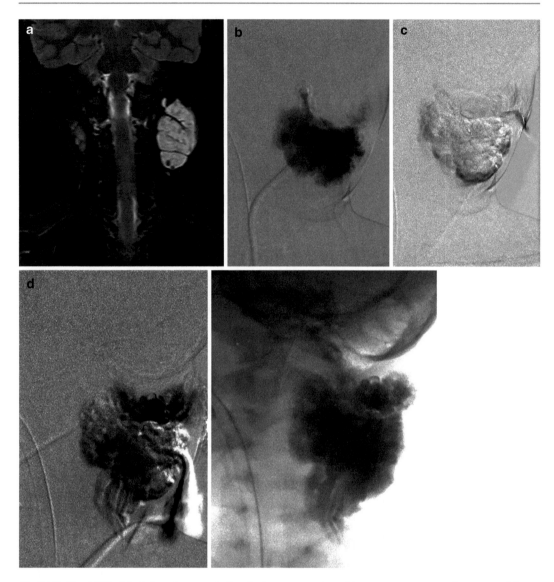

Fig. 31.1 Focal VM of the left neck recurred after single injection of small amount of STS. (**a**) Coronal STIR MRI shows the septated smooth-walled lesion containing phleboliths. No dilated veins adjacent to the mass. (**b**) Direct contrast injection fills the lower part of the mass. No draining veins. A second vent needle was placed. (**c**) Roadmap image during injection of 3% STS foam. Some penetration of the upper compartment has occurred due to the vent needle. (**d**) Roadmap image during injection of opacified bleomycin through the vent needle, filling the entire lesion. (**e**) Fluoroscopic image shows good filling of the entire lesion. The patient had a good response with almost complete regression after one procedure

a commercial polidocanol foam available in a convenient dispenser. Ethanol, STS, and polidocanol all cause intralesional thrombosis and inflammation, leading to significant swelling. A number of technical variations have been developed to enhance the effectiveness and safety of sclerotherapy procedures.

All of these agents can be effective in obliterating a blood vessel or venous lake, but cure of a venous malformation is usually not achieved, due to the genetic nature of the malformation and the regenerative ability of human tissue.

Sclerotherapy is usually performed with sedation or general anesthesia. Patients are often premedicated with IV fluids, antibiotics, and steroids. Ultrasound guidance can be used to access the lesion. Usually, the deep compartments are cannulated first. A variety of needles are used,

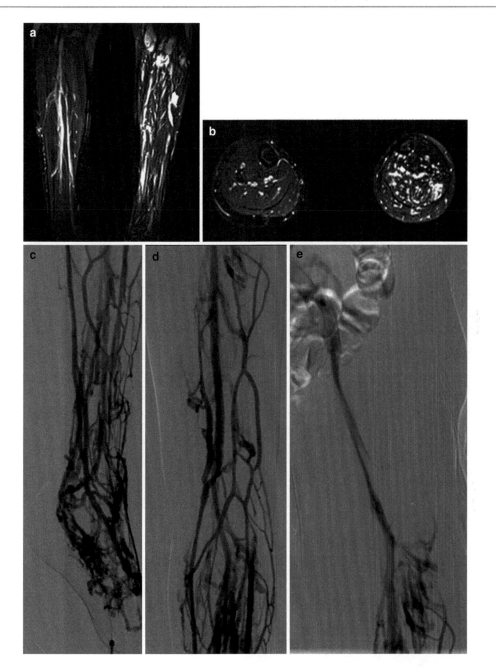

Fig. 31.2 Diffuse VM of the left lower extremity with undergrowth, dolichophlebectasia and progressive development of symptomatic venous lakes. See clinical photograph **a**. (**a, b**) Coronal and axial STIR images show smaller size of the left lower extremity, generalized prominence of venous channels, and some focal VMs. (**c–e**) Ascending venogram performed with the injector and step table digital subtraction technique shows generalized enlargement of deep and superficial veins from foot to pelvis. (**f**) Contrast injection in a focal VM of the foot, with connections to truncal vein. This was effectively sclerosed with foam. (**g**) Contrast injection in painful varicosities in gastrocnemius muscle, shows complex interconnecting varices draining to popliteal vein. This was embolized with n-BCA and foam. (**h**) Contrast injection into VM of the vastus lateralis, contributing to knee pain. This was embolized with n-BCA followed by foam. (**i**) Radiographic image after embolization of the vastus lateralis lesion and sclerosant injection [foam with Lipiodol] and superficial lesion below the patella. (**j**) Sagittal MRI of knee shows development of VM in the articular space and early degenerative changes. (**k**) T2-weighted MRI of pelvis showing numerous VMs in the left perirectal area and hip. (**l**) Percutaneous transperineal contrast injection shows that part of the VM seen on MRI is dilation of the left obturator internus vein. This was embolized with n-BCA and foam, preserving the rest of the internal iliac veins

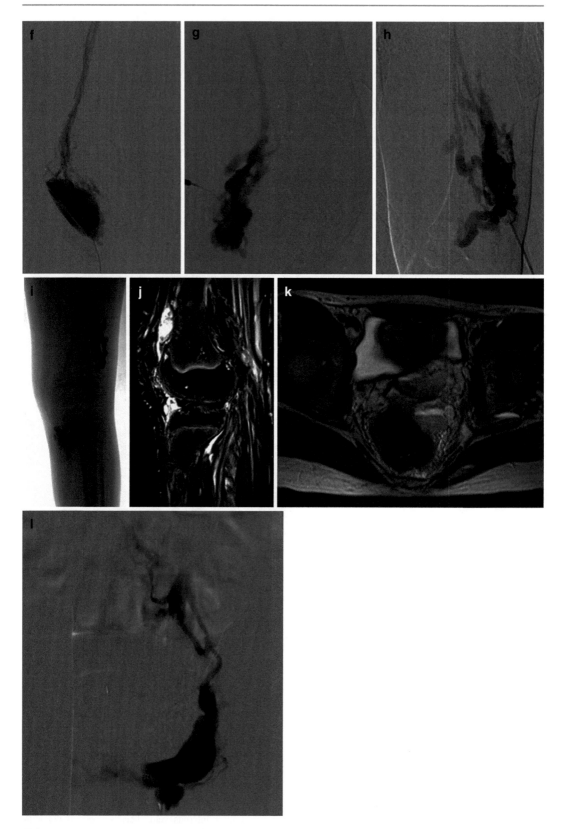

Fig. 31.2 (continued)

from tiny butterfly or hypodermic needles for superficial lesions, to larger [20gauge] sheathed needles, such as IV cannulas. After confirming needle placement and visualizing blood return through the needle, contrast medium is injected while fluoroscopic or radiographic acquisitions are obtained. Some types of angiographic equipment provide excellent image quality using the roadmap function, which uses a significantly lower radiation dose than regular digital subtraction angiography. The purpose of contrast injection is to confirm needle placement in the malformation, estimate the volume of the lesion, assess the venous drainage, and rule out the possibility of intra-arterial injection. The latter is the most important reason to always inject contrast medium as intra-arterial sclerosant injection can lead to catastrophic complications. All of the sclerosing agents used for VM, except for bleomycin, cause severe tissue necrosis when injected intra-arterially. The sclerosant injection can be monitored with roadmap imaging, as the unopacified agent, especially when foamed, displaces the previously injected contrast medium and appears white. When the lesion is filled with sclerosant, or when a draining vein is visualized, the injection is stopped. After waiting a few minutes, it is often possible to inject additional sclerosant, as the venous outflow may have occluded. Once contrast injection has shown favorable anatomy, it is also reasonable to monitor the injection by ultrasound, and the probe can be used to massage the agent into unfilled compartments.

Once there is rapid venous drainage, the draining vein should be controlled during the injection (Fig. 31.3). This can be done by manual compression, but it is my opinion that this technique has a higher rate of recanalization than when permanent outflow occlusion is used. This can be accomplished by placing coils in the draining vein or in the VM, or by injecting dilute embolization glue [n-BCA: Lipiodol 1:5] until it reaches the outflow vein, and then carefully injecting sclerosant behind it (Fig. 31.2). N-BCA injection into deep compartments of VM is generally well tolerated, but in superficial veins, especially in the presence of open skin lesions, there is a potential for infected thrombosis or prolonged foreign body reaction.

Endovenous or interstitial laser therapy using a diode or Nd:Yag laser fiber introduced into the lesion through a needle or cannula is sometimes helpful in shrinking the lesion or closing the outflow. Sclerosant can be injected after removing the laser fiber.

The double needle technique was devised to improve penetration of a VM with foam, while minimizing dilution and size of clot by allowing blood and excess sclerosant to escape. Two cannulas are placed, usually at opposite ends of a VM compartment. The distal cannula is kept open to drain, while the sclerosant is injected through the proximal one. Once the agent starts to drain through the vent cannula, the injection is stopped. Removal of blood from focal lesions and reinjection of sclerosant appears to achieve a better response with less swelling.

Most VMs consist of multiple compartments or channels. These are injected sequentially. If ultrasound guidance is being used, the more superficial part should be injected last, to maximize visualization with ultrasound. Injection of small cutaneous lesions is best done with direct observation of the skin rather than with imaging guidance, as it is important to note any color change that might lead to necrosis. If color change, such as blanching, occurs, the injection is stopped, and the skin is compressed gently with cold saline-soaked compresses.

Ethanol is an effective sclerosant for venous malformations, causing immediate necrosis of the endothelium and vein wall, and later causing intralesional thrombosis [7]. It is extremely painful on injection and thus is used with general anesthesia. Ethanol causes severe swelling, maximum about 24 h after the injection. Skin necrosis and peripheral neuropathy are relatively common complications. In most cases, nerve function recovers. A small percentage of patients receiving ethanol for ablation or sclerotherapy develop cardiopulmonary complications including severe hypoxia or electromechanical dissociation and cardiac arrest [8]. These complications are thought to be caused by microemboli and/or severe pulmonary vasospasm causing acute right heart failure. A number of studies have been undertaken to identify risks for this complication. A formula

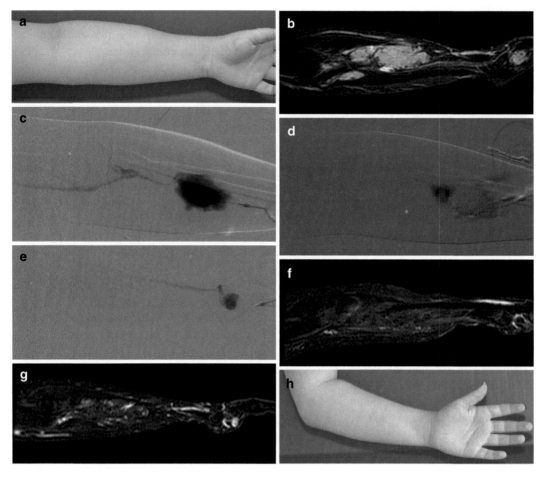

Fig. 31.3 Multifocal or diffuse VM of the forearm causing pain and weakness in a 10-year-old girl. (**a**) Photograph prior to treatment showing asymmetrical enlargement of the proximal forearm and base of thumb. (**b**) STIR coronal MRI of forearm shows multiple intramuscular VM's. (**c**) Percutaneous injection of one of the large focal VM's, showing minimal drainage. This was embolized with STS foam followed by bleomycin with double needle technique. (**d**) Roadmap image showing contrast injection in a second focal VM. (**e**) Contrast injection in a VM of the base of thumb. (**f**) STIR coronal MRI 2 months after the sclerotherapy procedure. Focal lesions are mainly closed, but there is still some swelling and thrombus. (**g**) STIR coronal MRI 6 months after the sclerotherapy procedure shows resolution of the focal lesions and decrease size of the soft tissues. (**h**) Photograph taken 2 months after sclerotherapy showing marked improvement in swelling. Patient was asymptomatic and able to return to sports

to inject no more than 0.1 mL per kilogram, no more frequently than every 10 min, has been proposed.

Total sclerosant volume per session is generally limited to 0.5 mL per kilogram. Diffusion through the wall of the VM into the surrounding tissue and skin is known to occur, and this can contribute to skin necrosis and nerve injury. Patients receiving a large amount of sclerosant need excellent hydration to avoid sequelae of hemoglobinuria.

Bleomycin is also an effective agent for treating VMs [9]. In addition to a mild sclerosing affect, bleomycin appears to recruit fibroblasts. It does not directly cause thrombosis, and therefore causes the least amount of swelling after injection. For these reasons, bleomycin is the most appropriate agent for treating sites where swelling is poorly tolerated, such as the orbit, airway, and some muscle compartments (Figs. 31.3 and 31.4). Disadvantages include the fact that treatment with bleomycin alone usually requires more procedures than with other sclerosants, and concern for pulmonary fibrosis. Injection of bleomycin after outflow occlusion with ethanol or foam is a good compromise [10] (Figs. 31.1, 31.3, and 31.4). This way, the bleomycin is retained in the VM, where it is more effective, and absorbed very slowly into the circulation. Bleomycin can also be "thickened" by foaming with an equal volume of albumin. The bleomycin dose is limited to 0.5 units/kg or 15 units per procedure, with the lifetime limit of 300 units. It should not be administered more frequently than every 2 weeks. When used as the sole

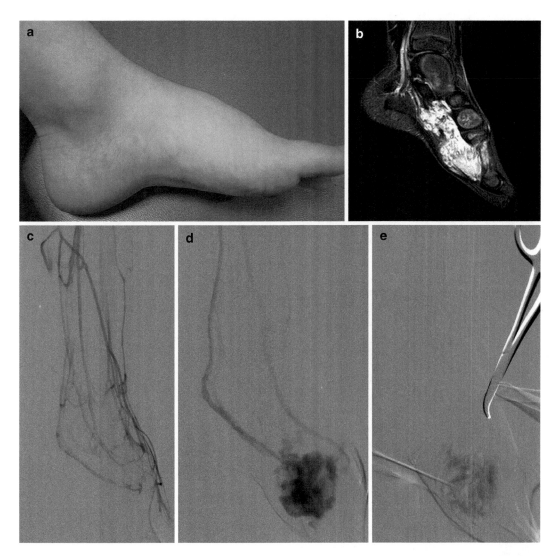

Fig. 31.4 Twelve-year-old boy with enlarging painful mass, sole of left foot. (**a**) Photograph prior to treatment showing soft tissue swelling in the arch. (**b**) Sagittal STIR image prior to treatment showing extensive intramuscular VM. (**c**) Ascending venogram through pedal IV shows normal anatomy. Cannula connected to heparinized saline infusion. (**d**) Contrast injection into anterior part of VM, shows direct drainage to plantar and dorsal veins. (**e**) Injection of STS foam using tourniquet control around the midfoot shows good retention within VM. Double needle technique with manual expression of blood after foam injection. (**f**) fluoroscopic image after injection of bleomycin/contrast mixture. (**g**) Sagittal STIR image 3 months after first sclerotherapy, shows residual VM, especially posteriorly. Patient was improved. (**h**) Contrast injection prior to the second sclerotherapy, posterior compartment of VM. (**i**) Sagittal T2-weighted image 3 months after second sclerotherapy. Good reduction of VM. (**j**) 3 months after treatment, patient has no pain or limitations

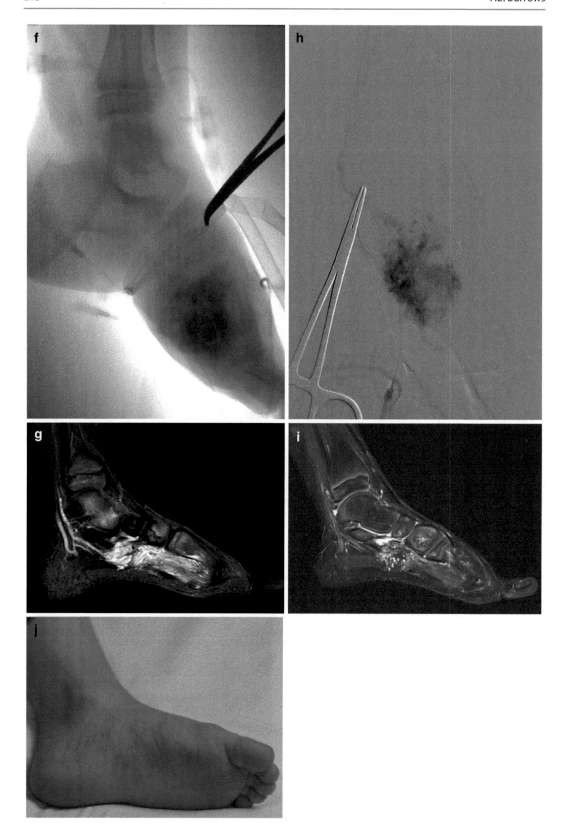

Fig. 31.4 (continued)

sclerosant, it works best when administered every 3 weeks. A study comparing ethanol and bleomycin showed that the bleomycin had similar efficacy in terms of symptom relief with less complications than ethanol, but required more procedures [11]. Pulmonary fibrosis has not yet been reported as a complication of sclerotherapy, although some patients have developed severe acute pulmonary reactions. More common side effects include severe nausea and vomiting and pigmentation of the skin.

Following completion of sclerotherapy, antibiotic ointment can be applied to the treated area to keep the skin moist. A loose dressing may be applied, but tight compression should be avoided. The treated area should be elevated, and ice is often helpful to control swelling and pain. Hydration, corticosteroids, and analgesics are prescribed.

Complications of ethanol and foam sclerotherapy are relatively common and include skin necrosis, peripheral nerve injury, compartment syndrome, deep vein thrombosis, pulmonary embolism, and cardiac arrest. Most of these can be avoided by using common sense. While ethanol is an effective sclerosant, it has the highest rate of serious complications, such as peripheral nerve injury and cardiac arrest. Foam sclerosant can also cause tissue necrosis and swelling, but nerve injury is much less common, and cardiac arrest is extremely rare [12]. Hemoglobinuria is caused by the lysis of blood cells that are in contact with sclerosant and drain into the systemic circulation. It can cause renal tubular obstruction and acute renal failure, if the patient is not very well hydrated.

In patients with extensive VM, sclerotherapy is usually repeated every 2–3 months. If only part of the lesion can be treated in one session, procedures can be spaced more closely. Patients with intramuscular VM should be encouraged to stretch the treated area or undergo physical therapy starting 2 weeks after the procedure, to prevent contractures.

For most patients with VM, sclerotherapy results in significant improvement in swelling and pain. However, extensive lesions usually are not cured, and symptoms will usually recur. The timing between completion of treatment and recurrence of symptoms depends on how thoroughly the lesion has been treated, and the biology of the VM. After staged treatment, many patients are asymptomatic for 7–10 years, although some VMs are more aggressive and recur faster than others. If the lesion is inadequately treated, symptoms are often improved initially, but recur after a few months. While surgical excision is helpful in specific cases, partial resection is often followed by rapid, sometimes more severe, recurrence.

Outcome of Endovascular Treatment of VMs

There are very few published series of long-term follow-up after treatment [13]. In the short term, almost all patients improve in terms of swelling and pain. Partial recurrence is common. Diffuse VMs of the lower extremities cannot be cured and become more symptomatic with reduced function over time.

Rapamycin has been used to treat a small number of patients with extensive VM, and appears to be effective in controlling pain and bleeding and improving coagulopathy [14].

Endovascular Treatment of Truncal Venous Malformations

Truncal VMs consist of dysplastic venous conducting channels, including the main conducting veins in patients with diffuse VM of a limb. Anomalous venous channels are most commonly seen in patients with combined slow flow vascular malformations, often with limb overgrowth. The anomalous veins in patients with CLVM or CLOVES syndrome are often tortuous, valveless channels that contribute to pooling of blood, resulting in pain, venous hypertension, thrombosis and pulmonary emboli, and sometimes orthostatic hypotension. Prior to closure of these channels, detailed venous mapping is necessary to evaluate the deep veins for adequacy. Often, the size of the anomalous superficial vein is inversely proportional to the size of the deep veins. In the

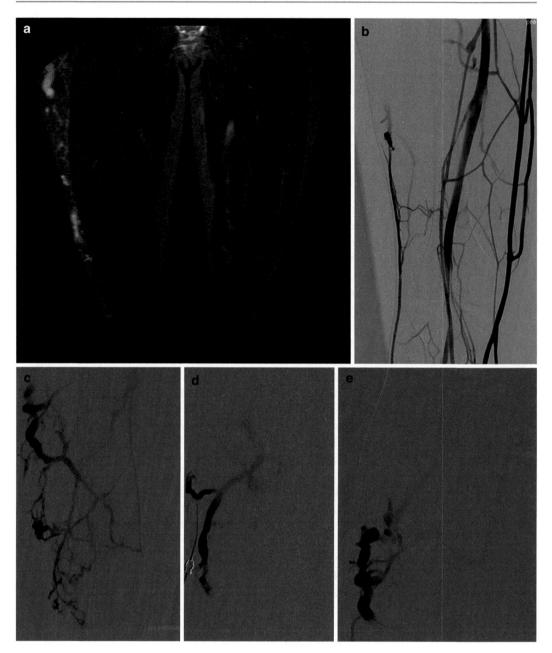

Fig. 31.5 Painful superficial varicosities of the right lateral thigh. (**a**) STIR coronal image shows tortuous veins in the subcutaneous fat of the right lateral thigh. (**b**) Ascending venogram right lower extremity, level of right thigh, shows normal femoral and saphenous veins, lateral marginal vein leading to the varicosities. (**c**) Contrast injection in one of the varicosities shows a network of subcutaneous veins communicating with the profunda femoral veins. (**d**) Selective cannulation of one of the draining channels. This was embolized with n-BCA followed by STS. (**e**) Contrast injection in a more superficial channel, also draining centrally. This was embolized with n-BCA, followed by STS. (**f**) Radiograph shows the n-BCA: lipiodol outlining the embolized veins. The center of the veins is more radiolucent, due to the presence of STS foam displacing the n-BCA. (**g**) Ascending venogram post embolization shows continued patency of the femoral and saphenous veins

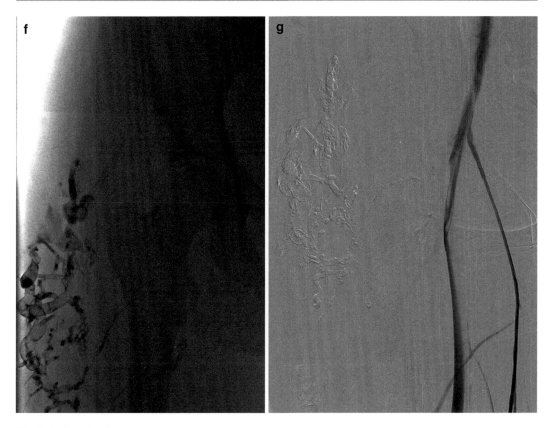

Fig. 31.5 (continued)

lower extremity, the deep veins must be imaged from the foot to the inferior vena cava. Care must be taken to avoid closing the main drainage pathways. Once the appropriate targets have been determined, the anomalous vein is usually catheterized distally, above the main communication between the foot and the deep veins. If the anomalous vein is amenable to catheterization throughout its length, it can be treated with endovenous laser ablation, or embolization. The technique for endovenous laser ablation is similar to that used for saphenous ablation [15, 16]. Two disadvantages of laser are the size of the anomalous vein, which may be several centimeters in diameter, and the location, which may be near a major nerve trunk. Laser should be avoided in the latter, due to the possibility of causing painful nerve injury. It may be necessary to combine endovenous laser and embolization or sclerotherapy to achieve safe and adequate occlusion. Extremely tortuous anomalous veins may need to be treated in seg-

ments. Embolization can be carried out with a combination of large fibered coils and sclerosant, or n-BCA. When using liquid agents, it is important to be aware of the perforators, to avoid damage to the deep veins (Fig. 31.5). Infusion of heparinized saline in a distal pedal vein is helpful to minimize the risk of DVT.

After performing ablation of conducting veins, compression stockings or wraps are usually applied. It may be appropriate to prescribe low molecular weight heparin for 2 weeks. If the veins are large, patients may need a second procedure to complete the ablation.

Summary

There are numerous endovascular techniques to treat symptomatic venous malformations. Most of these are effective in relieving symptoms, but patients with extensive disease typically require retreatment for many years, especially during periods of active growth. Because of the high potential for recurrence, techniques with the lowest chance of complications should be chosen.

References

1. Lee BB, Baumgartner I, Berlien P, Bianchini G, Burrows P, Gloviczki P, et al. Diagnosis and treatment of venous malformations. Consensus document of the international union of phlebology (IUP): updated 2013. Int Angiol: J Int Union Angiol. 2015;34(2):97–149.
2. Mazoyer E, Enjolras O, Laurian C, Houdart E, Drouet L. Coagulation abnormalities associated with extensive venous malformations of the limbs: differentiation from Kasabach-Merritt syndrome. Clin Lab Haematol. 2002;24(4):243–51.
3. Enjolras O, Ciabrini D, Mazoyer E, Laurian C, Herbreteau D. Extensive pure venous malformations in the upper or lower limb: a review of 27 cases. J Am Acad Dermatol. 1997;36(2 Pt 1):219–25.
4. Pireau N, Boon LM, Poilvache P, Docquier PL. Surgical treatment of intra-articular knee venous malformations: when and how? J Pediatr Orthop. 2016;36:316–22.
5. Burrows PE. Endovascular treatment of slow-flow vascular malformations. Tech Vasc Interv Radiol. 2013;16(1):12–21.
6. Jain R, Bandhu S, Sawhney S, Mittal R. Sonographically guided percutaneous sclerosis using 1 % polidocanol in the treatment of vascular malformations. J Clin Ultrasound. 2002;30(7):416–23.
7. Lee IH, Kim KH, Jeon P, Byun HS, Kim HJ, Kim ST, et al. Ethanol sclerotherapy for the management of craniofacial venous malformations: the interim results. Korean J Radiol. 2009;10(3):269–76.
8. Chapot R, Laurent A, Enjolras O, Payen D, Houdart E. Fatal cardiovascular collapse during ethanol sclerotherapy of a venous malformation. Interv Neuroradiol. 2002;8(3):321–4.
9. Zheng JW, Yang XJ, Wang YA, He Y, Ye WM, Zhang ZY. Intralesional injection of Pingyangmycin for vascular malformations in oral and maxillofacial regions: an evaluation of 297 consecutive patients. Oral Oncol. 2009;45(10):872–6.
10. Jin Y, Lin X, Li W, Hu X, Ma G, Wang W. Sclerotherapy after embolization of draining vein: a safe treatment method for venous malformations. J Vasc Surg. 2008; 47(6):1292–9.
11. Spence J, Krings T, TerBrugge KG, Agid R. Percutaneous treatment of facial venous malformations: a matched comparison of alcohol and bleomycin sclerotherapy. Head Neck. 2011;33(1):125–30.
12. Stuart S, Barnacle AM, Smith G, Pitt M, Roebuck DJ. Neuropathy after sodium tetradecyl sulfate sclerotherapy of venous malformations in children. Radiology. 2015;274(3):897–905.
13. Rautio R, Saarinen J, Laranne J, Salenius JP, Keski-Nisula L. Endovascular treatment of venous malformations in extremities: results of sclerotherapy and the quality of life after treatment. Acta Radiol. Stockholm, Sweden : 19872004;45(4):397–403.
14. Boscolo E, Limaye N, Huang L, Kang KT, Soblet J, Uebelhoer M, et al. Rapamycin improves TIE2-mutated venous malformation in murine model and human subjects. J Clin Invest. 2015;125(9):3491–504.
15. Gloviczki P, Driscoll DJ. Klippel-Trenaunay syndrome: current management. Phlebology. 2007;22(6):291–8. Venous Forum of the Royal Society of Medicine
16. King K, Landrigan-Ossar M, Clemens R, Chaudry G, Alomari AI. The use of endovenous laser treatment in toddlers. J vasc Interv Radiol: JVIR. 2013;24(6):855–8.

Endovascular Treatment of AVMs: Head and Neck

32

Wayne F. Yakes, Krasnodar Ivancev,
Robert L. Vogelzang, and Alexis M. Yakes

Vascular anomalies constitute some of the most difficult diagnostic and therapeutic enigmas that can be encountered in the practice of medicine, particularly in the complex anatomy of the head and neck region. Daunting functional anatomy and gross disfigurement are significant issues in the management of such anomalies in the head and neck area. Clinical presentations can be extremely varied, and attributing these symptoms that a patient may present with to a vascular malformation can be challenging to the most experienced physician. It is of paramount importance that a modern classification system, by way of identifying these lesions at the cellular histologic level in their common characteristics, eliminate the current confusion and allow all clinicians to speak the same language. Accurate terminology leads to precise identification of complex vascular entities and, thus, enhances patient care. It is for this reason that Mulliken, Glowacki, and

coworkers have provided us all with a classification system that, in my mind, is landmark in its impact [1–4]. This classification system has been adopted by the International Society for the Study of Vascular Anomalies (ISSVA).

Interventional radiology and interventional neuroradiology have pioneered a minimally invasive therapeutic specialty to treat a wide variety of vascular and nonvascular lesions of the body, the brain, spine, spinal cord, and head and neck areas. Interventional procedures routinely use minimally invasive, direct puncture, and transcatheter techniques to treat many conditions. In the head/neck area, the vast majority of entities that are treated are largely of vascular origin. The extensive array of catheters, guidewires, embolic agents, digital imaging systems, and the pharmaceutical products that are commonly used are a tribute to the hard work, insight, and imagination of the many dedicated investigators in this area. Because of significant laboratory research, clinical research, and extensive clinical experience, the judicious use of endovascular therapy is now commonplace in modern clinical practice. Now that it is firmly established as an essential therapeutic tool, its role will only continue to grow. In the head and neck, and paraspinal region, embolotherapy procedures have become an essential therapeutic modality that has assisted our colleagues in otolaryngology, plastic and reconstructive surgery, neurosurgery, ophthalmology,

W.F. Yakes, MD (✉) • A.M. Yakes, BM
The Yakes Vascular Malformation Center,
Englewood, CO 80113, USA
e-mail: Wayne.yakes@vascularmalformationcenter.com

R.L. Vogelzang, MD
Northwestern Medical Center, Chicago, IL, USA

K. Ivancev, MD, PhD
Division of Vascular Surgery,
University of Hamburg Medical Center,
Hamburg, Germany

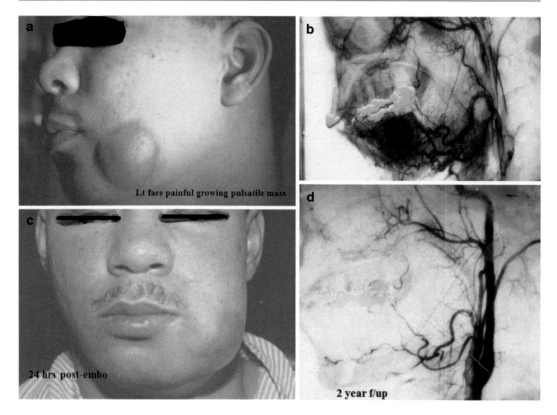

Fig. 32.1 (**a**) Left face painful pulsatile mass. (**b**) Left external carotid arteriogram demonstrating left face Yakes Type IIa AVM supplied from left facial artery. (**c**) Edema without tissue injury 24 h post-ethanol embolization. (**d**) Left common carotid DSA demonstrating cure of the AVM at 2-year follow-up

vascular surgery, and various pediatric surgical specialties. The scope of this chapter will deal with vascular malformations in the head and neck regions (Figs. 32.1, 32.2).

Vascular malformations were first treated by surgeons. The early rationale of proximal arterial ligation of arteriovenous malformations (AVMs) proved totally futile as the phenomenon of neovascular recruitment reconstituted arterial inflow to the AVM nidus. Microfistulous connections became macrofistulous feeders. Complete extirpation of an AVM nidus proved very difficult and extremely hazardous necessitating suboptimal partial resections, particularly in the head and neck.

The vast array of embolic agents that can be superselectively delivered with multiple catheter systems and direct puncture needles has blossomed due to the innovative ideas of numerous investigators and has led to improved quality and lower costs of care, quicker patient recuperation times, and the better outcomes that our patients deserve.

Particulate agents, coils, and detachable balloons dominated the early years of embolotherapy.

As catheter delivery systems and embolic agents improved, embolotherapy has since emerged as a primary mode of therapy in the management of vascular malformations. In many cases, these lesions are anatomically and surgically challenging or in surgically inaccessible areas.

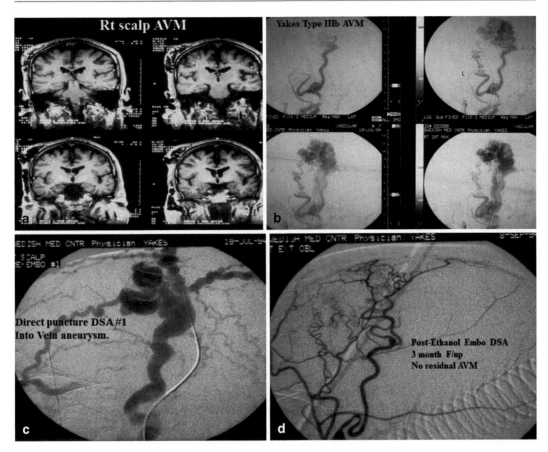

Fig. 32.2 (**a**) Head MR with coronal T1-weighted sequences demonstrating right scalp mass with flow-voids consistent with right scalp AVM. (**b**) Lateral right external carotid DSA demonstrating Yakes Type IIIb AVM. (**c**) Lateral direct puncture DSA into vein aneurysm demonstrating multiple out-flow veins diagnostic for Yakes Type IIIb AVM. The AVM "nidus" is the innumerable fistulae in the vein wall itself. Ethanol was injected into the vein aneurysm at this point. (**d**) Lateral right external carotid DSA demonstrating cure of the right scalp AVM

General Concepts

The main indication for Interventional Neuroradiologic procedures in the head and neck is largely as a preoperative measure to aid the surgeon in managing various clinical dilemmas. The various surgical specialties that have been served in the head and neck area are otolaryngology, plastic and reconstructive surgery, ophthalmology, neurosurgery, general surgery, maxillofacial surgery, and the various pediatric surgical specialists. Interventional procedures have been used to aid in the management of a wide variety of vascular lesions of the brain, head and neck, paraspinal area, and the upper thoracic region.

The various lesions managed include vascular neoplasms, congenital and post-traumatic vascular malformations, aneurysm disease, pseudoaneurysm disease, and epistaxis. Simply put, the goal of the endovascular approach in vascular lesions is to occlude or obliterate the abnormal vascular structures and retain all normal vascular structures. In those cases in which the carotid artery or vertebral artery may require sacrifice, preoperative test occlusion is performed. If the patient can tolerate the test occlusion procedure, these vessels are frequently sacrificed endovascularly prior to surgery to minimize the risks of postoperative stroke and intraprocedural hemorrhage. In extensive skull base tumors and other types of malignancies in which the risks of surgery are inherently high, interventional endovascular procedures have aided to allow a more complete resection and minimize the bleeding and the morbidity of the procedure.

In vascular tumors of the head and neck, preoperative embolization not only aids in the completeness of the surgical resection of the lesion, it reduces the surgical complication rate by providing an almost bloodless exposure with easier identification of important structures. Further, it can contribute to the shortening of the operation time which may be helpful in elderly patients.

Embolization procedures in the head and neck area should be performed only by interventionalists who are well trained and completely aware of the functional vascular anatomy. There are arterial anastomoses between the external carotid artery, internal carotid artery, and vertebral artery. If these collateral pathways are not recognized, then intracranial stroke can occur. Frequently encountered arterial anastomoses are those between the occipital artery and vertebral artery, the ascending pharyngeal artery and vertebral artery, the ascending pharyngeal artery and internal carotid artery, and the internal maxillary artery and internal carotid artery. Other primitive anastomoses may also be present that are retained from the fetal stage. These connections include the trigeminal artery, the otic artery, the hypoglossal artery, and the proatlantal intersegmental artery. Frequently during the course of an embolization, these anastomotic pathways are not visualized. However, as an embolization progresses and hemodynamics are altered, it can become very prominent, and this has to be recognized immediately. Techniques can be employed to avoid embolization risks despite such anastomoses being present. Superselective catheter and microcatheter placement, proximal temporary balloon occlusion to reverse flow from the major intracranial circulations, and protective embolization for temporary control of these anastomoses is needed. Not recognizing the sudden appearance of these anastomoses can result in disaster for the patient.

The cranial nerves and their extracranial segments are largely supplied by branches of the external carotid artery. Distal occlusion in these arteries could potentially cause a cranial nerve palsy. The type of embolic material used determines the degree of tissue ischemia and whether injured cranial nerves will recover or be permanently injured. Various external carotid arteries that supply the cranial nerves in the head and neck area are the ascending pharyngeal artery, the middle meningeal artery, the accessory meningeal artery, the stylomastoid branch occipital artery, the posterior auricular artery, the distal internal maxillary artery, and the transverse facial artery.

Whether cranial nerve palsy is permanent or transient can depend on several factors. If the artery is occluded proximal to the capillary bed level and the vasonervorum are intact, relative ischemia may occur that could cause transient nerve palsy. With revascularization by the collateral formations, clinical symptoms of cranial nerve injury may be improved though it does not return to normal. Embolic agents that can penetrate to the capillary bed level, such as liquid agents, are agents that exclude collateral circulation and can result in a temporary or permanent cranial nerve injury.

The cutaneous arterial branches of the external carotid artery that supply the scalp and overlying skin should be preserved. If these arteries do require embolization, then superselective catheter techniques can lessen the risks of causing ischemia and necrosis of the skin or scalp. This is particularly important in those groups of patients who will have scalp incisions, craniotomy, etc. If the arterial supply to that area is absent due to embolization, postoperative wound healing can be significantly retarded, infection can occur, and plastic surgery may be required to close the wound. The superficial temporal artery, deep temporal artery, posterior auricular artery, occipital artery, and muscular perforators from the vertebral artery all provide circulation to the scalp. If an entire distribution to a scalp area is occluded, scalp ischemia and necrosis can occur. Therefore, it is best when embolizing these vascular territories not to occlude large segments of these arteries. If one artery is occluded, collateral circulations will develop from contralateral side to overcome tissue ischemia. Too extensive of an embolization will not allow appropriate collateral artery formation.

In most cases, it is best to involve anesthesiology specialists to control the patient during these procedures. Consulting with the anesthesiologist will determine if a patient is to receive intravenous neuroleptic sedation or general anesthesia. If large doses of ethanol are thought to be used to treat a particular problem, then additional Swan-Ganz line and arterial line monitoring may be required. The Anesthesiology Pain Service can direct pain management strategies in the postoperative patient as well.

In those patients who have significant airway involvement with vascular malformation, whether it is a high-flow or a low-flow lesion, maintenance of the airway is an important consideration. In those unlucky patients who have involvement of the larynx, glottis, and vocal cords with vascular malformation, the mere act of intubation for endotracheal tube placement can cause swelling, and once the endotracheal tube is removed, the airway will occlude. It is extremely important to detect this possibility prior to contemplating endovascular therapy or general anesthesia. In this situation, a tracheostomy must be placed prior to any contemplated procedure. This will allow elective control of the airway and allow the malformation to be treated in a safe fashion. Thus, the multidisciplinary approach to complex problems in the head and neck is essential for optimal management of problematic lesions. Once the malformation is controlled and the tracheostomy is no longer needed, it can then be removed without incident. An emergent placement of a tracheostomy is always challenging, as opposed to an elective placement.

Concepts in Patient Management

After the diagnosis has been established, the next major decision is to determine whether therapy is warranted. The interventional radiologist/interventional neuroradiologist should plan and direct the patient's care with surgical specialists who are familiar with the management of hemangioma and vascular malformations and the problems with which they present. It is extremely important that appropriate surgical, medical, pediatric, and anesthesiologist specialists be involved for optimal patient care. They would function much like a tumor board team in the management of cancer.

With the use of intravascular ethanol, pain control is an issue. Anesthesiologists can greatly aid in solving this problem and determine whether general anesthesia or intravenous sedation is required for the proposed procedure. For children, general anesthesia is required. In patients with large vascular malformations, Swan-Ganz and arterial line monitoring are additionally performed. The maximum volume of ethanol used in treating patients with vascular malformations rarely exceeds 0.5 ml/kg body weight total dose. In some unusual instances, we will utilize up to 1 ml/kg body weight total dose. Most patients tolerate these total ethanol volumes very well. Exceeding these doses can lead to ethanol toxicity and is rarely needed in the head and neck area.

The area of vascular access, whether it is the groin, the arm, or other points of percutaneous catheter access, is prepped and draped in sterile fashion, as is the area of the malformation that is to be treated percutaneously. Fluoroscopy and/or CDI techniques are used in those patients requiring percutaneous access: Detailed arteriography is performed to determine the angioarchitecture of normal and abnormal arteries. In high-flow lesions, whereby the patient may have had prior therapy (surgical ligations, partial resections, coil placement, glue embolization, etc.), direct puncture techniques may be required to circumvent catheterization obstacles. Superselective placement of the catheter tip or the needle tip is a requirement. Only then can ethanol be injected into the malformation and all normal vascular structures be spared. To achieve superselectivity, coaxial and even triaxial systems may be required. In some instances, a long 6 or 8 French sheath may be placed at the groin into the abdominal aorta. Through this supporting sheath, 5 or 6

French catheter can be placed distally. Then through this 5 or 6 French distally placed catheter, a microcatheter can be triaxially placed in the even more distal positioning. Multiple arterial punctures may even be required to place additional catheters for distal embolization, or if necessary, occlusion balloon catheters to achieve some element of vascular stasis.

At times, even these complex maneuvers may fail and direct puncture of the malformation may be required. The area of percutaneous puncture is prepped and draped in sterile fashion. The needle, usually in the 18–23-gauge range, is advanced under real-time ultrasound guidance or by arterial contrast injections and fluoroscopic guidance. Once correct placement has been achieved with the direct puncture needle, contrast injections as well as ethanol injections may be performed through that needle. Proximal inflow occlusion may be necessary. Occlusion balloon catheters may be required to achieve vascular stasis. Bleeding is rarely a problem after removal of the direct puncture needle. However, if there is concern, as the needle is being retracted, a simple injection of Avitene (Alcon Laboratories, Ft. Worth, TX, USA), a topical hemostatic agent which can be injected (mixed with contrast) as the needle is retracted. This can be done in the direct puncture of high-flow malformations but usually is not required in the direct puncture of low-flow malformations.

After ethanol injection, I typically wait 10–15 min before performing another direct puncture angiogram or catheter angiogram. Frequently, additional compartments of vascular malformation will fill as others become thrombosed. The procedure is terminated when the maximum amount of ethanol is reached, if a significant amount of malformation is successfully treated, or if a complication occurs requiring the termination of the procedure.

After the procedure, the patient is revived from anesthesia and sent to the recovery room for observation. From there the patient is usually placed in a routine hospital ward for 4 h observation. It is unusual for patients to require placement in the intensive care unit (ICU). Postoperative management consists of intrave-nous Decadron, intravenous fluids, and IV Inapsine (droperidol injection, Janssen Pharmaceuticals, Inc., Titusville, NJ, USA) as needed to control nausea. Oral or intramuscular Toradol (Ketorolac Tromethamine, Syntex Laboratories, Palo Alto, CA, USA) is helpful for controlling pain and swelling in adult patients. Pain after a vascular malformation treatment is unusual; however, oral and IV pain medications may be given additionally if needed. Patients with GI sensitivity to steroids can also be placed on Zantac (Ranitidine Hydrochloride, Glaxo Inc., Research Triangle Park, NC, USA) to protect against gastric and duodenal ulcer development. If no complications have occurred that require management, the patient can be discharged the same day. Discharge medications usually include a tapering dose of steroids over 5–7 days, Zantac or Prilosec management to prevent ulcer development and pain medications, if required.

Patients always develop focal swelling in the area of malformation that is treated. In most patients, this swelling will resolve within 1–2 weeks. Usually after 4 weeks' time, all swelling is resolved and the patient, now at their new baseline, is ready for follow-up therapy as required. After serial ethanol endovascular therapy, MR and CDI can be used to document the efficacy of therapy. CDI spectral analysis gives accurate information in treated and untreated high-flow AVMs. AVMs demonstrate high-velocity and low-resistance waveforms on ultrasonographic examination. As the high-flow malformation serially becomes ablated, the waveform will normalize and the resistive indexes and flow volumes that can be calculated will become normalized as well.

MR is also an important follow-up modality. MR is excellent for evaluating high-flow and low-flow lesions as well as pediatric hemangioma. After serial ablation of a high-flow or low-flow lesion, alterations in the MR signal characteristics become obvious. In high-flow lesions on the T1 sequences, flow voids become absent, and thrombosed vessels are identified. Gradient echo sequences demonstrate decreased arterial vascularity because of the AVM thrombosis. In low-flow lesions, the T2-weighted fast spin-echo fat-suppressed imaging sequence and STIR sequences are important. Residual venous malformation will demonstrate markedly increased signal. Thrombosed and treated malformation will have a much-diminished signal. Our patients are evaluated with noninvasive and angiographic studies annually. After several years of persistent AVM closure, noninvasive imaging modalities can be sufficient follow-up.

Complications

Various complications can occur with any interventional procedure. Because vascular malformations are historically one of the most problematic lesions to ever be treated by any branch of medicine, complications must be expected. In our initial series, I reported a total complication rate of 30% (10% major, 20% minor), with more experience our complication rate has dropped overall to less than 10% [5]. Complications are related to the tissues that are being embolized. Nontarget embolization with ethanol will lead to tissue necrosis as capillary beds of normal arteries will be totally destroyed. The tissues that are being fed by these capillary beds will be devitalized and necrotic. Therefore, it is essential that superselective catheter positioning and superselective needle positioning be achieved before ethanol can be considered to be injected.

Vascular spasm, edematous tissues, and venous thrombosis can lead to complications. Localized skin blisters may occur, usually a minor annoyance that heals uneventfully. Injury to adjacent muscles, organs, or other tissues is possible. Motor or sensory nerve injuries can occur. We have found that most neural injuries have been related to the swelling with resultant nerve compression rather than nontarget embolization of the vasa nervorum. Aggressive Decadron therapy is essential to minimize the effects of the swelling and to allow the nerve to recover more quickly. It is unusual for nerve injuries to be permanent. Intense venous thrombosis can cause sufficient edema to initiate arterial thrombosis. The arterial thrombosis, coupled with the venogenic edema, can lead to extensive tissue necrosis. If suspected, then arteriography and fibrinolytic infusion must be performed to revascularize the tissues.

Bleeding is an uncommon complication of peripheral vascular malformations, unlike those of the brain and spinal cord whose propensity to bleed is their main presenting symptom. Vascular malformations will cause bleeding only if they involve the alimentary canal or in high-flow lesions that may cause superficial tissue ulceration related to arterial steel from normal tissues and venous hypertension of those tissues causing them to act in a pathologic fashion. In these situations, the malformation requires primary treatment. Only then will the tissues become normal, heal, and discontinue the hemorrhagic or necrotic process. Attempts at skin grafting without treating the underlying malformation are doomed to failure.

Involvement of the appropriate clinical specialists in the management of complications is essential to minimize the morbidity of that complication. A multidisciplinary team of specialists is required in the management of vascular malformations. Each specialist brings important knowledge and experience to the table in the management of these problematic lesions. It is important for this team of physicians to be involved routinely with patients with vascular malformations so that when a complication occurs, they are familiar with the underlying pathology, the complications that can result from treating that pathology, and to manage the complication appropriately to minimize its morbidity.

Summary

Head and neck vascular malformations are extremely challenging because of the complex soft tissue neuroanatomy, complex vascular anatomy, intracranial to extracranial arterial connections, sensitive neural structures particularly of the 7th nerve, orbital injuries, and the potential for intracranial stroke. Another significant issue is choice of embolic agents used to endovascularly manage head and neck AVMs.

If the goal of the procedure is a preoperative embolization, then most embolic agents are possible to use. Particulate agents such as polyvinyl alcohol particles (PVA; Biodyne, El Cajon, CA), Contour Emboli (Boston Scientific Corp, Marlborough, MA), Ivalon (i valon, San Diego, CA), and Embosphere Microspheres (Merit Medical Systems, South Jordan, UT) are excellent nonpermanent embolic preoperative agents that cause little inflammation. The literature is solid that particle embolic agents are never curative in AVM management [6, 7]. Polymerizing embolic agents such as the tissue adhesives isobutyl-2-cyanoacrylate and n-butyl-cyanoacrylate (Histoacryl Blau, B Braun Medical, Sempach, Schweiz) and Onyx (ELOS Medtech, Memphis, TN) are used in the preoperative management of AVMs, but the medical literature and the clinical experience prove that nBCA and Onyx are only rarely curative, alone without surgical resection [7–12]. However with the use of ethanol as an embolic agent to treat AVMs, many authors from all over the world repeatedly prove its curative potential [5, 13–45].

References

1. Mulliken JB, Glowacki J. Hemangiomas and vascular malformations in infants and children: a classification based on endothelial characteristics. Plast Reconstr Surg. 1982;69:415.
2. Mulliken JB, Zetter BR, Folkman J. In vitro characteristics of endothelium from hemangiomas in vascular malformations. Surgery. 1982;92:348.
3. Glowacki J, Mulliken JB. Mast cells in hemangiomas and vascular malformations. Pediatrics. 1982;70:48.
4. Finn MC, Glowacki J, Mulliken JB. Congenital vascular lesions: clinical application of a new classification. J Pediatr Surg. 1983;18:894.
5. Yakes WF, Haus DK, Parker SH, Gibson MD, Hopper KD, Mulligan JS, Pevsner PH, Johns JC Jr, Carter TE. Symptomatic vascular malformations: ethanol embolotherapy. Radiology. 1989;170:1059–66.
6. Sorimachi T, Koike T, Takeuchi T, Minakawa T, Abe H, Nishimaki K, Ito Y, Tanaka R. Embolization of cerebral AVMs achieved with PVA particles: angiographic reappearance and complications. AJNR Am J Neuroradiol. 1999;20:1323–8.
7. White RI Jr, Pollack J, Persing J, Henderson KJ, Thompson JG, Burdge CM. Long-term outcome of embolotherapy and surgery for high-flow extremity AVMs. J Vasc Interv Radiol. 2000;11:1285–95.
8. Rao VR, Mandalam KR, Gupta AK, Kumar S, Joseph S. Dissolution of isobutyl-2-cynaoacrylate on long-term follow-up. AJNR Am J Neuroradiol. 1989;10:135–41.
9. Dickey KW, Pollack JS, Meier GH, Denny DF, White RI Jr. Management of large high-flow AVMs of the shoulder and upper extremity with transcatheter embolotherapy. J Vasc Interv Radiol. 1995;6:765–73.
10. Rosen RJ, Contractor S. The use of cyanoacrylate adhesives in the management of congenital vascular malformations. Semin Interv Radiol. 2004;21:59–66.
11. Jahan R, Murayama Y, Gobin YP, Duckwiler GR, Vinters HV, Vinuela F. Embolizations with onyx clinicopathological experience in 23 patients. Neurosurgery. 2001;48:984–95.
12. Bruno CA Jr, Meyers PM. Endovascular management of AVMs of the brain. Interv Neurol. 2013;1:109–23.
13. Rak KM, Yakes WF, Ray RL, et al. MR imaging of peripheral vascular malformations. AJR Am J Roentgenol. 1992;159:107–12.
14. Yakes WF. Endovascular management of high-flow arteriovenous malformations. Semin Interv Radiol. 2004;21:49–58.
15. Vogelzang RL, Yakes WF. Vascular malformations: effective treatment with absolute ethanol. In: Pearce WH, Yao JST, editors. Arterial surgery: management of challenging problems. Stanmford: Appleton and Lange publishers; 1997. p. 553–60.
16. Yakes WF, Krauth L, Ecklund J, Swengle R, Dreisbach JN, Seibert CE, Baker R, Miller M, VanderArk G, Fullagar T, Prenger E. Ethanol endovascular management of brain arteriovenous malformations: initial results. Neurosurgery. 1997;40:1145–54.
17. Yakes WF, Luethke JM, Parker SH, Stavros AT, Rak KM, Hopper KD, Dreisbach JN, Griffin DJ, Seibert CE, Carter TE, Guilliland JD. Ethanol embolization of vascular malformations. Radiographics. 1990;10:787–96.
18. Yakes WF, Pevsner PH, Reed MD, Donohue HJ, Ghaed N. Serial embolizations of an extremity arteriovenous malformation with alcohol via direct percutaneous puncture. AJR Am J Roentgenol. 1986;146:1038–40.
19. Kerber C. Balloon catheter with a calibrated leak: a new system for superselective angiography and occlusive catheter therapy. Radiology. 1976;120:547–50.
20. Yakes WF, Parker SH, Gibson MD, Haas DK, Pevsner PH, Carter TE. Alcohol embolotherapy of vascular malformations. Semin Interv Radiol. 1989;6:146–61.
21. Park KB, Do YS, Kim DI, Kim YK, Shin BS, Park HS, et al. Predictive factors for response of peripheral arteriovenous malformations to embolization therapy: analysis of clinical data and imaging findings. J Vasc Interv Radiol. 2012;23:1478–86.
22. Keljo DJ, Yakes WF, Andersen JM, Timmons CF. Recognition and treatment of venous malformations of the rectum. J Pediatr Gastroenterol Nutr. 1996;23:442–6.
23. Do YS, Yakes WF, Shin SW, Lee BB, Kim DI, Liu WC, Shin ES, Kim DK, Choo SW, Choo LW. Ethanol

embolization of arteriovenous malformations: interim results. Radiology. 2005;235:674–82.

24. WFJ Y. Endovascular management of high flow arteriovenous malformations. Chin J Stomatol. 2008;43:327–32.

25. Vinson AM, Rohrer DB, Wilcox CW, et al. Absolute ethanol embolization for peripheral arteriovenous malformation: report of 2 cures. South Med. 1988;381:1052–5.

26. Yakes WF, Haas DK, Parker SH, Gibson MD, Hopper KD, Mulligan JS, Pevsner PH, Johns JC, Carter TE. Symptomatic vascular ethanol embolotherapy. (RSNA – SCVIR special series I). Radiology. 1989;170:1059–66.

27. Mourao GS, Hodes JE, Gobin YP, Casasco A, Aymard A, Merland JJ. Curative treatment of scalp arteriovenous fistulas by direct puncture and embolization with absolute alcohol. J Neurosurg. 1991;75:634–7.

28. Yakes WF, Rossi P, Odink H. Arteriovenous malformation management: how I do it. Cardiovasc Intervent Radiol. 1996;19:65–71.

29. Yakes W, Baumgartner I. Interventional treatment of arterio-venous malformations. Gefasschirurgie. 2014;19:325–30.

30. Yakes WF, Luethke JM, Merland JJ, Rak KM, Slater DD, Hollis HW, et al. Ethanol embolization of arteriovenous fistulas: a primary mode of therapy. J Vasc Interv Radiol. 1990;1:89–96.

31. Cho SK, Do YS, Kim DI, Kim YW, Shin SW, Park KB, Ko JS, Lee AR, Choo SW, Choo IW. Peripheral arteriovenous malformations with a dominant outflow vein: results of ethanol embolization. Korean J Radiol. 2008;9:258–67.

32. Yakes WF. Extremity venous malformations: diagnosis and management. Semin Interv Radiol. 1994;11:332–9.

33. Yakes WF. Diagnosis and management of venous malformations. In: Savader SJ, Trerotola SO, editors. Venous interventional radiology with clinical perspectives. New York: Thieme Medical Publishers Inc; 1996. p. 139–50.

34. Levardi AM, Mangiri M, Vaghi M, Cazzulari A, Carrafiello G, Mattassi R. Sclerotherapy of peripheral venous malformations: a new technique to pre-

vent serious complications. Vasc Endovasc Surg. 2010;44:282–8.

35. Bisdorff A, Mazighi M, Saint-Maurice JP, Chapot R, Lukaszuricz AC, Houdart E. Ethanol threshold doses for systemic complications during sclerotherapy of superficial venous malformations: a retrospective study. Neuroradiology. 2011;53:891–4.

36. Hyun D, Do YS, Park KB, Kim DI, Kim YW, Park HS, Shin SW, Song YG. Ethanol embolotherapy of foot AVMs. J Vasc Surg. 2013;58:1619–26.

37. Park HS, Do YS, Park KB, Kim DI, Kim YW, Kim MJ, Shin BS, Choo IW. Ethanol embolotherapy of hand AVMs. J Vasc Surg. 2011;53:725–31.

38. Do YS, Park KB, Park HS, Cho SK, Shin SW, Moon JW, Kim DI, Kim YW, Chang IS, Lee SH, Hwang HY, Choo IW. J Vasc Interv Radiol. 2010;21:807–16.

39. Jin Y, Lin X, Chen H, Hu X, Fan X, Li W, Ma G, Yang C, Wang W. Auricular AVMs: potential success of superselective ethanol embolotherapy. J Vasc Interv Radiol. 2009;20:736–43.

40. Fan XD, Su LX, Zheng LZ, Zhang ZY. Ethanol embolization of AVMs of the mandible. AJNR Am J Neuroradiol. 2009;30:1178–83.

41. Pekkola J, Lappalainen P, Vuola T, Klockars P, Salminen P, Pitkaranta A. Head and neck AVMs: results of ethanol sclerotherapy. AJNR Am J Neuroradiol. 2013;34:198–204.

42. Settecase F, Hetts SW, Nicholson AD, Amans MR, Cooke DJ, Dowd CF, Higashida RT, Halbach VV. Superselective intra-arterial ethanol sclerotherapy of feeding artery and nidal aneurysms in ruptured cerebral arteriovenous malformations. AJNR Am J Neuroradiol. 2015;37:692–7. Published online 12 Nov 2015

43. Vogelzang RL, Attasi R, Vouchi M. Ethanol embolotherapy of vascular malformations: clinical outcomes at a single center. J Vasc Interv Radiol. 2014;25:206–13.

44. Lee BB, Do YS, Yakes WF. Management of AVMs: a multidisciplinary approach. J Vasc Surg. 2004;39:590–600.

45. Yakes WF. Arteriovenous malformations – how i treat them: alcohol. Ces Radiol. 2008;62:146–52.

Endovascular Treatment of AVM: Trunk and Extremity

Young Soo Do and Kwang Bo Park

General Overview

The common clinical manifestations of the trunk and extremity AVM are pulsating mass, pain, ulceration, bleeding, tissue necrosis, enlargement of draining vein, and venous hypertension and/or cardiac failure. Patients with hand or foot AVM have more ischemic pain, ulceration, and/or necrosis. But around 40% of patients with pelvis AVM with huge dilated vascular lesions have no symptoms due to deep location of the lesion and wide space of the pelvis. In the extremity, bone involvement of AVM is not rare about 18%.

Because of its biologic nature and the high-flow shunting of the AVM, AVMs have a more aggressive behavior and are more often associated with life- or limb-threatening complications than other types of CVM. Therefore, early aggressive treatment of AVM is recommended. Inappropriate treatment strategy (e.g., partial excision, ligation, or endovascular occlusion of the feeding artery) only stimulates the AVM lesion to a proliferative state, resulting in massive growth with uncontrollable complications. Surgical resection of AVM lesions carries the risk of a massive intraoperative hemorrhage, incomplete removal of the AVM nidus, surrounding organ or tissue injury, and

Y.S. Do, MD (✉) • K.B. Park, MD (✉)
Department of Radiology, Samsung Medical Center,
Sungkyunkwan University School of Medicine,
Seoul, South Korea
e-mail: ys.do@samsung.com

high recurrence rates. Therefore, endovascular treatment using a variety of embolic and sclerosing agents, independently or combined with surgical treatment, has become an accepted therapeutic option for the management of AVM.

Indications for treatment of trunk and extremity AVM are the presence of subjective clinical symptoms that make daily life uncomfortable (e.g., subjective pain, disfiguring mass), patients with complicating signs of AVMs (e.g., ulcer, skin necrosis, secondary infection, hemorrhage, secondary varicosities, and/or limited joint movement), patients with progressively enlarging AVMs over time, and patients with or expecting to have cardiopulmonary complications (e.g., dyspnea, cardiomegaly, or overt heart failure) [1–6].

Embolic and Sclerosing Agents

Embolic Agents

Particle Embolic Agents
Particle embolic agents, which include polyvinyl alcohol particles, microspheres, and Gelfoam, have been used to treat AVM. Their use, alone or in combination with other agents, is well documented, and symptom improvement right after treatment is good, but treatment effect does not last long, and early recurrence of AVM is always a problem. Because we have better embolic agents for treatment of peripheral AVM, their

© Springer-Verlag Berlin Heidelberg 2017
Y.-W. Kim et al. (eds.), *Congenital Vascular Malformations*, DOI 10.1007/978-3-662-46709-1_33

primary use is to alter the hemodynamics of the lesion to improve the effectiveness of other therapies [7].

N-Butyl Cyanoacrylate (NBCA)

NBCA is a clear free-flowing adhesive liquid that will polymerize in contact with any ionic solution. NBCA must be combined with ethiodized oil to reduce the polymerization time and to add radiopacity. The acute inflammatory response and glue casting may play a role in the success of vascular obliteration.

Embolization with NBCA may result in proximal feeder occlusion, or the mixture may pass through arteriovenous shuts and embolize the lung. It is difficult to control the level of occlusion, and it has been reported that lesions treated with NBCA can recanalize on long-term follow-up causing AVM recurrence. Immediate technical success rate is good with symptomatic improvement, but clinical result is not long-lasting. The mass effect by injected NBCA is not problematic in deep lesion, but mass can be troublesome if located in pressure area [7–10].

Onyx

Onyx is a copolymer of ethylene and vinyl alcohol dissolved in dimethyl sulfoxide (DMSO). Compared to NBCA, this agent is more controllable due to the specific slow flow behavior dynamics and slow polymerization process from the outside to the inside of the Onyx cast. This results in penetration of different portions of the nidus until a satisfactory result is obtained. Onyx with higher concentration of copolymer (8 or 20%) should be used for embolization of high-flow AVM.

Onyx has been widely used in the management of cerebral AVM, but there are a few reports of transarterial or retrograde transvenous embolization of peripheral AVM with Onyx. Wohlgemuth et al. [13] reported retrograde transvenous embolization with Onyx after preparatory transarterial-flow reduction or venous-flow reduction with Amplatzer Vascular Plug in eleven peripheral AVM patients with dominant outflow (angiographic type II AVM). Cure was achieved in ten patients and partial remission in one patient. Compared to ethanol, there are less procedure-related complications, but there is no long-term follow-up data of clinical success and recurrence. Because Onyx is mechanically occlusive but not adherent to vascular tissues, there is a risk of recanalization and recurrence. Because a large amount of Onyx-18 is usually necessary to treat peripheral AVM, the high cost and remained palpable or visible Onyx through the tissue and skin can be another disadvantage [11–13].

Coils

Coil embolization of the proximal feeding artery has the same problems associated with surgical ligation of the proximal feeding artery. Right after embolization of the feeding artery with coils, new collateral vessels supplying the AVM develop immediately from surrounding arteries. When this is done, effective treatment through the feeding artery is not possible. It is never clinically appropriate to use coils to occlude the primary feeding arteries except emergency patients with uncontrollable heart failure or bleeding.

Coils can be used in the fistula of type I or type IIIb AVM or outflow vein of type II AVM to reduce the amount of ethanol and to stabilize the thrombosis within the large venous component and to reduce the risk of tissue injury from arterial embolization. Coil embolization can be used in combination with ethanol to secure definitive treatment. Once flow has been slowed by the coils, the injection of ethanol can induce permanent occlusion of the AVM. Do et al. [2] reported ethanol embolotherapy of pelvis AVM after preparatory flow reduction with coils in twelve pelvis AVM patients with dominant outflow (angiographic type II AVM). Cure was achieved in ten patients and partial remission in two patients. Using coils in the fistula or draining vein can reduce the complications.

Sclerosing Agent

Ethanol

Ethanol has proven its efficacy in the management of peripheral AVM. Ethanol has the unique ability to induce protein denaturation of the endothelial cells with subsequent vessel wall denudation and

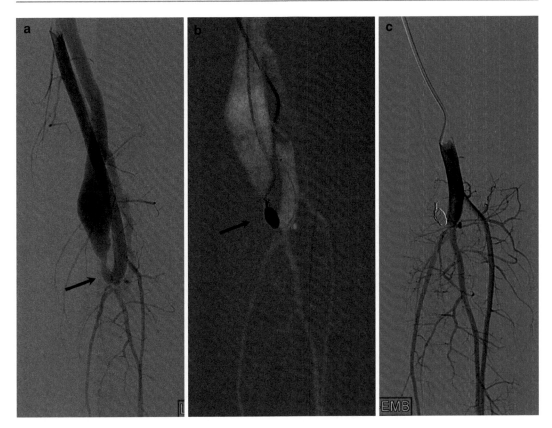

Fig. 33.1 A 3-year-old boy with type I AVM. (**a**) Pretreatment angiography shows the fistula (*arrow*) between the tibioperoneal trunk and femoral vein. (**b**) Microcoils (*arrow*) were inserted to occlude the fistula. (**c**) Completion angiography shows total occlusion of the fistula

thrombus formation, resulting in the complete obliteration of the vessel lumen rather than simple obstruction, and does not allow recanalization by permanently damaging the endothelium of the AVM nidus.

The treatment approach can be different according to the angiographic type of AVM. The angiographic classification of peripheral AVM is well described in Chap. 10. The main target of type I AVM is the fistula between the artery and vein. This fistula can be occluded with coils with or without additional ethanol injection (Fig. 33.1). The main target of type II AVMs is the venous component of the nidus. Therefore, the mainstay therapeutic approaches are transvenous or direct puncture. Before ethanol injection, coil embolization of the venous component of the nidus through a transvenous or direct puncture approach is often required to reduce the

amount of ethanol and to stabilize the thrombosis within the large venous component. Only the transarterial approach and ethanol injection are available for type IIIa AVMs because the fistula is too fine for direct puncture. Type IIIb AVMs can be treated properly via transarterial and direct puncture approaches. However, if there are no obstacles in terms of access and safe embolization, the transarterial approach is preferred because of familiarity with arterial angiographic findings, the ease of detecting a normal artery arising near an AVM, and the direct puncture hazard whereby ethanol can leak into adjacent soft tissues. The treatment of type III AVMs via a transvenous approach is contraindicated. The approaches used for mixed types are combinations of those used to treat the individual types, but an approach that simultaneously treats all types present is preferred. Figure 33.2 briefly

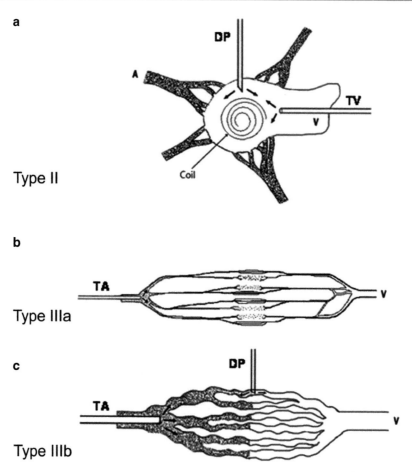

Fig. 33.2 A diagram presenting approaches to ethanol embolotherapy according to the angiographic type. *A* artery, *DP* direct puncture, *TV* transvenous, *V* vein (**a**) The main target of type II AVMs is the venous component of the nidus. The mainstay therapeutic approaches are transvenous or direct puncture. (**b**) Only the transarterial approach and ethanol injection are available for type IIIa AVMs because the fistula is too fine for direct puncture. (**c**) Type IIIb AVMs can be treated via transarterial and direct puncture approaches

describes the therapeutic approaches used by angiographic type. During this procedure, compression of the draining vein by means of pneumatic compression bands or hand can reduce the total amount of ethanol [14].

Ethanol may be diluted with a nonionic contrast medium when used to treat superficial AVMs which carry a high risk of skin necrosis. Multiple sessions are often required in order to reduce the risk of nontarget embolization of normal surrounding tissue and to obtain a cure of the AVM. In high-flow AVM lesions, sometimes, injection of high-concentration ethanol into the AVM lesion is not effective due to rapid clearance of the ethanol by fast-moving blood. To prolong the contact time between the ethanol and the endothelium of the target AVM nidus, a tourniquet or a pneumatic cuff can be used in extremity AVM, and an intravascular occlusion balloon or coil embolization of the dominant draining vein, not feeding artery, can be used in the trunk or pelvis AVM (Figs. 33.2, 33.3 and 33.4) [1, 2].

Park et al. [1] reported the largest series (*n*=176) of ethanol embolotherapy for peripheral AVM. Ethanol embolotherapy was effective in 91% of patients with cure in 39% of patients. Angiographic classification and AVM extent were significant predictive factors for overall clinical outcome. Localized AVM and type I or II AVM had a high probability for excellent final outcomes compared with diffuse AVM and type III or combined AVM.

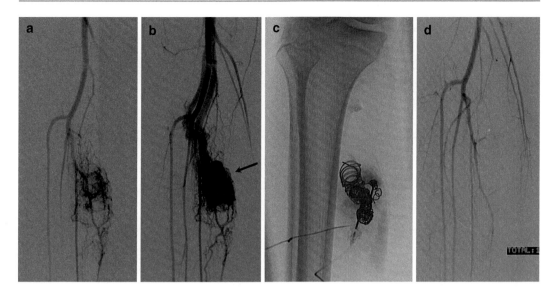

Fig. 33.3 A 21-year-old male with type II AVM in the calf. (**a**, **b**) Pretreatment angiography (arterial, venous phase) shows multiple small feeding arteries connected to the single enlarged draining vein (*arrow*). (**c**) Multiple coils (*arrow*) were inserted after direct puncture of the enlarged draining vein, and 12 cc of pure ethanol was injected through the needle. (**d**) Completion angiography shows complete obliteration of the AVM

However, despite its excellent results with promising outcomes of an increased chance of cure, cardiopulmonary collapse requiring resuscitation has been reported as very rare. Pulmonary hypertension is a potential fatal complication associated with ethanol embolotherapy and occurs when a significant amount of ethanol is injected. The etiology of pulmonary hypertension is related to either precapillary pulmonary artery spasm or extensive micro-thromboembolism. The development of pulmonary hypertension can lead to subsequent cardiopulmonary arrest if not controlled effectively. To reduce the risk of cardiopulmonary complications during ethanol embolotherapy, appropriate measures should be taken which include administration of general anesthesia and close cardiopulmonary monitoring. When high volume of ethanol injection (more than 0.5 ml/kg) is planned, pulmonary artery Swan-Ganz line and arterial line monitoring are recommended to minimize the possibility of this event occurring. When the mean PAP is elevated by more than 25 mmHg, infusion of nitroglycerine is recommended as a bolus injection (50–100 μg) and then as a continuous infusion (0.3–3.0 μg/kg/min) through the Swan-Ganz line [1–5].

A total dose of ethanol which is less than 1 ml/kg is the maximum volume that can be safely given during a procedure since the volumes higher than this can result in toxicity. In Samsung Medical Center, limiting ethanol injections (total volume less than 0.5 ml/kg of body weight, single bolus injection less than 0.1 ml/kg of body weight) every 10 min will be able to obviate the need of pulmonary artery monitoring [15, 16].

Ethanol embolotherapy is sufficient to eliminate or improve symptoms of AVMs in a high percentage of patients, but with substantial risk of minor and major complications. Reported complication rates of ethanol embolotherapy range from 10% to 61%, and most of them are minor complications like skin blisters, focal skin necrosis, and/or transient nerve injury. In major complications (less than 10%), skin necrosis required skin graft, amputation for tissue necrosis, thrombolysis for distal embolism, permanent nerve injury, acute pancreatitis from ethanol use, and acute renal failure were reported [1–5].

Stent Graft

Use of a stent graft in the treatment of AVMs will have the same problems associated with surgical ligation or endovascular occlusion of the proximal feeding artery, leaving the "nidus" (surviving

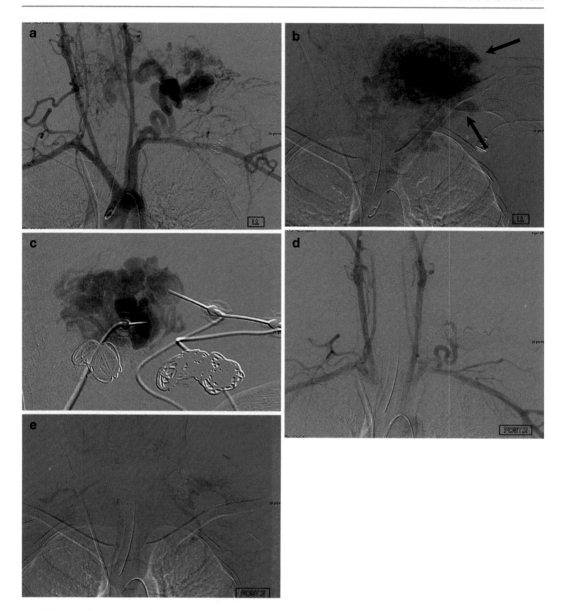

Fig. 33.4 A 37-year-old male with type IIIb AVM in the left shoulder. (**a**, **b**) Pretreatment angiography (arterial, venous phase) shows multiple hypertrophied feeding arteries and draining veins (*arrows*). (**c**) Ethanol and coil embolotherapy was performed after direct puncture of the fistula. (**d**, **e**) After four sessions of ethanol and coil embolotherapy, completion angiography (arterial, venous phase) shows near-complete obliteration of the shoulder AVM

primitive mesenchymal lesion) intact, and will result in recurrence or aggravation of the AVM. Therefore, stent graft should not be used in the treatment of AVMs with rare exceptions of uncontrollable cardiac failure, bleeding, or others.

Conclusion

At present, the first choice of therapy for the management of the trunk and extremity AVM is endovascular treatment using liquid embolic agents (e.g., NBCA, Onyx, ethanol) not particles. Symptomatic improvement of NBCA is good, but clinical result is not long-lasting. Onyx is a better controllable agent, but the reported data using Onyx is limited, and there is a risk of recanalization and recurrence. The high cost and remained palpable or visible Onyx through the tissue and skin can be another disadvantage. Ethanol embolotherapy is sufficient to eliminate or improve symptoms of AVMs in a high percentage of patients, but with substantial risk of minor and major complications. Selection of the right embolic agents can be determined by several factors: physician's experience of using embolic agents, availability of general anesthesia, multidisciplinary team, lesion location, and clinical circumstances.

References

1. Park KB, Do YS, Kim DI, Kim YW, Shin BS, Park HS, et al. Predictive factors for response of peripheral arteriovenous malformations to embolization therapy: analysis of clinical data and imaging findings. J Vasc Interv Radiol. 2012;23:1478–86.
2. Do YS, Kim YW, Park KB, Kim DI, Park HS, Cho SK, et al. Endovascular treatment combined with embolosclerotherapy for pelvic arteriovenous malformations. J Vasc Surg. 2012;55:465–71.
3. Park HS, Do YS, Park KB, Kim DI, Kim YW, Kim MJ, et al. Ethanol embolotherapy of hand arteriovenous malformations. J Vasc Surg. 2011;53:725–31.
4. Lee BB, Baumgartner I, Berlien HP, Bianchini G, Burrows P, Do YS, et al. Consensus document of the international union of angiology (IUA)-2013. Current concept on the management of arterio-venous malformations. Int Angiol. 2013;32(1):9–36.
5. Do YS, Park KB, Park HS, Cho SK, Shin SW, Moon JW, et al. Extremity arteriovenous malformations involving the bone: therapeutic outcomes of ethanol embolotherapy. J Vasc Interv Radiol. 2010;21:807–16.
6. Flye MW, Jordan BP, Schwartz MZ. Management of congenital arteriovenous malformations. Surgery. 1983;94:740–7.
7. Tan KT, Simons ME, Rajan DK, Terbrugge K. Peripheral high-flow arteriovenous vascular malformations: a single-center experience. J Vasc Interv Radiol. 2004;15:1071–80.
8. Natarajan SK, Born D, Ghodke B, Britz GW, Sekhar LN. Histopathological changes in brain arteriovenous malformations after embolization using onyx or N-butyl cyanoacrylate. Laboratory investigation. J Neurosurg. 2009;111:105–13.
9. Sofocleous CT, Rosen RJ, Raskin K, Fioole B, Hofstee DJ. Congenital vascular malformations in the hand and forearm. J Endovasc Ther. 2001;8:484–94.
10. White RI, Pollak J, Persing J, Henderson KJ, Thomson JG, Burdge CM. Long-term outcome of embolotherapy and surgery for high-flow extremity arteriovenous malformations. J Vasc Interv Radiol. 2000;11:1285–95.
11. Castaneda F, Dodwin SC, Swischuk JL, Wong GC, Bonilla SM, Wang MJ, et al. Treatment of pelvic arteriovenous malformations with ethylene vinyl alcohol copolymer. J Vasc Interv Radiol. 2002;13:513–6.
12. Numan F, Ömeroglu A, Kara B, Cantasdemir M, Adaletli I, Kantarci F. Embolization of peripheral vascular malformations with ethylene vinyl alcohol copolymer (Onyx). J Vasc Interv Radiol. 2004;15:939–46.
13. Wohlgemuth WA, Müller-Wille R, Teusch VI, Dudeck O, Cahill AM, Alomari AI, et al. The retrograde transvenous push-through method: a novel treatment of peripheral arteriovenous malformations with dominant venous outflow. Cardiovasc Intervent Radiol. 2015;38:623–31.
14. Cho SK, Do YS, Shin SW, Kim DI, Kim YW, Park KB, et al. Arteriovenous malformations of the body and extremities: analysis of therapeutic outcomes and approaches according to a modified angiographic classification. J Endovasc Ther. 2006;13:527–38.
15. Shin BS, Do YS, Cho HS, Kim DI, Hahm TS, Kim CS, et al. Effects of repeat bolus ethanol injections on cardiopulmonary hemodynamic changes during embolotherapy of arteriovenous malformations of the extremities. J Vasc Interv Radiol. 2010;21:81–9.
16. Ko JS, Kim JA, Do YS, Kwon MA, Choi SJ, Gwak MS, et al. Prediction of the effect of injected ethanol on pulmonary arterial pressure during sclerotherapy of arteriovenous malformations: relationship with dose of ethanol. J Vasc Interv Radiol. 2009;20:39–45.

Kurosh Parsi

Introduction

Lymphatic malformations (LMs) are congenital anomalies of the lymphatic system occurring in 1 in 2000–4000 births. These anomalies are present at birth but may not be apparent until later in life. Other congenital vascular malformations include venous malformations (VMs), capillary malformations (CMs) and arteriovenous malformations (AVMs). VMs are the most common vascular malformations followed by LMs and CMs. Fortunately, AVMs are the least common but the most aggressive and the most difficult to treat.

Vascular malformations including LMs may be classified into truncular and extra-truncular subcategories. Truncular LMs arise at later stages (>3 weeks) of embryogenesis and hence involve mature lymphatic vessels. These anomalies present with primary lymphoedema.

Extra-truncular LMs arise earlier (<3 weeks) than truncular LMs during the reticular phase of vasculogenesis and result in cystic deformities. Extra-truncular lesions are further characterised

into macrocystic (cysts >1 cm), microcystic (cysts <1 cm) or mixed cystic lesions (Table 34.1).

LMs are further discussed in chapters 17 (extra-truncular LMs) and 18 (truncular LMs). In this chapter, we revise these anomalies and discuss management strategies and treatment options.

Embryologic Basis of the Classification

LMs are errors of morphogenesis involving the lymphatic vessels. These errors can occur during various stages of embryogenesis. The reticular phase of vasculogenesis occurs during the first 3 weeks of development. At this stage the circulation consists of unstructured tangled small vessels actively growing from mesenchymal cells (angioblasts). Abnormalities occurring at this stage of vasculogenesis will not involve lymphatic trunks or other mature lymphatic vessels and morphologically will result in lymphatic cysts. These anomalies are termed extra-truncular LMs. After about 3 weeks, the vessels differentiate to form vascular trunks adjacent to major nerves. Abnormalities occurring at this stage of vasculogenesis will involve the lymphatic trunks and mature vessels. These anomalies present with lymphoedema and are defined as truncular LMs.

K. Parsi
Department of Dermatology, St. Vincent's Hospital, Sydney, Australia

University of New South Wales, Sydney, Australia
e-mail: kparsi@sydneyskinandvein.com.au

Table 34.1 Basic classification of lymphatic malformations (LMs)

	Extra-truncular LMs	Truncular LMs
Stage of embryogenesis	Early (<3 weeks)	Late (>3 weeks)
Clinical presentation	Cystic deformity	Primary lymphoedema
Sub-classification	Macrocystic (>1 cm) Microcystic (<1 cm) Mixed cystic	

Measurements in cm refer to cyst diameter

Clinical Presentation

Truncular Lymphatic Malformations

Truncular LMs present with primary lymphoedema. This can be associated with secondary cutaneous changes such as hyperkeratosis, induration and verrucous change. Lymphoedema can be complicated by secondary dermatophyte or bacterial infections. When associated with morbid obesity, chronic lymphoedema can progress to elephantiasis nostras verrucosa complicated by severe cellulitis and sepsis.

Extra-truncular Lymphatic Malformations

Macrocystic, Microcystic and Mixed Lesions

Extra-truncular LMs are fluid-filled spaces forming macrocysts, microcysts or mixed lesions. These lesions can be solitary or diffuse and can infiltrate other tissues. They are most commonly found on the lymphatic-rich areas such as the head and neck and can affect any site with the exception of the brain. LMs can cause significant complications such as dysphagia, nerve compression, organ compression and respiratory failure. Airway involvement is more common in childhood. LMs can compromise the airways by intrinsic involvement or extrinsic compression. Acute haemorrhage in a macrocystic lesion may require early intervention or even tracheostomy. LMs can occur in bones resulting in vanishing bone disease (*Gorham–Stout syndrome*). This condition results in near-complete resorption of the affected bones.

Macrocystic lesions present as a soft tissue mass or deformity, whereas microcystic lesions present as fluid-filled or blood-filled vesicles and may even have a warty appearance. The vesicles normally contain a yellow colour lymphatic fluid, but bleeding from the fragile cystic walls into the lesion will result in a blood-stained appearance (Fig. 34.1). Events such as infection, trauma or bleeding into the lesion can cause a rapid and painful enlargement of the cysts. Depending on the chronicity of the lesion and the site, secondary cutaneous hyperkeratosis and verrucous change may be present (Fig. 34.2). Secondary cutaneous changes are more likely with microcystic and mixed cystic lesions.

Combined and Complex Malformations

Patients with LMs may have co-existing CMs, VMs or AVMs. Syndromic conditions such as Klippel–Trenaunay (KTS) and Parkes Weber (PWS) syndromes can present with a combination of LMs, VMs, CMs (KTS) and AVMs (PWS). Venolymphatic malformations (VLMs) are a collection of aberrant venous and lymphatic channels with disorganised endothelial cells in various proportions.

LMs may also be a finding in other conditions such as the Turner syndrome, Proteus syndrome, Milroy disease and CLOVES syndrome (congenital, lipomatous, overgrowth, vascular malformations, epidermal nevi and spinal/skeletal abnormalities).

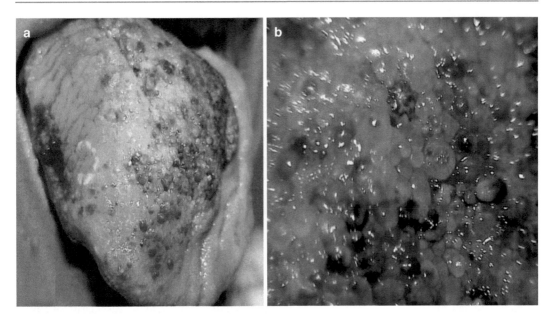

Fig. 34.1 (**a**) Microcystic lymphatic malformation of the tongue. (**b**) Close-up view. Note clear lymphatic fluid in some vesicles and haemorrhage in others

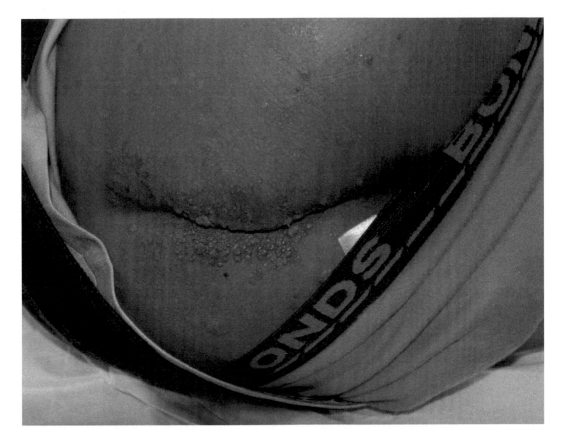

Fig. 34.2 Secondary cutaneous changes of a mixed cystic lymphatic malformation. Note the verrucous appearance

Lymphangiectasia

Lymphangiectasias are the lymphatic equivalent of venulectasias and telangiectasias of the venous system. These are saccular dilations of the superficial lymphatic vessels and appear as translucent vesicles that can enlarge to form small bullae and nodules. Some lesions may be pedunculated and develop a hyperkeratotic verrucous surface. Lymphangiectasias develop secondary to increased intra-lymphatic pressure that results from lymph accumulation in the superficial lymphatic vessels. Lymphangiectasias may be caused by an underlying lymphoedema or be secondary to an LM. *Lymphangioma circumscriptum* refers to lymphangiectasias involving the skin and the subcutaneous tissues secondary to an LM.

Investigations

A number of basic investigations are required to confirm the clinical diagnosis of a congenital anomaly, define the extent of the lesion, detect any associated structural, syndromic or secondary abnormalities and plan treatment.

Duplex Ultrasound

Every patient with a vascular anomaly should receive a duplex ultrasound (DUS) study. Such studies should be undertaken at dedicated phlebology/vascular laboratories familiar with vascular tumours and malformations. This will avoid the need for repeat studies, unnecessary expenses and runaround for patients and parents.

Diagnosis of an LM can be made in utero via routine ultrasound or foetal magnetic resonance imaging (MRI) performed in the late second to third trimesters. Prenatal detection will allow planning for treatment outside the uterus during delivery (ex utero intrapartum treatment – EXIT) [1].

DUS is the first line of investigation to confirm the diagnosis of a congenital anomaly such as an LM. This is due to its non-invasive nature, low cost, availability and ability to exclude a wide range of differential diagnoses.

Vascular Tumour Versus Malformation

The aim of the DUS study is to confirm the clinical diagnosis of an LM, exclude other causes and detect co-existing venous or arteriovenous anomalies. The first question to address is whether the presenting mass is a soft tissue mass, a vascular tumour or a malformation. The majority of soft tissue masses have a non-specific ultrasound appearance. Vascular tumours are primarily a soft tissue mass, whereas malformations are primarily formed of vascular spaces. B-mode can readily make the distinction based on the echogenic morphology of a tumour as against the anechoic vascular spaces of a malformation [2]. Doppler studies will demonstrate the vascularity of a proliferating tumour such as a haemangioma but will be negative if the haemangioma has already involuted. Hence, B-mode characteristics are very important in making the distinction between tumours and malformations, and Doppler should only be used to confirm the B-mode findings.

Lymphatic Malformation Versus Arteriovenous Malformation

On B-mode ultrasound, macrocystic LMs appear as noncompressible anechoic cystic spaces containing and separated by thin echogenic septae. AVMs are also noncompressible and may have a 'honeycomb' appearance that can be confused with the cystic structure of LMs (Fig. 34.3a, b). AVMs however have thicker walls compared to the thin septae of LMs, and the surrounding tissue may show echogenic fibrosis due to chronic trauma. Doppler studies will further characterise an AVM by demonstrating a low resistance high velocity arterial flow pattern. By contrast, LMs will show no spontaneous flow. Importantly, vascularity (pulsatile arterioles) will be evident in the septae of an LM and in the surrounding tissues, and this should not be interpreted as high flow within the lesion (Fig. 34.3c). This is why it is important to obtain adequate B-mode information before proceeding to and be confused by a Doppler study.

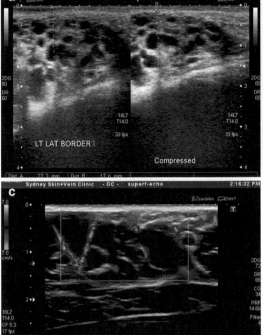
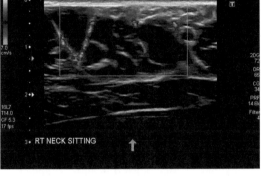

Fig. 34.3 (**a**) B-mode image of an arteriovenous malformation. While the gross morphology may resemble an LM, the walls are thicker and there is associated soft tissue fibrosis. (**b**) B-mode image of a macrocystic lymphatic malformation. Note the thin septae. (**c**) Colour Doppler demonstrating the vascularity within the lymphatic septae. This should not be interpreted as flow within the lesion

Lymphatic Malformation Versus Venous Malformation

VMs can be differentiated from macrocystic LMs by their relatively thicker walls and compressibility. Wall thickening may be even more prominent secondary to recurrent thrombophlebitis and localised intravascular coagulopathy (LIC), a common finding in larger VMs. Venous wall thickness in contrast to thin lymphatic septae is an important distinguishing feature on B-mode ultrasound. Compressibility is another important useful B-mode feature. Patent VMs are compressible, whereas LMs are relatively noncompressible. On Doppler examination, small VMs may show no detectable flow, while larger patent VMs would demonstrate flow induced by compression. By contrast, no flow would be detected within the cystic spaces of an LM.

Previously Treated or Thrombosed Lesions

The difficulty may arise when a VM or LM has been previously treated with sclerotherapy or if a VM lesion is thrombosed. History of previous treatment or recent thrombophlebitis should be obtained before proceeding with a DUS examination. Thrombosed or sclerosed VMs will be non- or partially compressible depending on the extent of the intra-luminal occlusion. With high-resolution B-mode imaging, thrombus within a VM would appear slightly hypoechoic. Sclerosed VMs should appear echogenic unless they contain intra-luminal haemolysed blood which would appear hypoechoic or anechoic. Treated LMs with no discernable cyst will also be echogenic on DUS.

Microcystic and Mixed Lymphatic Malformations

B-mode examination may also be used to investigate microcystic and mixed LMs. These lesions will demonstrate an echogenic soft tissue abnormality with ill-defined borders and diffuse involvement of the adjacent anatomic structures.

Magnetic Resonance Imaging (MRI)

While DUS is very useful in confirming the diagnosis of an LM, the two-dimensional interrogation of the lesion by standard ultrasound systems is currently incapable of defining the three-dimensional morphology of a vascular anomaly, the extent of the lesion and its precise relationship with adjacent structures. MRI is therefore considered mandatory in all patients with vascular malformations. Macrocystic LMs show hyperintense signal in T2 images and low intensity signal in T1 images, with post-contrast enhancement of the septa. Microcystic lesions generally appear as T2 images with homogeneous hyperintense signal [3]. VLMs can be assessed on MRI and computerised tomography (CT) using contrast [4]. Enhancement of the vascular space, presence of phleboliths and accompanying venous channels would define the venous components. Non-enhancement and fluid–fluid levels from intracystic haemorrhages are features of the lymphatic components.

Other Imaging Modalities

Lymphoscintigraphy is used to assess lymphoedema in truncular LMs and is usually not required for extra-truncular LMs. Lymphangiography is an obsolete method abandoned from current clinical practice (please see Chap. 18).

Other Investigations

A biopsy may be required for mixed or microcystic lesions to exclude skin lesions with a similar verrucous appearance or to detect malignancy.

A cutaneous angiosarcoma may develop secondary to lymphoedema referred to as *Stewart–Treves syndrome*. Squamous cell carcinoma (SCC) may arise at sites of co-existing chronic venous hypertension and venous ulceration. Acroangiodermatitis (pseudo-Kaposi's sarcoma) can develop in patients with underlying AVMs.

Genetic studies may be required when there is a family history of vascular anomalies or in the presence of syndromic conditions. Family screening may be required in such patients. A full blood count and in particular a white cell count needs to be obtained as some patients with LMs demonstrate lymphopenias rendering them prone to cellulitis.

Treatment

General Measures

The most important and often neglected step in the management of patients with vascular malformations is the general measures aimed at improving the quality of life. Given the confusing terminology and general lack of knowledge within the wider medical community, patients, parents or carers often understand little about these conditions and have limited resources and ability to cope with the chronicity, cosmetic disfigurement and social stigma. There may be a constant threat of losing a digit, a limb or a body part and amputation may have been suggested as a treatment option. Hence, general measures aiming at improving the patient education and quality of life should be proactively taught and implemented. These measures can be classified under the following headings:

1. *Explain the diagnosis.* The diagnosis of a vascular malformation, its subtype (LM, truncular vs. extra-truncular) and its course and prognosis should be explained. A clear explanation will encourage the patient to be more compliant with treatment instructions. A clear and unambiguous diagnosis using the current terminology should be documented and appear on all correspondence with other

healthcare professionals involved in the patient's care. Obsolete terms such as *lymphangioma, cavernous lymphangioma, cystic hygroma, cystic lymphangioma* and *lymphangioma circumscriptum* should be avoided.

2. *Stop triggers.* LMs are prone to infection, bleeding and trauma. Infections may require oral antibiotics such cephalexin but recurrent infections and cellulitis may require long-term antibiotic treatment. Trauma to the lesion should be avoided.

3. *Treat the associated conditions and comorbidities.* A complete medical assessment and system review is required and may need to be repeated on a regular basis. Patients with primary lymphoedema and syndromic conditions may have significant comorbidities such as diabetes and obesity. Patients with associated VMs need to be assessed for coagulopathies. Psychiatric assessment and treatment may be required especially in teenage patients affected by cosmetic disfigurement.

4. *Supportive measures.* This includes compression garments and stockings. Class II (20–30 mmHg) compression is usually adequate in the preoperative and post-operative management of extra-truncular LMs. Higher compressions (30–40 mmHg) may be used for primary lymphoedema provided the arterial pressures are normal.

5. *Patient education and support.* Adequate time should be spent to explain the diagnosis and ensure compliance with post-operative measures. Education is especially important to manage and prevent secondary complications such as infection and bleeding. Local or web-based support groups may help patients, parents or carers cope with a chronic condition.

6. *Team approach.* Referral to other specialists and management in a multidisciplinary team environment is highly recommended. Relevant specialists with adequate knowledge of vascular malformations should be involved in the management of the patient. A typical team may include phlebologists, surgeons, dermatologists, interventional radiologists, paediatrician, vascular/phlebology trained nurses, physiotherapists, occupational therapists, social workers, psychologists, speech pathologists and dieticians. Although a team approach may be necessary, it is essential that a single physician takes charge of the patient management and coordinates all efforts.

7. *Genetics and family member screening.* Referral to genetics and family screening is required when dealing with primary lymphoedema or when LM is part of a syndrome.

8. *Treatment plan.* Patients with vascular malformations typically require multiple interventions. These interventions should be planned in advance with no longer than 4 weeks interval between the procedures. Longer intervals can result in earlier recurrence especially in mixed veno-lymphatic lesions.

Specific Measures

Truncular LM are managed as for lymphoedema and are discussed in Chap. 18.

Here, we focus on specific measures to treat extra-truncular LMs. Treatment modalities for extra-truncular LMs include conservative measures, medical treatments, percutaneous drainage, sclerotherapy, laser therapy, radiofrequency ablation and surgery. These different modalities may be used in various combinations. During the consultation process, all treatment options should be discussed irrespective of whether or not those treatments are provided by the individual practitioner or centre. This is to ensure transparency and to allow the patients to seek a second opinion from other practitioners or centres that provide the alternative treatment options. Pros and cons for each modality should be discussed in detail before embarking on interventions or surgery. Treatment modalities are best described as a spectrum of options ranging from the least to the most invasive. One way of presenting this information is as follows:

- Conservative measures
- Medical treatments
- Interventions – sclerotherapy, laser and radiofrequency ablation
- Surgery

Conservative Measures

LMs may spontaneously resolve without any therapy in 15–70% of cases [5]. For patients with no symptoms or functional impairment, general measures described above, observation and monitoring may be offered as the first option. Patients should be reassessed on a regular basis, measurements and serial photographs obtained. A diary of recurrent complications such as infection, bleeding and rapid expansion should be maintained. Serial imaging with ultrasound and MRI may be required to determine progression in size and involvement of important adjoining structures. By contrast, lesions with severe life-threatening functional impairment should be treated early.

Medical Treatment

Medical treatment is relatively new and is being assessed in multiple trials. Medical treatment may play an adjunctive role to endovascular interventions or may be the only treatment option for extensive mixed or microcystic LMs. Antiproliferative agents, such as sirolimus (rapamycin), seem to be effective in very extensive, diffuse malformations, especially in new born infants with extensive cervicofacial lesions. A number of clinical trials are underway investigating the role of sirolimus in the management of diffuse LMs, and the results are so far promising [6, 7]. Other drugs and in particular sildenafil and propranolol are of limited benefit. Sildenafil has shown mixed results demonstrating efficacy in some trials but no benefits in others. [8–10] Propranolol is possibly useful in the presence of a co-existing haemangioma [11]. Antiangiogenic measures are further discussed in detail in Chaps. 17 and 45.

Interventions for Macrocystic Lesions

The choice of intervention should be individualised, and more than one type of intervention can be planned and performed based on the anatomical location, lesion characteristics, indications and contraindications.

Sclerotherapy

A whole range of sclerosing agents and other injectables have been used to treat LMs. These have included ethanol, doxycycline, OK-432, detergent sclerosants, sodium morrhuate, dextrose, tetracycline, hypertonic saline, acetic acid, cyclophosphamide, interferon, fibrin glue, corticosteroids and even boiling water. Ethanol followed by doxycycline, detergent sclerosants, bleomycin and OK-432 has been the most popular agent, and the use of other agents listed has been unsuccessful.

Sclerotherapy is effective in treating macrocystic LMs but is less useful in treating microcystic lesions. Sclerotherapy is significantly less invasive than surgery and in general shows better efficacy and lower recurrence rates. In one study comparing surgery with sclerotherapy, 95% of patients had an excellent to fair response with sclerotherapy, while only 67% had complete resolution after surgery [12]. In another study, surgery and sclerotherapy showed a similar effectiveness in the treatment of head and neck LMs at 1-year follow-up [13]. The published reports are influenced by the operator's experience, choice of the sclerosing agent, surgical or interventional techniques and the preferred methods of treatment in individual centres. Techniques of sclerotherapy and a description of sclerosing agents are described in the next section.

Endovascular Laser Ablation (EVLA)

Ablation methods are relatively new and not assessed in large studies. The anecdotal experience with laser ablation shows effectiveness in treating difficult macrocystic LMs and VLMs. Since 2008, the author has employed endovascular laser ablation (EVLA) for very large and diffuse macrocystic LMs as well as large VMs including the embryonic marginal vein. An infrared 980 nm laser was initially utilised, later replaced by 1470 and 1500 nm systems. All these wavelengths are effective but the higher wavelengths are less painful and cause less bruising.

Care should be taken to preserve critical neurovascular structures. This requires optimal ultrasound visualisation and identification of all significant structures, use of adequate volumes of tumescent anaesthesia to separate the target lesion from adjacent structures and use of the lowest possible effective energy settings.

Radiofrequency Ablation (RFA)

Radiofrequency ablation (RFA) has been described to treat VLMs [4]. A report by Koo et al. found ultrasound-guided RFA and ethanol ablation to be safe and effective in treating VLMs of the head and neck [4]. The authors followed a meticulous protocol that involved a comprehensive pretreatment evaluation of the cranial nerves and parotid duct with CT or MRI and performed all procedures under ultrasound guidance. RFA was performed at 15 W using a 19G, 0.5-cm active-tip internally cooled electrode. Seventeen patients were treated, sixteen of whom showed >50% volume reduction. There were no significant complications. Postoperative heat and swelling was experienced by most patients but managed by applying ice packs. The procedure was repeated within 2–4 weeks until all accessible components were ablated.

Interventions for Microcystic and Mucosal Lesions

Radiofrequency Ablation (RFA)

RFA has been used to treat microcystic and mixed LMs and mucosal lesions [14]. Here, RFA is used to vaporise the tissue. The author uses a cutaneous RF system to treat microcystic LMs. When used on cutaneous lesions, RFA can cause hypopigmentation and scarring.

RFA has been successfully used to reduce the size of oral cavity LMs [14]. This approach provides symptom relief and reduces the risk of bleeding and infection [14]. RFA can be delivered in high-frequency or low-frequency modes to treat oral lesions. The high-frequency mode is used to destroy deeper tissues and induces fibrosis. In the low-frequency mode, the energy is transmitted through a conductive medium such as isotonic saline. This method protects the nearby tissues and removes a thin superficial layer. Low-frequency mode is ideal for removal of airway lesions.

Lasers

Resurfacing lasers such as carbon dioxide (CO_2, 10, 600 nm far infrared) and fractionated erbium as well as Nd:YAG (1064 nm, near infrared) and pulsed dye lasers have been used to vaporise the tissues non-selectively to treat microcystic LMs [15].

Surgery

Surgery for LMs has been associated with a mortality rate of 6%, complications rate of 19–33% and a recurrence rate of up to 53% [5]. Not all patients with LM are suitable for surgery and patients should be selected carefully.

Surgical Resection

Surgical resection of LMs can be associated with significant morbidity including major blood loss, iatrogenic injury and deformity [15]. Surgical resection aims to provide a definitive treatment and is indicated in lesions larger than 3 cm, in patients with airway compromise, dyspnoea, dysphagia, bone erosion or significant deformity [16]. Surgical resection is best reserved for lesions suitable for a complete excision such as well-circumscribed macrocystic LMs of the neck (cystic hygroma) or localised microcystic lesions. Surgical resection may also be indicated after failed sclerotherapy.

Endoscopic Laser Resection

Endoscopic laser resection with CO_2 or YAG lasers has been used to treat mucosal lesions. This method allows a more accurate lesion removal, without functional impairment. Large lesions may require other treatments such as sclerotherapy. Endoscopic laser resection may also be used as an alternative treatment for palliative cases.

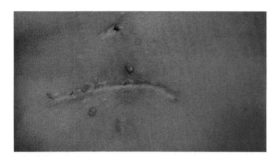

Fig. 34.4 Scarring after surgical debulking of a mixed lymphatic malformation

Surgical Debulking

Complete surgical resection may not always be an option due to the size or anatomical location of the malformation or extensive infiltration of other tissues. In such circumstances, surgical debulking may be attempted. This may require large incisions prone to complicated wound healing, infection and extensive scarring (Fig. 34.4). Surgical debulking may not be curative and further sclerotherapy may be required after debulking.

Liposuction

Liposuction and ultrasound-assisted liposuction have been used to debulk tissues infiltrated with LMs. Ultrasound-assisted liposuction is a procedure that uses high-frequency ultrasound to liquefy fat before it is removed. This procedure has been used as an alternative to surgical debulking and has been found particularly useful in areas with significant fibrofatty tissue. [17, 18] Liposuction has also been used in conjunction with sclerotherapy to treat macrocystic LMs of the neck by rupturing the cysts [19].

Sclerotherapy

Techniques

Sclerotherapy for macrocystic LMs is performed by accessing the cystic cavity with a direct puncture under ultrasound guidance, aspirating and discarding the cystic fluid and introducing the sclerosant. The aim should be to maximise the exposure of the cystic wall to the active sclerosing agent, minimise dilution and deactivation of the sclerosant by the cystic fluid and approximate the vessel walls to allow for adhesion and ultimately endoluminal fibrosis. Procedures are scheduled every 4–6 weeks, and success is determined by ultrasound or MR imaging.

This procedure can be divided into the following steps:

Setting

Given the risk of infection, sclerotherapy for LMs should be performed under sterile conditions. Patients may require monitoring especially when ethanol is being employed, and hence the procedure should be performed in an operating theatre, a hybrid theatre or an angiography suite. Adequate anaesthesia (general anaesthesia or intravenous sedation) and pain management especially when ethanol is being used are required.

Image Guidance

Sclerotherapy of LMs should be performed under image guidance. Extravasation of irritant sclerosants such as ethanol can result in significant tissue loss. Inadvertent intraarterial injection of most sclerosants will result in significant tissue necrosis. DUS guidance is the best modality for peripheral LMs. Less commonly, fluoroscopy, CT and MR are used to provide guidance and quantitative image-based evaluation of treatment outcome [20].

Access

Access can be obtained by direct puncture using a needle or by cannulation under ultrasound guidance. The author performs all procedures under ultrasound guidance and prefers to access the lesion using two short cannulas, each connected to short extension tubes. One cannula is used to drain (exit) and the other is used to inject (entry).

Drainage

An important step in the treatment of macrocystic LMs is drainage of the cystic fluid. This is a protein-rich fluid containing lymphocytes and macrophages and may be blood-stained

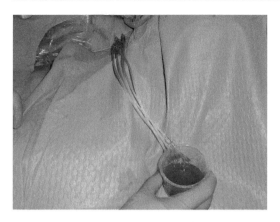

Fig. 34.5 Lymphatic fluid drained from the cyst. Note the fluid is blood-stained

(Fig. 34.5). [21] Mixing the sclerosing agent with the cystic fluid will result in a number of negative outcomes. Other than the dilution effect of the fluid, detergent sclerosants are deactivated by the protein-rich fluid resulting in reduced potency [22, 23]. By draining the fluid, sclerosants gain direct access to the cystic wall while maintaining the original potency.

Saline Flush

The author uses a saline irrigation technique where normal saline is injected into the lesion to ensure the cavity is completely emptied of the lymphatic fluid. Saline will enter via the entry cannula and exit via the exit cannula ensuring complete removal of the lymphatic fluid.

Local Anaesthetic

Perivascular Tumescent Anaesthesia

The author employs a technique of infiltrating the tissue surrounding the vascular anomaly with perivascular tumescent anaesthetic fluid to collapse the lesion, reduce post-operative pain and maintain the lesion internally compressed for the ensuing few hours. The fluid contains normal saline, lignocaine, adrenalin and sodium bicarbonate. This is done after the lesion has been accessed and fluid has been drained. This technique allows approximation of the vessel wall and helps with management of the post-operative pain.

Intralesional Lignocaine

Intralesional lignocaine has been used prior to ethanol embolisation [4]. This is done to minimise post-operative pain and, if applicable, to test the presence of a cranial nerve through the temporary paralysis of the corresponding innervated site. The technique involves injecting lignocaine (2%) for 30 s and then aspirating the anaesthetic solution before injecting ethanol.

Sclerosant

The sclerosant is introduced using the entry cannula or directly via a needle depending on the technique employed. When using the two-cannula system, a circuit is formed where the fluid enters the cavity via one cannula and exits via the second. The author uses this technique for detergent sclerosants and doxycycline.

Ethanol is injected slowly with little pressure to avoid extravasation [4]. Ethanol is then retained inside the lesion for 5 min and then aspirated and discarded [24]. The dwell time of 5 min is ideal to avoid systemic absorption of ethanol. The allocated procedure time should be at least 1 h to avoid rapid injection and rapid systemic absorption of ethanol [24].

Post-operative Compression

There is no consensus regarding the use of compression after sclerotherapy for LMs. It is the authors' practice to apply compression garments specific to the site of the lesion for 7 days on average after the procedure. Garments are made to measure beforehand.

Post-operative Antibiotics

To minimise the risk of infection, prophylactic antibiotics may be prescribed in high-risk patients.

Sclerosing Agents

Agents used to treat LMs include doxycycline, detergent sclerosants, bleomycin, ethanol and OK-432 (picibanil). Less commonly, acetic acid and hypertonic saline have been used.

Doxycycline

Doxycycline is a tetracycline antibiotic classified as a chemical irritant when used as a sclerosing agent. It inhibits matrix metalloproteinases and cell proliferation. Doxycycline is used at 10 mg/mL to a max of 400 mg per treatment session. The lyophilised (freeze-dried) preparation contains ascorbic acid and mannitol as excipients. This agent is primarily used for macrocystic LMs but has also been tried in microcystic lesions. [25] The author employs the two-cannula technique described above when using doxycycline.

Doxycycline and STS are the author's preferred sclerosants to treat LMs. In a study reporting on treatment of 29 children with head and neck LMs, doxycycline showed similar efficacy to STS with 51.7% demonstrating complete resolution and 27.6% moderate improvement [26]. In a systematic review of the use of doxycycline in treatment of paediatric head and neck LMs, the overall success rate was reported to be 84.2% [27]. In a study comparing doxycycline with OK-432, the administration time for OK-432 was found to be shorter than that for doxycycline, but OK-432 required more treatments overall to achieve clinical success.

Doxycycline in general is a very safe sclerosant. It may cause mild post-operative pain due to its inflammatory effect. The use of peri-lesional tumescent anaesthesia minimises discomfort in the post-operative period. Being a tetracycline-related compound, doxycycline can form a stable calcium complex in bone-forming tissues and teeth. This is reported when tetracyclines are used systemically and not injected locally in an LM. Nonetheless, there remains a theoretical risk of tooth discolouration when doxycycline is used to treat children younger than 7 years of age.

Sodium Tetradecyl Sulphate (STS)

Sodium tetradecyl sulphate (STS) is an anionic sulphated surfactant. Given its negative charge, STS can denature proteins and is considered a harsh detergent. STS is manufactured by STD Pharmaceutical Products Ltd. (Hereford, UK) and available in Australia as FIBRO-VEIN. At 3%, each mL of FIBRO-VEIN contains 30 mg of STS and 2% benzyl alcohol as a bactericidal excipient. Clinically, STS is used in a foam format with a 1 + 4 liquid plus gas composition to sclerose veins. STS is strongly deactivated by circulating blood cells and proteins [22]. The main advantage of foam over liquid is displacement of intravenous blood and reducing the mixing of active STS with blood components. Given the cystic nature of LMs, the foam does not seem to have a theoretical advantage over liquid although no studies have investigated this. Therefore, STS is commonly used in the liquid format to treat LMs. STS has been found to have a similar efficacy to doxycycline in treating LMs [26, 28, 29].

Liquid STS is used at 3% to treat macrocystic LMs. Maximum dose per session is 4 mL of 3% STS liquid. Higher volumes injected can cause toxicity. When used in the foam format, the max volume used to treat veins is 20 mL (Australasian College of Phlebology Standards) [30]. When treating LMs, it is important to drain the cystic fluid first before injecting STS to prevent its deactivation by proteins. It is also important to ensure STS is not mixed with cystic fluid in the tubing or needles used. The two-cannula system described above minimises such mixture.

STS is associated with a number of adverse effects including rare cases of anaphylaxis [30]. Extravasation of liquid STS at 3% (as against foam) can result in tissue necrosis. In addition, an intraarterial injection or even a high-pressure/rapid intravenous injection can result in skin and tissue necrosis. Injections should be performed under ultrasound guidance and delivered at low speed and with little pressure. Most other reported adverse effects such as the small risk of venous thrombosis are associated with intravenous use and not relevant to LMs.

Polidocanol (POL)

Polidocanol (POL) is a nonionic surfactant. POL is a polyethylene glycol ether of lauryl alcohol and classified as a local anaesthetic although has doubtful anaesthetic properties [31]. As a sclerosing agent, POL is available in Australia as Aethoxysklerol 3% (Chemische Fabrik Kreussler & Co GmbH, Wiesbaden, Germany). At 3%, each ml of Aethoxysklerol contains 30 mg of

POL in water for injection with 5% (v/v) ethanol. POL at 0.1–0.5% is used to treat telangiectasias and reticular veins and at 1–3% to treat varicose veins. It is typically used in a foam format to treat veins. POL is 2–3× less potent than STS.

POL has been used to treat VMs and VLMs but less commonly to treat LMs [32, 33]. Similar to STS, there is no theoretical advantage for using POL in foam format when treating LMs. When used intravenously, the max dose is 2 mg/kg of body weight. Higher doses are associated with local anaesthetic toxicity. When used intravenously, POL has been linked with rare cases of anaphylaxis, and similar to STS, extravasation and intraarterial injection can result in tissue necrosis.

Bleomycin

Bleomycin is a cytotoxic antibiotic isolated from the gram-positive bacteria *Streptomyces verticillus*. Bleomycin inhibits DNA synthesis and is used as a chemotherapy agent to treat lymphomas, testicular carcinomas, squamous cell carcinomas and malignant pleural effusion [34–37]. When used as a sclerosant, it induces an inflammatory reaction which subsequently causes fibrosis. Intralesional injection of bleomycin is used to treat cutaneous warts and macrocystic LMs. It has also been used to sclerose VMs [38, 39]. In the author's opinion, bleomycin is best reserved for LMs, and safer procedures such as foam sclerotherapy and EVLA/RFA are excellent choices for patients with VMs [40].

The sclerosant is prepared by dissolving 8 mg of bleomycin A5 (pingyangmycin) powder in 5 mL of normal saline with addition of 2 mL of lignocaine 2% and 1 mL of dexamethasone (5 mg) [15]. The dosage per injection is 1 mL/cm^2 of the lesion as determined by clinical measurement. The maximal dose for one injection is 8 mg, and the total dose should not exceed 40 mg in an adult patient. The cystic fluid should be completely drained before the injection of bleomycin. Multiple injections may be needed at different sites for larger or more extensive lesions. After injection, the lesion is compressed for 5 min to prevent bleeding and effusion of the sclerosant. The procedure is repeated in 3–4 weeks.

Pulmonary fibrosis is the most severe toxicity associated with bleomycin. The most frequent presentation is pneumonitis progressing to pulmonary fibrosis. Pulmonary toxicities occur in 10% of treated patients. In approximately 1%, the non-specific pneumonitis induced by bleomycin progresses to pulmonary fibrosis and death. Pulmonary toxicity has been observed in all age groups including the younger patients and those treated with lower doses, but the risk of pulmonary fibrosis is higher in elderly patients and in those exceeding the total cumulative dose of 400 units. A unit of bleomycin is equal to the formerly used milligram activity.

Bleomycin doses used in sclerotherapy are much smaller in comparison, typically 1–5% of the lowest dose associated with possible pulmonary fibrosis [37]. Bleomycin A5 (pingyangmycin) concentration used to treat LMs can range from 0.5 to 4 mg/mL, and the dose per treatment session can range from 2 to 16 mg or 0.3 mg/kg body weight. [21] The maximum cumulative dose per patient has been reported to be 70 mg [21].

In a systematic review and meta-analysis, outcome of intralesional bleomycin injections for LMs was reported in 20 studies with a total of 631 patients, and VMs were studied in 12 articles including 690 patients. Good to excellent size reduction was reported in 84% of LMs and 87% of VMs [41]. Pulmonary fibrosis or nerve injury was never encountered. In this meta-analysis, a 2% incidence of facial nerve paralysis (2%) was observed in patients treated with ethanol but not with bleomycin [41]. Electromyography and motor nerve conduction studies have shown no abnormality in facial nerve function when intralesional bleomycin was used in the maxillofacial region [42].

Following intralesional use, bleomycin can cause post-operative pain, erythema and swelling. The pain usually lasts 72 h [43]. Bleomycin can cause local skin necrosis, ulceration and eschar formation at the site of injection [44] and infection in 1% [41]. Fever, chills and vomiting may occur soon after the intralesional administration.

OK-432 (Picibanil)

OK-432 (picibanil) is a biologic preparation of lyophilised (freeze-dried) powder containing *Streptococcus pyogenes Su* strain cells (group A, type 3) treated with benzylpenicillin potassium. This agent is thought to provoke an immune response resulting in cytokine production by leukocytes. It was initially used in the treatment of malignant tumours, especially for malignant hydrothorax as a non-specific immunostimulant. The use of OK-432 to treat LMs was reported by Ogita et al. in 1987 [45]. It is thought to stimulate lymphatic endothelial proliferation resulting in obliteration of lymphatic channels with minimal local fibrosis.

OK-432 is prepared at 0.1 mg/10 mL. It is usually injected into the cystic space from different entry points and directions until the lesion is expanded. The dose should not exceed 20 mL per application. If the lesion is not reduced at 4–6 weeks after the procedure, a second treatment can be performed, and the dose may be increased to 0.3 mg (30 mL) [15].

OK-432 is associated with risk of anaphylaxis. Skin prick test for penicillin allergy should be performed prior to treatment. Crash trolley containing drugs, equipment and a defibrillator to manage anaphylaxis should be available. The author is aware of one case of mortality possibly due to cardiac arrest when the agent was used to treat a VLM involving the airways. More commonly, a low-grade fever of up to 39 °C occurs within 6 h of the procedure which goes away after 2–4 days with the use of antipyretic drugs. Localised erythema, pain and swelling will last up to 5 days [35].

Ethanol

Ethanol has lost its popularity for treating VMs and LMs given its potential for significant complications and availability of safer alternative treatment options. Ethanol preparations suitable for sclerotherapy include 95% or 98% dehydrated forms, generally available through hospital pharmacies for neurolysis. Ethanol is a non-specific chemical irritant that rapidly denatures proteins. The damage is transmural and not contained within the vessel lumen. Extravasation can cause tissue necrosis including significant nerve damage.

Systemic adverse effects include CNS depression, hypoglycaemia, hypertension, hyperthermia, cardiac arrhythmias, pulmonary vasoconstriction and pulmonary hypertension and electromechanical dissociation. Cardiovascular collapse, sometimes fatal, can result from effects on the pulmonary vasculature or myocardium.

Ethanol sclerotherapy requires supervised training and should only be performed by experienced practitioners. To minimise systemic adverse effects, ethanol should be administered in small aliquots, with adequate time for recovery between injections. Total dose of 1 ml/kg or 60 mL should not be exceeded in one procedure. The volume limitation is partially responsible for ethanol's failure in effectively treating extensive LMs.

Conclusion

Congenital vascular malformations including lymphatic anomalies and malformations are chronic diseases requiring careful long-term management plans. Intervention should form part of the overall management of the patient, carefully planned and executed. A number of treatment options are available for LMs but sclerotherapy has been most effective in the management of macrocystic LM. Superficial, localised and well-circumscribed lesions can be surgically excised. Microcystic lesions can be treated with surgery, RF or laser ablation.

Acknowledgements I am grateful to Dr. David Connor for his assistance with the preparation of the manuscript.

References

1. Perkins JA, Manning SC, Tempero RM, Cunningham MJ, Edmonds Jr JL, Hoffer FA, et al. Lymphatic malformations: review of current treatment. Otolaryngol Head Neck Surg. 2010;142(6):795–803. e1
2. Parsi K, Myers KA. Tumours and fistulae. In: Myers KA, Clough AM, editors. Practical vascular ultrasound: an illustrated guide. Boca Raton: CRC Press; 2014. p. 215–28.
3. Sierre S, Teplisky D, Lipsich J. Vascular malformations: an update on imaging and management. Arch Argent Pediatr. 2016;114(2):167–76.

4. Koo HJ, Lee JH, Kim GY, Choi YJ, Baek JH, Choi SH, Nam SY, Kim SY, Suh DC. Ethanol and/or radiofrequency ablation to treat venolymphatic malformations that manifest as a bulging mass in the head and neck. Clin Radiol. 2016;71(10):1070.e1–7.

5. Ha J, Yu YC, Lannigan F. A review of the management of lymphangiomas. Curr Pediatric Rev. 2014;10(3):238–48.

6. Adams DM, Trenor 3rd CC, Hammill AM, Vinks AA, Patel MN, Chaudry G, et al. Efficacy and safety of sirolimus in the treatment of complicated vascular anomalies. Pediatrics. 2016;137(2):e20153257.

7. Hammill AM, Wentzel M, Gupta A, Nelson S, Lucky A, Elluru R, et al. Sirolimus for the treatment of complicated vascular anomalies in children. Pediatr Blood Cancer. 2011;57(6):1018–24.

8. Danial C, Tichy AL, Tariq U, Swetman GL, Khuu P, Leung TH, et al. An open-label study to evaluate sildenafil for the treatment of lymphatic malformations. J Am Acad Dermatol. 2014;70(6):1050–7.

9. Koshy JC, Eisemann BS, Agrawal N, Pimpalwar S, Edmonds JL. Sildenafil for microcystic lymphatic malformations of the head and neck: a prospective study. Int J Pediatr Otorhinolaryngol. 2015;79(7):980–2.

10. Rankin H, Zwicker K, Trenor 3rd CC. Caution is recommended prior to sildenafil use in vascular anomalies. Pediatr Blood Cancer. 2015;62(11):2015–7.

11. Ozeki M, Kanda K, Kawamoto N, Ohnishi H, Fujino A, Hirayama M, et al. Propranolol as an alternative treatment option for pediatric lymphatic malformation. Tohoku J Exp Med. 2013;229(1):61–6.

12. Gilony D, Schwartz M, Shpitzer T, Feinmesser R, Kornreich L, Raveh E. Treatment of lymphatic malformations: a more conservative approach. J Pediatr Surg. 2012;47(10):1837–42.

13. Balakrishnan K, Menezes MD, Chen BS, Magit AE, Perkins JA. Primary surgery vs primary sclerotherapy for head and neck lymphatic malformations. JAMA otolaryngol Head Neck Surg. 2014;140(1):41–5.

14. Goswamy J, Penney SE, Bruce IA, Rothera MP. Radiofrequency ablation in the treatment of paediatric microcystic lymphatic malformations. J Laryngol Otol. 2013;127(3):279–84.

15. Zhou Q, Zheng JW, Mai HM, Luo QF, Fan XD, Su LX, et al. Treatment guidelines of lymphatic malformations of the head and neck. Oral Oncol. 2011;47(12):1105–9.

16. Manning SC, Perkins J. Lymphatic malformations. Curr Opin Otolaryngol Head Neck Surg. 2013;21(6):571–5.

17. Francis CS, Rommer EA, Kane JT, Iwata K, Panossian A. Limited-incision surgical debulking of lymphatic malformations using ultrasound-assisted liposuction. Plast Reconstr Surg. 2012;130(6):920e-2e.

18. Tavakkolizadeh A, Wolfe KQ, Kangesu L. Cutaneous lymphatic malformation with secondary fat hypertrophy. Br J Plast Surg. 2001;54(4):367–9.

19. Mitsukawa N, Satoh K. New treatment for cystic lymphangiomas of the face and neck: cyst wall rupture and cyst aspiration combined with sclerotherapy. J Craniofac Surg. 2012;23(4):1117–9.

20. Harmoush S, Chinnadurai P, El Salek K, Metwalli Z, Herce H, Bhatt A, et al. Multimodality image-guided sclerotherapy of low-flow orbital vascular malformations: report of single-center experience. J Vasc Interv Radiol. 2016;27:987–95.

21. Schook CC, Mulliken JB, Fishman SJ, Grant FD, Zurakowski D, Greene AK. Primary lymphedema: clinical features and management in 138 pediatric patients. Plast Reconstr Surg. 2011;127(6): 2419–31.

22. Connor DE, Cooley-Andrade O, Goh WX, Ma DD, Parsi K. Detergent sclerosants are deactivated and consumed by circulating blood cells. Eur J Vasc Endovasc Surg. 2015;49(4):426–31.

23. Parsi K, Exner T, Connor DE, Herbert A, Ma DD, Joseph JE. The lytic effects of detergent sclerosants on erythrocytes, platelets, endothelial cells and microparticles are attenuated by albumin and other plasma components in vitro. Eur J Vasc Endovasc Surg. 2008;36(2):216–23.

24. Furukawa H, Sasaki S, Oyama A, Hayashi T, Funayama E, Saito N, et al. Ethanol sclerotherapy with 'injection and aspiration technique' for giant lymphatic malformation in adult cases. J Plastic Reconstruct Aesthetic Surg. 2011;64(6):809–11.

25. Shiels 2nd WE, Kenney BD, Caniano DA, Besner GE. Definitive percutaneous treatment of lymphatic malformations of the trunk and extremities. J Pediatr Surg. 2008;43(1):136–9. ; discussion 40

26. Farnoosh S, Don D, Koempel J, Panossian A, Anselmo D, Stanley P. Efficacy of doxycycline and sodium tetradecyl sulfate sclerotherapy in pediatric head and neck lymphatic malformations. Int J Pediatr Otorhinolaryngol. 2015;79(6):883–7.

27. Cheng J. Doxycycline sclerotherapy in children with head and neck lymphatic malformations. J Pediatr Surg. 2015;50(12):2143–6.

28. Kiratli H, Tarlan B. Total clinical regression of an orbital macrocystic lymphatic malformation following intralesional sodium tetradecyl sulphate injection. J AAPOS. 2015;19(1):78–80.

29. Kok K, McCafferty I, Monaghan A, Nishikawa H. Percutaneous sclerotherapy of vascular malformations in children using sodium tetradecyl sulphate: the Birmingham experience. J Plastic Reconstruct Aesthetic Surg. 2012;65(11):1451–60.

30. Cavezzi A, Parsi K. Complications of foam sclerotherapy. Phlebology. 2012;27(Suppl 1):46–51.

31. Parsi K. Interaction of detergent sclerosants with cell membranes. Phlebology. 2015;30(5):306–15.

32. Cabrera J, Redondo P. Sclerosing treatment of vascular malformations. An Sist Sanit Navar. 2004;27(Suppl 1):117–26.

33. Blaise S, Charavin-Cocuzza M, Riom H, Brix M, Seinturier C, Diamand JM, et al. Treatment of low-flow vascular malformations by ultrasound-guided sclerotherapy with polidocanol foam: 24 cases

and literature review. Eur J Vasc Endovasc Surg. 2011;41(3):412–7.

34. Burrows PE, Mason KP. Percutaneous treatment of low flow vascular malformations. J Vasc Interv Radiol. 2004;15(5):431–45.

35. Ogita S, Tsuto T, Nakamura K, Deguchi E, Iwai N. OK-432 therapy in 64 patients with lymphangioma. J Pediatr Surg. 1994;29(6):784–5.

36. Alomari AI, Karian VE, Lord DJ, Padua HM, Burrows PE. Percutaneous sclerotherapy for lymphatic malformations: a retrospective analysis of patient-evaluated improvement. J Vasc Interv Radiol. 2006;17(10): 1639–48.

37. Orford J, Barker A, Thonell S, King P, Murphy J. Bleomycin therapy for cystic hygroma. J Pediatr Surg. 1995;30(9):1282–7.

38. Jia R, Xu S, Huang X, Song X, Pan H, Zhang L, et al. Pingyangmycin as first-line treatment for low-flow orbital or periorbital venous malformations: evaluation of 33 consecutive patients. JAMA Ophthalmol. 2014;132(8):942–8.

39. Spence J, Krings T, KG t B, LB d C, Agid R. Percutaneous sclerotherapy for facial venous malformations: subjective clinical and objective MR imaging follow-up results. AJNR Am J Neuroradiol. 2010;31(5):955–60.

40. Lee BB, Baumgartner I, Berlien P, Bianchini G, Burrows P, Gloviczki P, et al. Diagnosis and treatment of venous malformations. Consensus Document of the International Union of Phlebology (IUP): updated 2013. Int Angiol. 2015;34(2):97–149.

41. Horbach SE, Rigter IM, Smitt JH, Reekers JA, Spuls PI, van der Horst CM. Intralesional bleomycin injections for vascular malformations: a systematic review and meta-analysis. Plast Reconstr Surg. 2016;137(1):244–56.

42. Karavelioglu A, Temucin CM, Tanyel FC, Ciftci AO, Senocak ME, Karnak I. Sclerotherapy with bleomycin does not adversely affect facial nerve function in children with cervicofacial cystic lymphatic malformation. J Pediatr Surg. 2010;45(8):1627–32.

43. Saitta P, Krishnamurthy K, Brown LH. Bleomycin in dermatology: a review of intralesional applications. Dermatol Surg. 2008;34(10):1299–313.

44. Kirby JS, Miller CJ. Intralesional chemotherapy for nonmelanoma skin cancer: a practical review. J Am Acad Dermatol. 2010;63(4):689–702.

45. Ogita S, Tsuto T, Nakamura K, Deguchi E, Tokiwa K, Iwai N. OK-432 therapy for lymphangioma in children: why and how does it work? J Pediatr Surg. 1996;31(4):477–80.

Complications of Endovascular Treatment of Peripheral Congenital Vascular Malformations

35

Kurosh Parsi and Young Soo Do

Introduction

Interventional procedures in the management of congenital vascular malformations (CVMs) have enjoyed rapid advances in the past two decades. This has followed advances in related fields such as diagnostic ultrasound, magnetic resonance imaging (MRI), histopathology and molecular genetics. Endovascular procedures using a variety of embolic and sclerosing agents have replaced surgery as the preferred treatment option. The new interventional techniques have shown superior results to excisional surgery and have significantly reduced the need for aggressive surgical procedures. Interventional techniques are performed under fluoroscopic and/or duplex ultrasound (DUS) guidance, and advances in these imaging modalities have tremendously helped with a better management of vascular anomalies.

In this chapter, we present an overview of complications associated with embolization and sclerotherapy of *peripheral* vascular malformations. Cerebrospinal lesions are not covered in this chapter, but the basic principles discussed here apply to all vascular malformation.

Factors Influencing the Risk of Complications

Interventional techniques have evolved in the past 20 years, performed in different centres around the world where the focus and operator's training and skills have been quite variable. In addition, there are no evidence-based guidelines or widely accepted consensus to help with selection of the best treatment approach. Consequently, variable efficacy and complication rates have been reported in association with what may appear to be the same procedure. In general, older publications report a higher incidence of complications, morbidity and mortality and lower efficacy rates. When interpreting older reports, one must be mindful that agents such as ethanol are associated with a higher complication rate, which is not true for the more recently deployed foam sclerosants. Significant complications such as tissue necrosis, nerve damage, anaphylaxis, thromboembolism and cerebrovascular events are significantly less common with foam sclerosants.

Other than the choice of embolic/sclerosing agent, factors such as the type of malformation, anatomical location, patient selection, procedural technique and postoperative management can influence the outcome.

K. Parsi (✉)
Department of Dermatology, St. Vincent's Hospital, University of New South Wales, Sydney, Australia
e-mail: kparsi@sydneyskinandvein.com.au

Y.S. Do (✉)
Sungkyunkwan University, School of Medicine and Samsung Medical Center, Seoul, South Korea
e-mail: ys.do@samsung.com

© Springer-Verlag Berlin Heidelberg 2017
Y.-W. Kim et al. (eds.), *Congenital Vascular Malformations*, DOI 10.1007/978-3-662-46709-1_35

These factors may be classified into the following eight categories:

1. *Type of malformation.* High-flow arteriovenous malformations (AVMs) predispose a higher risk of postoperative necrosis and nerve damage irrespective of the treatment method and the choice of embolic agent. Low-flow lesions of venous malformations (VMs) and lymphatic malformations (LMs) pose less risk. Injection of embolic agents into AVMs may block smaller vessels downstream causing necrosis of the affected tissues. Furthermore, the intimate association of nerves with arteries in neurovascular bundles predisposes the treatment of AVMs to a higher risk of nerve damage. VMs communicate with and drain into the venous system. Sclerotherapy of VMs can predispose to occlusion or thrombophlebitis of the adjoining normal veins. Treatment of LMs carries the risk of postoperative infection due to intimate communication between these lesions and the lymphatic system. Hence, the type of CVM predisposes the procedure to risks specific to that particular type.

2. *Choice of sclerosing/embolic agents.* Physiochemical and pharmacological properties of sclerosing/embolic agents influence both the efficacy and complications associated with their use. The chemical nature of the agent determines the mode of action and the type of injury imposed on the vessel and the surrounding structures. For example, chemical irritants such as ethanol penetrate beyond the intimal layer of target lesions causing a transmural injury that extends beyond the target vessel. This may result in injury to adjacent vital structures. By contrast, detergent sclerosants only remove the endothelial layer, and hence the injury is in general contained unless thrombophlebitis sets in postoperatively. Viscous embolic agents act by physically blocking the target lesions and depend on the subsequent fibrosis to achieve permanent occlusion. Detergent sclerosants get deactivated by blood components and hence carry very little systemic adverse effects, whereas ethanol causes significant systemic effects [4].

3. *Anatomical location of the lesion.* This is often the most important factor in determining which embolic/sclerosing agent to use.
   - *Proximity to vital or neurologic structures.* Chemical irritants such as ethanol are associated with a high risk of damage to adjacent structures. This is especially important when the lesion is diffuse, poorly localized and infiltrative.
   - *Proximity to the normal deep venous drainage.* Direct drainage of VMs into the adjoining deep veins can potentially increase the risk of sclerosis or thrombosis of the adjoining veins. This can cause significant risks, for example, when treating VM lesions on the neck draining into the jugular or subclavian veins.
   - *Hands, feet and digits.* Endovascular treatment of AVMs of the hand/fingers has a significantly higher risk of complications including fingertip ischaemia and necrosis (Fig. 35.1) [1].
   - *Superficial location.* Superficial lesions with dermal involvement are at a higher risk of skin necrosis.

4. *Patient-related factors.* Co-morbidities, concurrent coagulopathy, hypercoagulable states, thrombophilia or bleeding disorders, drugs and supplements such as anticoagulants, platelet inhibitors and oestrogen supplementation may adversely influence the treatment outcomes.

5. *Management strategy.* Prior to commencing interventions, a management plan should be generated to include the number of proposed treatments and follow-up intervals. Any such plans should ensure the proposed procedures are in line with long-term strategies. For example, ligation or coil embolization of arteries feeding an AVM can block future vascular access. This approach can also provoke an AVM to recruit collateral vessels that may enlarge and feed the nidus.

6. *Imaging.* Optimal imaging is essential to allow vascular access and guide the catheterization and embolization procedures. This is

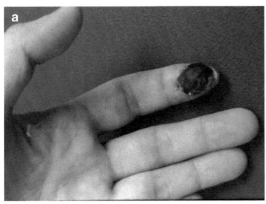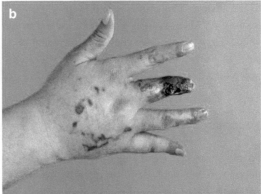

Fig. 35.1 (**a, b**) Fingertip necrosis and ischaemia following ethanol embolization (Courtesy of Prof. BB Lee)

especially relevant to ultrasound-guided procedures. Inadvertent intraarterial injections can result in significant tissue necrosis. In one case of a combined veno-lymphatic malformation of the neck, inadvertent injection of the venous component with the lymphatic embolic agent has resulted in a cardiac arrest and death mostly attributed to poor imaging (private communication with author, KP).

7. *Adjunctive procedures and postoperative care.* Adjunctive undertakings such as delivery of tumescent anaesthesia to reduce the size of the vessel and application of postoperative compression can make a substantial difference in treatment outcomes.

8. *Operator experience.* Currently, physicians with variable training and experience provide vascular interventions to treat CVM. Given the lack of standardization, an apparent 'same' procedure can result in varying efficacy and complication rates.

Sclerosing and Embolic Agents

A variety of embolic and sclerosing agents have been used in the management of CVM. Ethanol and the detergent sclerosant sodium tetradecyl sulphate (STS) are the most commonly used agents. Another detergent agent, polidocanol (POL), is less frequently used. Detergent sclerosants are commonly used in the foam format.

Arteriovenous Malformations (AVMs)

Absolute alcohol (ethanol 95–100%) is used in embolization of high-flow AVMs and to a much lesser degree in the treatment of low-flow lesions. Ethanol is a non-specific chemical irritant that acts by causing cellular lysis, protein denaturation and ultimately chemical necrosis of target lesions. This agent is also used in endoscopic ablation of oesophageal varices and renal cysts. Ethanol can result in significant complications such as acute pulmonary hypertension, right heart failure and arrhythmias.

Highly viscous agents, n-butyl cyanoacrylate (nBCA – 'glue') and Onyx, are embolic agents used to focally occlude AVMs. nBCA is an adhesive liquid that will polymerize in contact with any ionic solution. nBCA needs to be combined with ethiodized oil to reduce the polymerization time and to add radio-opacity. Other than its adhesive effects, nBCA induces an inflammatory response, which helps with vessel obstruction. A less adhesive liquid, Onyx, is a liquid polymerizing embolic agent. Its active component is a copolymer of ethylene and vinyl alcohol (EVOH) dissolved in dimethyl sulfoxide (DMSO). Onyx is administered slowly, which allows a more controlled approach to penetrate the lesion and reach the nidus.

Use of coils in the treatment of AVMs is not recommended as coils placed in feeding arteries can induce the development of collateral circulation. In addition, coils will block future access to the lesion. The only role coils may play in treating AVMs is to focally occlude the draining veins. This may reduce the flow rates and can act as an adjunct to the embolization procedure.

Venous Malformations

Foam sclerosants are the agents of choice when treating VMs and less frequently to treat AVMs. Ethanol has been mostly superseded by foam sclerosants in the management of VMs and should only be used discriminately. STS and POL foam are the most commonly used agents. VMs and subtypes such as glomuvenous malformations (GVMs) and blue rubber bleb (BRB) lesions respond very well to percutaneous sclerotherapy [2].

Detergent sclerosants act by disrupting the endothelial lining of blood vessels, exposing the underlying collagen to induce endovascular fibrosis. These agents are less harsh than chemical irritants such as ethanol. Detergent sclerosants may be used in the liquid or foam format. Foams are created by mixing the liquid detergent with a gas such as room air or carbon dioxide (CO_2). Sclerosants are delivered to the target vessels either by direct injection under ultrasound guidance or using various catheter techniques. Foam sclerosants are x100,000 more viscous than liquid sclerosants and ethanol and hence less likely to be washed away in high-flow lesions [3]. Foam sclerosants displace the intravascular blood hence decreasing the deactivation and dilution of the active sclerosing agent. Therefore, foam sclerosants are approximately x4 more effective than liquid agents [4]. Complications of foam sclerosants have been previously reviewed [5].

In the past 10 years, the author (KP) has been using endovenous laser ablation (EVLA) in the management of selected vascular malformations and in particular the embryonic marginal vein, large intramuscular VMs and large subcutaneous VMs. Complex VMs may require a combined strategy involving surgery and open access sclerotherapy [6].

Lymphatic Malformations

Doxycycline, bleomycin and OK-432 are the most commonly used agents in the treatment of macrocystic LMs. Ethanol has a limited role and should only be used discriminately. The cystic fluid is usually aspirated and discarded first before the lesion is injected.

Doxycycline is a tetracycline antibody classified as a chemical irritant when used as a sclerosing agent.

Bleomycin is a cytotoxic glycopeptide antibiotic isolated from a strain of *Streptomyces verticillus*. It is used as a chemotherapy agent to treat malignant lymphoma. Intralesional injection of bleomycin is used to treat cutaneous warts and LMs.

OK-432 (Picibanil) is a lyophilized incubation mixture of group A *Streptococcus pyogenes* of human origin with antineoplastic activity.

Localized Complications

Pain and Swelling

Foam Sclerosants

Most patients experience very little pain following foam sclerotherapy. Application of adequate compression following treatment is important to prevent significant postoperative thrombophlebitis, which can result in pain and swelling. Pain a few days or weeks following treatment may be due to retained coagulum within the treated VMs. Aspiration of such coagulum and use of non-steroidal anti-inflammatory agents (NSAIDs) are usually enough to relieve the pain.

Ethanol

Pain and substantial swelling are considered expected sequelae of ethanol embolization [7]. Depending on the location of the lesion, the swelling may obstruct vital structures such as the airway [8]. Use of systemic steroids may be required to prevent significant postoperative swelling.

Viscous Embolic Agents and Coils

Depending on the anatomical site of the lesion, nBCA and Onyx can induce significant postoperative pain. For instance, embolization of AVM of a digit may result in significant postoperative neuropathic pain that can last for weeks. Drugs such as pregabalin (Lyrica) may be used to treat such neuropathic pain but may be ineffective (author's experience). Measures to reduce the postoperative swelling may help alleviate the pain. Amputation of the affected digit may be required. Similarly, coils when employed to treat AVMs can induce significant postoperative ischemic pain.

Lymphatic Agents

Doxycycline may cause some mild postoperative pain due to its inflammatory effect. Bleomycin can cause postoperative pain, erythema and swelling. The pain usually lasts 72 h but is relieved with analgesia [9]. OK-432 can cause local swelling and pain secondary to its inflammatory action [10].

Skin and Soft Tissue

Foam Sclerosants

The foam preparation of sclerosing agents is less toxic to the surrounding tissues mostly due to its significant gas composition and the smaller active liquid content. In a clinical study of foam sclerotherapy of VMs, the incidence of skin necrosis was less than 2%, and skin complications were managed with conservative treatment [11, 12]. STS is a harsher agent compared with POL and is best reserved for deeper and larger lesions. Malformations with a dermal involvement or a very superficial location should be best treated with lower concentrations of foam sclerosants. Author's (KP) preference is to use a 0.5% concentration of POL 1 + 4 foam for superficial lesions and a 1.5% STS foam for deeper and larger vessels. Inadvertent intraarterial injection into a nontarget artery with resultant embolization of normal capillary beds will result in cutaneous necrosis [13]. In addition, using STS to treat lesions with cutaneous involvement may

trigger the veno-arteriolar reflex (VAR) vasospasm resulting in skin necrosis [14]. Given the detergent nature of these agents, infection is a very rare complication.

Ethanol

Ethanol is associated with a higher incidence of soft tissue injuries, skin necrosis and amputation especially when treating lesions with skin or subcutaneous soft tissue involvement (Figs. 35.1, 35.2 and 35.3). In a large clinical study of embolo/sclerotherapy of CVMs using ethanol in most cases, skin necrosis occurred in 29% (42 of 143) of the AVM patients and 8% (22 of 273) of the VM patients. In the AVM patients with skin necrosis, conservative treatment, such as applying a simple dressing, was enough in most patients (57%), but escharectomy (24%), skin graft (10%) or amputation (9%) was required in the patients with deep tissue injury. In the VM patients with skin necrosis, conservative treatment was enough in most patients (59%), but escharectomy (32%) or skin graft (9%) was

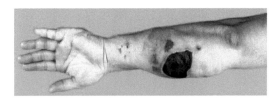

Fig. 35.2 Skin necrosis following ethanol embolization of an arteriovenous malformation (AVM). (Courtesy of Prof. BB Lee)

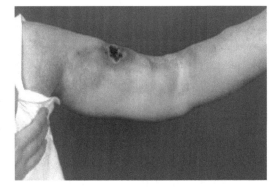

Fig. 35.3 Skin necrosis following alcohol embolization of a venous malformation (Courtesy of Prof. BB Lee)

required in patients with deep tissue injury. Ethanol always causes the skin to split as it is extruded. Prophylactic antibiotics are advised when treating LMs as they tend to become infected quite frequently.

Viscous Embolic Agents and Coils

nBCA and Onyx are associated with a low frequency of skin complications [15, 16]. However, Onyx creates a black mass that will show through the skin and may require surgical excision for cosmetic reasons. Coils can induce tissue necrosis when used to occlude arteries feeding superficial AVMs.

Lymphatic Agents

Doxycycline is a chemical irritant, and hence its extravasation can rarely cause soft tissue or skin necrosis [17]. Bleomycin can cause local skin necrosis, ulceration and eschar formation at the site of injection [18] and infection in 1%. [19] OK-432 can cause local oedema, an inflammatory response and rarely abscess formation. The inflammatory reaction does not cause damage to the overlying skin and does not lead to ulceration [20].

Nerve Injury

Foam Sclerosants

Nerve injury is a very unlikely complication of foam sclerotherapy. In a clinical study of foam sclerotherapy of VMs, the incidence of nerve injury was less than 1% [11]. Extravasation of a high concentration of STS preparation especially in the liquid format or a direct injection into a nerve can cause nerve damage. Meticulous imaging and in particular ultrasound guidance are required to avoid this complication.

Ethanol

Nerve injuries occur frequently with ethanol. In a large clinical study of embolo/sclerotherapy of CVMs with ethanol in most cases, nerve palsy occurred in 9% (13 of 143) of the AVM patients and 11% (30 of 273) of the VM patients [15].

All nerve palsy of the AVM patients and most nerve palsy of the VM patients recovered completely at an average of 5.3 months (range, 1–24 months), but seven palsies in VM group did not resolve. The most common site of nerve palsy was in the upper extremity. No specific management was needed, but four patients with permanent motor nerve palsy received an orthosis.

Viscous Embolic Agents and Coils

When using nBCA or Onyx as embolic agents for AVMs, nerve palsy is quite rare [14, 16]. Coil embolization can result in nerve palsy either by inducing an ischemic effect or by a direct space-occupying effect. This is especially reported when coils are packed to treat AV fistulae.

Lymphatic Agents

In a review of 27 studies including 1406 patients treated with intralesional bleomycin, nerve injury was not documented. In this meta-analysis, a 2% incidence of facial nerve paralysis (2%) was observed in patients treated with ethanol, but was never reported after intralesional bleomycin injections [19]. Facial nerve function in patients treated with intralesional bleomycin injections in the maxillofacial region has been studied [21]. Electromyography and motor nerve conduction studies were within normal ranges in all patients.

Major and Systemic Complications

Cardiovascular and Pulmonary

Foam Sclerosants

Detergent sclerosants rarely cause cardiovascular adverse effects, although there has been at least one report of a reversible cardiac arrest following the use of POL [22]. POL is classified as a local anaesthetic and hence an overdose can cause bradycardia. Safe dose of POL as a sclerosant liquid is 2 mg/kg of body weight. When used in foam format, a max limit of 20 mL of foam per session should be respected (see below).

Ethanol

Ethanol has proven its efficacy in the management of CVMs; however, its use has been associated with significant complications and in particular cardiopulmonary collapse requiring resuscitation [23]. Pulmonary hypertension is a potentially fatal complication of ethanol embolotherapy and occurs when large volumes of ethanol are injected that eventually reach the lungs. The aetiology of pulmonary hypertension and cardiopulmonary complications is described in Chap. 32. To reduce this risk, appropriate measures should be taken which include administration of general anaesthesia and close cardiopulmonary monitoring. When high volume of ethanol injection (more than 0.5 ml/kg) is planned, pulmonary artery Swan-Ganz line and arterial line monitoring are recommended. When the mean pulmonary artery pressure (PAP) is elevated by more than 25 mmHg, infusion of nitroglycerine is recommended as a bolus injection ($50–100 \mu g$) and then as a continuous infusion ($0.3–3.0 \mu g/kg/min$) through the Swan-Ganz line [24–28]. In one animal study, milrinone was superior to nitroglycerine in maintaining increased cardiac output and reducing significant increases in pulmonary artery hypertension in reaction to repeat bolus injections of absolute ethanol [29]. When an elevated PAP is sustained at the end of the treatment, keeping the patient at the intensive care unit for close PAP monitoring and for the continuous administration of nitroglycerine is recommended.

A total dose of ethanol, which is less than 1 ml/kg, is the maximum volume that can be safely delivered during a procedure since higher volumes can result in toxicity. The dose of the single bolus injection is also important in preventing cardiovascular collapse. In one prospective study, a significant increase of the right ventricular end-diastolic volume index and right ventricular end-systolic volume index was observed at a dose of more than 0.14 ml/kg of body weight for a single bolus injection of absolute ethanol. Based on this study, the single bolus injection of absolute ethanol less than 0.1 ml/kg of body weight is strongly recom-

mended to prevent cardiovascular collapse in clinical practice.

In Samsung Medical Center, limiting ethanol injections (total volume less than 0.5 ml/kg of body weight, single bolus injection less than 0.1 ml/kg of body weight) every 10 min has obviated the need of pulmonary artery monitoring [30, 31]. When we use ethanol for the treatment of VMs, we use limiting ethanol injections every 10 min without pulmonary artery monitoring. By contrast, we monitor the PAP in most AVM patients undergoing ethanol embolisation.

Viscous Embolic Agents and Coils

nBCA and Onyx are not associated with cardiopulmonary complications. Coils can dislodge and embolize to lungs.

Lymphatic Agents

Bleomycin when used in large doses may produce toxic effects such as pulmonary fibrosis. Pulmonary fibrosis has been associated with intravenous bleomycin administration exceeding the total cumulative dose of 400 mg. Bleomycin doses used in sclerotherapy are small in comparison, typically 1–5% of the lowest dose associated with possible pulmonary fibrosis [32]. In 27 studies enroling 1325 patients, no pulmonary fibrosis was reported [19]. OK-432 and doxycycline are not associated with cardiopulmonary complications.

Cerebrovascular Events

Foam Sclerosants

Yamaki et al. reported the superiority of foam versus liquid sclerotherapy in a prospective comparative randomized study of VM treatment [12]. Foam sclerotherapy delivers good relief of symptoms and clinical improvement with minimal risk of complications in the VMs. However, after foam sclerotherapy, there are well-documented but rare reports of significant neurological events including major stroke, seizures and transient ischaemic attacks by the cerebrovascular air embolism of bubbles through right-to-left shunt (e.g. patent foramen ovale). Immediate treatment with hyperbaric O_2 (100% O_2) was recommended to overcome neurological events [15, 33].

The overall frequency of neurological complications of foam sclerotherapy for the treatment of varicose veins is reported to be from 0% to 2%. To reduce the cerebrovascular air embolism during foam sclerotherapy of VMs, the volume of injected foam should be limited. European guideline suggests limiting the injected volume of foam sclerosants to less than 10 mL. The Australasian College of Phlebology (ACP) consensus recommendations have set this limit at 20 mL per session. But these guidelines apply to the treatment of varicose veins and not VMs. In a high proportion (around 30%) of VMs, there is an isolated VM without draining vein. For those patients, higher foam volume may be applicable with less risk of air embolism. CO_2 is approximately 20 times more soluble in blood than oxygen and nitrogen is the least soluble gas. At higher volumes, CO_2-based foam sclerosants cause fewer complications compared with air-based foam [34]. Finally, tumescent anaesthetic may be employed to 'lock' the injected foam in place, reducing its distal drainage. In addition to neurovascular complications associated with the foam format, overdosage of POL beyond the prescribed 2 mg/kg dosage can cause anaesthetic toxicity.

Ethanol

Ethanol is associated with significant neurological adverse events but these are mostly of a localized nature. Ischaemic or haemorrhagic strokes have not been reported as a complication of ethanol sclerotherapy when this agent is used to treat *peripheral* vascular malformations.

Viscous Embolic Agents

nBCA and Onyx are routinely used to treat cerebral AVMs. In this setting, both can cause ischaemic and haemorrhagic cerebrovascular events [35]. In one study, 14% patients showed procedure-related neurological deficit with 2%

showing permanent disabling deficits and 1% treatment-related mortality [36].

Coils and Lymphatic Agents

When used to treat peripheral lesions, these agents are not associated with an increase of neurovascular adverse events.

Thrombotic Complications

Foam Sclerosants

In a clinical study of foam sclerotherapy of VM, there was no deep vein thrombosis (DVT) during follow-up [11]. These agents however can cause thrombophlebitis of the target lesions and the adjoining veins. The use of compression after treatment can alleviate the risk of this complication.

Ethanol

Significant DVT occurs very rarely after embolo/sclerotherapy of CVM (less than 1%). In a large clinical study of ethanol embolotherapy of AVMs ($n = 176$) and VMs ($n = 158$), the reported incidence of DVT was 1.1% and 0%, even though immediate DUS imaging study was performed the day after treatment to rule out DVT [15]. It has been suggested that the use of larger volumes can increase the risk of DVT [11, 24, 37].

Viscous Embolic Agents, Coils and Lymphatic Agents

This complication has not been reported as a direct effect of these procedures; however, postoperative immobility may predispose patients to DVT.

Haemoglobinuria

Foam Sclerosants

Haemoglobinuria may develop as a consequence of the haemolysis that follows any sclerosant injection. This is a rare complication of foam sclerotherapy and will only occur if excessively high doses of agents have been used. This complication is extremely rare but possible given their lytic effect on red blood cells (RBC) [4, 38].

Based on the manufacturer's recommendation, the max dose of STS 3% used in one sitting should be limited to 4 mL (Australia) and 10 mL (USA). This dose should be adjusted when treating children with a lower body mass. The maximum dose of POL is 2 mg/kg of body weight. Good hydration and monitoring of urine output may be required [8].

Ethanol

Haemoglobinuria is a common finding following ethanol embolo/sclerotherapy of VMs or AVMs, especially when using doses greater than 0.5 mL/kg of body weight. It is caused by the haemolytic effect of ethanol. No renal impairment due to haemoglobinuria has been reported [25]. Post-op hydration with intravenous saline may be required.

Viscous Embolic Agents, Coils and Lymphatic Agents

These agents have no lytic properties and hence not associated with this complication.

Distal Embolism

The incidence of distal embolism is quite low (less than 1%). Distal embolism related to embolotherapy of AVMs may result either from the obliteration of an affected normal artery by reflux of embolic or sclerosing agents into the adjacent normal artery or from simple arterial occlusion due to reflux of a thrombus formed at the lesion site. Thrombolysis with urokinase or tissue plasminogen activator is quite effective for treatment of distal embolism due to reflux of a thrombus, but ineffective due to reflux of sclerosing agents [24].

Anaphylaxis

Anaphylaxis is an extremely rare complication of sclerotherapy constituting an emergency situation. If anaphylaxis is suspected, stopping the injection immediately and standard emergency procedures including the administration of epinephrine is required [34].

Other Complications

Less common but significant other adverse events include severe swelling with progression to compartment syndrome, arterial embolization, coil embolization and organ ischaemia.

Complications Secondary to Anaesthesia

Complications can occur secondary to anaesthesia. In patients with VM involving the head and neck, the process of intubation or even a laryngeal mask combined with a positive pressure ventilation can result in excessively high venous pressures. This can result in bleeding into airways.

Mortality

Ethanol and OK-432 have been associated with mortality following their use in treatment of vascular malformations. Fortunately, the incidence remains very low.

Conclusion

Foam sclerosants enjoy a lower complication rate compared with ethanol. Adequate imaging, careful treatment strategy and planning and careful postoperative care can help with reducing the risk of complications and increasing the success rate.

Acknowledgements The authors thank Prof. BB Lee for providing the figures used in this chapter.

References

1. Upton J, Taghinia A. Special considerations in vascular anomalies: operative management of upper extremity lesions. Clin Plast Surg. 2011;38:143–51.
2. Parsi K, Kossard S. Multiple hereditary glomangiomas: successful treatment with sclerotherapy. Australas J Dermatol. 2002;43:43–7.
3. Wong K, Chen T, Connor DE, Behnia M, Parsi K. Basic physiochemical and rheological properties of detergent sclerosants. Phlebology. 2015;30:339–49.

4. Connor DE, Cooley-Andrade O, Goh WX, Ma DD, Parsi K. Detergent sclerosants are deactivated and consumed by circulating blood cells. Eur J Vasc Endovasc Surg. 2015;49:426–31.

5. Cavezzi A, Parsi K. Complications of foam sclerotherapy. Phlebology. 2012;27(Suppl 1):46–51.

6. Kim B, Somia N, Pereira J, Parsi K. Open access sclerotherapy: an alternative technique to treat complex venous malformations. Dermatol Surg. 2014;40:802–5.

7. Donnelly LF, Bisset 3rd GS, Adams DM. Marked acute tissue swelling following percutaneous sclerosis of low-flow vascular malformations: a predictor of both prolonged recovery and therapeutic effect. Pediatr Radiol. 2000;30:415–9.

8. Burrows PE, Mason KP. Percutaneous treatment of low flow vascular malformations. J Vasc Interv Radiol. 2004;15:431–45.

9. Saitta P, Krishnamurthy K, Brown LH. Bleomycin in dermatology: a review of intralesional applications. Dermatol Surg. 2008;34:1299–313.

10. Ogita S, Tsuto T, Nakamura K, Deguchi E, Iwai N. OK-432 therapy in 64 patients with lymphangioma. J Pediatr Surg. 1994;29:784–5.

11. Park HS, Do YS, Park KB, et al. Clinical outcome and predictors of treatment response in foam sodium tetradecyl sulfate sclerotherapy of venous malformations. Eur Radiol. 2016;26:1301–10.

12. Yamaki T, Nozaki M, Sakurai H, et al. Prospective randomized efficacy of ultrasound-guided foam sclerotherapy compared with ultrasound-guided liquid sclerotherapy in the treatment of symptomatic venous malformations. J Vasc Surg. 2008;47:578–84.

13. Parsi K, Hannaford P. Intra-arterial injection of sclerosants: report of three cases treated with systemic steroids. Phlebology. 2015;31:241–50.

14. Tran D, Parsi K. Veno-arteriolar reflex vasospasm of small saphenous artery complicating sclerotherapy of the small saphenous vein. Austr N Z J Phleb. 2007;10:29–32.

15. Lee KB, Kim DI, Oh SK, et al. Incidence of soft tissue injury and neuropathy after embolo/sclerotherapy for congenital vascular malformation. J Vasc Surg. 2008;48:1286–91.

16. Tan KT, Simons ME, Rajan DK, Terbrugge K. Peripheral high-flow arteriovenous vascular malformations: a single-center experience. J Vasc Interv Radiol. 2004;15:1071–80.

17. Shergill A, John P, Amaral JG. Doxycycline sclerotherapy in children with lymphatic malformations: outcomes, complications and clinical efficacy. Pediatr Radiol. 2012;42:1080–8.

18. Kirby JS, Miller CJ. Intralesional chemotherapy for nonmelanoma skin cancer: a practical review. J Am Acad Dermatol. 2010;63:689–702.

19. Horbach SE, Rigter IM, Smitt JH, et al. Intralesional bleomycin injections for vascular malformations: a systematic review and meta-analysis. Plast Reconstr Surg. 2016;137:244–56.

20. Ogita S, Tsuto T, Nakamura K, et al. OK-432 therapy for lymphangioma in children: why and how does it work? J Pediatr Surg. 1996;31:477–80.

21. Karavelioglu A, Temucin CM, Tanyel FC, et al. Sclerotherapy with bleomycin does not adversely affect facial nerve function in children with cervicofacial cystic lymphatic malformation. J Pediatr Surg. 2010;45:1627–32.

22. Marrocco-Trischitta MM, Guerrini P, Abeni D, Stillo F. Reversible cardiac arrest after polidocanol sclerotherapy of peripheral venous malformation. Dermatol Surg. 2002;28:153–5.

23. Cordero-Schmidt G, Wallenstein MB, Ozen M, et al. Pulmonary hypertensive crisis following ethanol sclerotherapy for a complex vascular malformation. J Perinatol. 2014;34:713–5.

24. Park HS, Do YS, Park KB, et al. Ethanol embolotherapy of hand arteriovenous malformations. J Vasc Surg. 2011;53:725–31.

25. Do YS, Kim YW, Park KB, et al. Endovascular treatment combined with emboloscleorotherapy for pelvic arteriovenous malformations. J Vasc Surg. 2012;55:465–71.

26. Do YS, Park KB, Park HS, et al. Extremity arteriovenous malformations involving the bone: therapeutic outcomes of ethanol embolotherapy. J Vasc Interv Radiol. 2010;21:807–16.

27. Lee BB, Baumgartner I, Berlien HP, et al. Consensus Document of the International Union of Angiology (IUA)-2013. Current concept on the management of arterio-venous management. Int Angiol. 2013;32:9–36.

28. Park KB, Do YS, Kim DI, et al. Predictive factors for response of peripheral arteriovenous malformations to embolization therapy: analysis of clinical data and imaging findings. J Vasc Interv Radiol. 2012;23:1478–86.

29. Kim JS, Nam MH, Do YS, et al. Efficacy of milrinone versus nitroglycerin in controlling pulmonary arterial hypertension induced by intravenous injections of absolute ethanol in anesthetized dogs. J Vasc Interv Radiol. 2010;21:882–7.

30. Ko JS, Kim JA, Do YS, et al. Prediction of the effect of injected ethanol on pulmonary arterial pressure during sclerotherapy of arteriovenous malformations: relationship with dose of ethanol. J Vasc Interv Radiol. 2009;20:39–45. quiz 45

31. Shin BS, Do YS, Cho HS, et al. Effects of repeat bolus ethanol injections on cardiopulmonary hemodynamic changes during embolotherapy of arteriovenous malformations of the extremities. J Vasc Interv Radiol. 2010;21:81–9.

32. Orford J, Barker A, Thonell S, King P, Murphy J. Bleomycin therapy for cystic hygroma. J Pediatr Surg. 1995;30:1282–7.

33. Bush RG, Derrick M, Manjoney D. Major neurological events following foam sclerotherapy. Phlebology. 2008;23:189–92.

34. Rabe E, Breu FX, Cavezzi A, et al. European guidelines for sclerotherapy in chronic venous disorders. Phlebology. 2014;29:338–54.
35. Lv X, Wu Z, Jiang C, et al. Complication risk of endovascular embolization for cerebral arteriovenous malformation. Eur J Radiol. 2011; 80:776–9.
36. Hartmann A, Pile-Spellman J, Stapf C, et al. Risk of endovascular treatment of brain arteriovenous malformations. Stroke. 2002;33:1816–20.
37. Yun WS, Kim YW, Lee KB, et al. Predictors of response to percutaneous ethanol sclerotherapy (PES) in patients with venous malformations: analysis of patient self-assessment and imaging. J Vasc Surg. 2009;50:581–9. 589 e581
38. Parsi K, Exner T, Connor DE, et al. The lytic effects of detergent sclerosants on erythrocytes, platelets, endothelial cells and microparticles are attenuated by albumin and other plasma components in vitro. Eur J Vasc Endovasc Surg. 2008;36:216–23.

Surgical Treatment of Low-Flow CVM

Raul Mattassi

Summary

Low-flow CVM are truncular or extratruncular type. Truncular superficial dilated dysplastic veins can be removed surgically if deep veins are normal. Venous aneurysm needs treatment because pulmonary embolism may happen. Tangential resection or vein transplant are the best treatment. Extratruncular forms, limited or infiltrating, may be sited in every part of the body. Often they are intramuscular. Treatment options are surgical removal, sclerosis by direct puncture with foam or alcohol injection, and laser treatment. According to great variability in site and extension, treatment strategy should be decided at a multidisciplinary discussion.

Low-flow CVM are dysplasias of veins and can be divided in defects of the main trunks (*truncular malformations*) and areas of dysplastic vessels sited in the tissues (*extratruncular malformations*) [1]. They are the most common CVM. In our recent series, collected between 2011 and 2015, the majority of defects are sited in the lower limbs, followed by the head and neck, in a group of 624 patients (Table 36.1).

Before deciding treatment strategy, a complete and correct diagnostic procedure should be done, as CVM are extremely variable and a complete hemodynamic and morphologic data about the defect is mandatory [2, 3].

Treatment options are surgical approach; sclerosant treatment, including alcohol procedure; and laser. Due to the great variability of CVM, treatment strategy and technique should be decided individually. Incidence of surgery, once the only treatment available, beside sclerosis, is now lesser done because of the introduction of alcohol sclerosis (much more effective than the old classical sclerosis in VM) and superficial and interstitial laser procedure. However, surgery is still a crucial technique for treatment of VM and has a specific role that should be always considered by planning treatment strategy.

Surgical Treatment of Truncular Defects

Venous truncular defects include aplasia, hypoplasia, and congenital dilatation of veins. Approach to main vein aplasia and hypoplasia as well as persistence of marginal vein will be discussed in Chap. 37.

Superficial dilated dysplastic veins of the lower limbs can be removed surgically. However, a precise diagnostic hemodynamic study of the limb should be performed before operation in order to rule out dysplasia of the deep system; deep vein aplasia excludes surgical treatment, while hypoplasia does not (see Chap. 39). Dilated

R. Mattassi
Center for Vascular Malformations "Stefan Belov",
Clinical Institute Humanitas "Mater Domini",
Castellanza, Varese, Italy
e-mail: raulmattassi@gmail.com

Y.-W. Kim et al. (eds.), *Congenital Vascular Malformations*, DOI 10.1007/978-3-662-46709-1_36

superficial dysplastic veins may look like varicose veins. However, it is much more common atypical aspects, like abnormal dilated areas; atypical sites, like the lateral edge of the limb or the foot; and the presence of nevus (Fig. 36.1). Diffuse, superficial dilated dysplastic veins are best treated by step-by-step surgical removal, avoiding exten-

Table 36.1 Distribution of venous malformations in the body 624 cases (2011–2015)

Site	Cases
Lower limbs	323 (52%)
Head and neck	126 (20%)
Upper limbs	103 (16.5%)
Thorax	32 (5%)
Abdomen and pelvis	26 (4%)
Gluteus	9 (2%)
Multiple locations	5 (1.5%)
Total	624

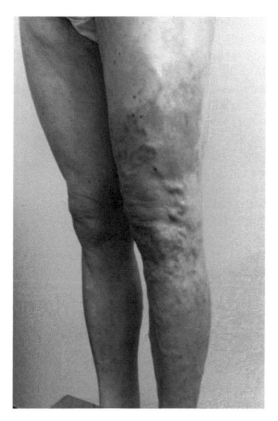

Fig. 36.1 Superficial venous malformation in the left lower limb with skin nevus and dysplastic veins, located in an atypical area

sive, long-lasting operations that may complicate by bleeding and infection of wounds [4].

Venous aneurysms are sometimes symptomatic, like in the lower limbs, originating pain by stasis and compression of near sited structures. Common is the location on jugular, portal vein, saphena magna, poplitea, superficial and common femoral, azygos, and vena cava superior. Pulmonary embolism has been reported [5]. Surgical removal is possible in collateral veins, like great saphenous or jugular vein. Aneurysms of main veins can be treated by tangential resection of the malformation and plastic or resection with a great saphenous graft transplant [6]. Tangential resection has a better outcome, as saphenous transplant can be sometimes complicated by thrombosis (Fig. 36.2).

Surgical Treatment of Extratruncular VM

Extratruncular VM may be sited in every part of the body. Intramuscular location is common. Every muscle can be involved. Extension of the defect may vary from small, limited to large, extensively infiltrating malformations [7].

Limited intramuscular VM can be removed by surgery, even if percutaneous alcohol treatment is often the procedure of choice [8]. A correct localization of the defect is required before operation. Duplex scan and MR examination are necessary to establish clearly site and extension of the defect. A duplex scan mapping is recommended before beginning surgery. Limited, intramuscular CVM can be removed easily, especially if the location is superficial, just under the muscular fascia. A longitudinal incision of muscular fascia at the site of malformation allows exposing the defect. Pathological muscular fibers, without contractile function, are recognizable by a different, pale color at the periphery of the malformation and can be resected. Deeper in the muscle, sited defects may be difficult to recognize; an intraoperative echographic study may be helpful in order to avoid extensive muscle dissection. Resection with complete removal and closure of the fascia is the correct procedure. Stitches on

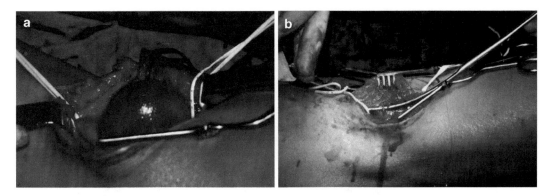

Fig. 36.2 (**a**) Popliteal venous aneurysm exposed (**b**) after tangential clamping and resection

muscular fibers in the resected area are not necessary.

Diffuse, intramuscular infiltrating malformations are not a good indication for surgery as diffuse, difficult-to-control bleeding is possible. Those extended malformations may cause a limited, local intravascular coagulopathy (LIC) with elevated D-dimer and fibrinogen consumption [9, 10]. In some diffuse cases, operation may increase that phenomenon with development of a disseminated intravascular coagulopathy (DIC) and diffuse, uncontrollable bleeding. D-dimer and fibrinogen dosage before surgery is highly recommended in those cases. If low fibrinogen level exists before surgery, a treatment with low-molecular heparin is recommended until fibrinogen is normalized. If surgery is performed, tourniquet is recommended in locations like limbs. By release of tourniquet after completion of the resection, extensive bleeding is possible. Postoperative strict control of fibrinogen is also necessary to prevent bleeding, as fibrinogen, normalized by heparin treatment before operation, may reduce again in the postoperative period.

VM localized outside muscles can also be resected avoiding damage to other important structures, like nerves and tendons. VM that include nerves inside the defect should be approached by a step-by-step procedure. The nerve should be prepared first and completely exposed *through* the malformation. Only after that step, the malformation itself can be removed. Intraoperative nerve stimulator to find out nerve location can be useful.

Diffuse, infiltrating extratruncular VM that are not completely removable by surgery can be partially reduced by transfix stitches in the context of the dysplastic mass. Tangential clamping with a Satinsky clamp followed by suture just below the clamp and resection of the excluded mass is another effective surgical technique to reduce the hemodynamic impact of extensive infiltrating, not completely resectable VM [11].

VM in the head can be treated often by nonsurgical techniques: laser, foam, and ethanol sclerosis [12]. In some limited superficial defects, surgical removal may be indicated. Surgery on superficial defects should be preferably performed by plastic surgeon to avoid anesthetic scars (Fig. 36.3). In the oral cavity, resection of the tongue VM is possible, but laser or alcohol treatment is less invasive and with good results. A location that may create specific treatment difficulties is *airway involvement*. VM in that area, especially if protruding in the airway, may be very fragile and can bleed severely during intubation: that bleeding can be very difficult to control. Moreover, if sclerosis is planned, obstruction of airways by edema is a real danger. Airway survey with flexible fiber-optic laryngoscopy in the office setting is required every time an involvement in that area is suspected. MR exam will confirm that data. A temporary tracheostomy is recommended in those cases [13].

VM on the neck are often limited and superficial. Surgical removal is often possible with good results. Intramuscular VM can be also removed by surgery. In our experience, alcohol sclerosis is

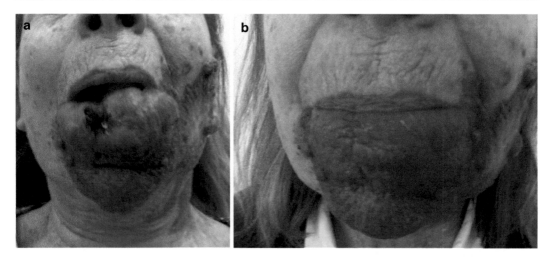

Fig. 36.3 (a) Patient with an extended VM of the lower lip with repeated bleeding. (b) After surgical removal of a large part of the defect, treatment continues in a step-by-step laser and alcohol procedure

an excellent alternative to operation. VM located on the scalp should be approached with caution. A direct intracranial connection should be excluded by duplex scan and MR exam. Surgery is a good option in VM located on the scalp, as alcohol occlusion may create permanent hair loss.

Thorax location of VM is possible. Superficial, limited defects can be easily removed by surgery. Intramuscular forms, especially infiltrating, can be a difficult task for the surgeon, as thorax muscles are formed of different oriented layers that makes surgery complex, highly destructive, and with elevated risk of recurrence. A step-by-step radical procedure is the best surgical approach [14].

Abdominal superficial location can be treated surgically if the defect is limited. However, alcohol procedure is often preferred, especially if the defect is intramuscular and of the infiltrating form. Surgery can be combined as the last step to complete removal of the remaining defect. In the *pelvis*, involvement of perineum, especially labia majora in females, is common [15]. Intramuscular location of VM is possible, like in the psoas muscle. Alcohol sclerosis approach is preferred, but surgical treatment is also possible, even if difficult. Diffuse, infiltrating VM of pelvis may fill out the whole space between pelvic organs, like rectum, vagina, bladder, prostate, and uterus.

Infiltration of that structures by the malformation is common, especially the rectum, which may be the cause of rectal bleeding. Bladder infiltration may cause intermittent hematuria. Surgical approach to that infiltrating forms is very complex, difficult, and with a high risk of severe bleeding. Other treatment options, according to the single case, like endoscopic laser or alcohol treatment, should be considered and, if possible, preferred to surgery [16].

Surgical removal of *superficial VM of the limbs* is possible. In extensive malformations, we prefer a step-by-step procedure to avoid wound complication [4]. Location on *the hand* is best treated by surgery in our experience, as foam sclerosis is little effective and alcohol treatment has a high probability to damage hand nerves. Operation may be long lasting and difficult in diffuse forms, as infiltration may be extensive and bleeding control not always easy. A step-by-step strategy, with several operations instead of a single one, is preferred. A tourniquet should be always applied in that surgery, and a team-based approach with a hand specialist is highly recommended (Fig. 36.4) [17].

Lower limbs are the most common location of extratruncular VM. Intramuscular location is frequent and should be approached as discussed above [4]. *Intraarticular* malformations, most frequent on the knee, is a severe, permanent function-limiting disease. It is often erroneously named "synovial hemangioma" in the orthopedic literature [18]. Venous malformations destroy joint cartilage diffusely until removal of the defect is performed. As that location exists since birth, it should be early recognized in order to remove the defect as soon as possible to stop that progressive damage. Surgical approach in team with orthopedic specialist is our preferred strategy (Fig. 36.5). Radical removal of affected synovia together with the malformations is the best approach. Some authors suggest arthroscopic approach [19].

Intraosseous VM location may be an extension of soft tissue infiltration. That VM site rarely needs treatment except in case of extensive bone destruction and thinning with increased risk of pathologic fracture which is a severe complication as bone healing is difficult due to the malformation. Surgical removal of the surrounding malformation and strengthening of bone with cement injection is possible but rarely necessary. Percutaneous alcohol intraosseous and periosteal treatment is preferred in our experience.

In conclusion, surgery can be applied in truncular and extratruncular VM, limited or infiltrating. Technique may vary according to the specific case. Combination with other techniques and timing of the procedures should be decided on an individual basis, adapting the treatment to the specific patient [20].

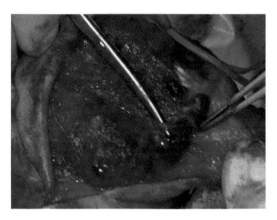

Fig. 36.4 Surgical resection of venous malformations of the hand. A nerve is prepared and isolated from the dysplastic veins to be removed

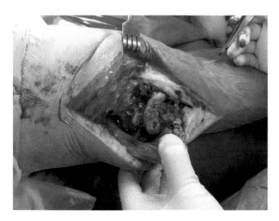

Fig. 36.5 Intraoperative image of infiltrating venous malformations inside the knee joint

References

1. Lee BB, Laredo J, Lee TS, Huh S, Neville R. Terminology and classification of congenital vascular malformations. Phlebology. 2007;22(6):249–52.
2. Lee BB, Antignani PL, Baraldini V, Baumgartner I, Berlien P, Blei F, Carrafiello GP, Grantzow R, Ianniello A, Laredo J, Loose D, Lopez Gutierrez JC, Markovic J, Mattassi R, Parsi K, Rabe E, Roztocil K, Shortell C, Vaghi M. ISVI-IUA consensus document diagnostic guidelines of vascular anomalies: vascular malformations and hemangiomas. Int Angiol. 2015) Aug;34(4):333–74.
3. Lee BB, Baumgartner I, Berlien P, Bianchini G, Burrows P, Gloviczki P, Huang Y, Laredo J, Loose DA, Markovic J, Mattassi R, Parsi K, Rabe E, Rosenblatt M, Shortell C, Stillo F, Vaghi M, Villavicencio L, Zamboni P. Diagnosis and treatment of venous malformations consensus document of the International Union of Phlebology (IUP): updated 2013. Int Angiol. 2015;34(2):97–149.
4. Mattassi R. Vascular malformations of the limbs: treatment of venous and arteriovenous malformations. In: Mattassi R, DA L, Vaghi M, editors. Hemangiomas and vascular malformations. An atlas of diagnosis and treatment. 2nd ed. Milan: Springer; 2015. p. 417–30.
5. Tomko T, Malý R, Jiska S, Chovanec V. Popliteal venous aneurysm as a cause of recurrent pulmonary embolism. Vasc Endovascular Surg. 2011;47(2):155–8. doi:10.1177/1538574412473185. Epub 2013 Jan 10
6. Johnstone JK, Fleming MD, Gloviczki P, Stone W, Kalra M, Oderich GS, Duncan AA, De Martino RR, Bower TC. Surgical treatment of popliteal venous aneurysms. Ann Vasc Surg. 2015;29(6):1084–9. doi:10.1016/j.avsg.2015.02.009. Epub 2015 May 22
7. Mattassi R, Vaghi M. Intramuscular venous malformations. Int Angiol. 2004;23(suppl I):23.

8. Rivas S, López-Gutiérrez JC, Díaz M, Andrés AM, Ros Z. Venous malformations. Diagnosis and treatment during the childhood. Cir Pediatr. 2006;19(2):77–80.

9. Dompmartin A, Acher A, Thibon P, Tourbach S, Hermans C, Deneys V, Pocock B, Lequerrec A, Labbé D, Barrellier MT, Vanwijck R, Vikkula M, Boon LM. Association of localized intravascular coagulopathy with venous malformations. Arch Dermatol. 2008;144(7):873–7. doi:10.1001/archderm.144.7.873.

10. Mazoyer E, Enjolras O, Bisdorff A, Perdu J, Wassef M, Drouet L. Coagulation disorders in patients with venous malformation of the limbs and trunk: a case series of 118 patients. Arch Dermatol. 2008;144(7):861–7. doi:10.1001/archderm.144.7.861.

11. Loose DA. Surgical management of venous malformations. Phlebology. 2007;22(6):276–82.

12. Su L, Fan X, Zheng L, Zheng J. Absolute ethanol sclerotherapy for venous malformations in the face and neck. J Oral Maxillofac Surg. 2010;68(7):1622–7. doi:10.1016/j.joms.2009.07.094. Epub 2009 Dec 4

13. Teresa O, Waner M. Upper airway congenital vascular lesions. In: Mattassi R, Loose DA, Vaghi M, editors. Hemangiomas and vascular malformations. An atlas of diagnosis and treatment. 2nd ed. Milan: Springer; 2015. p. 343–55.

14. Arneja JS, Gosain AK. An approach to the management of common vascular malformations of the trunk. J Craniofac Surg. 2006;17(4):761–6.

15. Wang S, Lang JH, Zhou HM. Venous malformations of the female lower genital tract. Eur J Obstet Gynecol Reprod Biol. 2009;145(2):205–8.

16. Burrows P. Vascular malformations involving the female pelvis. Semin Intervent Radiol. 2008 Dec;25(4):347–60. doi:10.1055/s-0028-1102993.

17. Di Giuseppe P. Treatment of vascular malformations in the hand. In: Mattassi R, Loose DA, Vaghi M, editors. Hemangiomas and vascular malformations. An atlas of diagnosis and treatment. 2nd ed. Milan: Springer; 2015. p. 379–86.

18. Lopez-Oliva CL, Wang EH, Cañal JP. Synovial hemangioma of the knee: an under recognized condition. Int Orthop. 2015;39(10):2037–40. doi:10.1007/s00264-015-2930-4. Epub 2015 Jul 31

19. Hauert J, Loose DA. Orthopedic problems. In: Mattassi R, Loose DA, Vaghi M, editors. Hemangiomas and vascular malformations. An atlas of diagnosis and treatment. Milan: Springer; 2015. p. 369–78.

20. Dompmartin A, Vikkula M, Boon L. Venous malformations: update on etiopathogenesis, diagnosis & management. Phlebology. 2010;25(5):224–35.

Surgical Treatment for High-Flow CVM

37

Dirk A. Loose

The term fast-flow or high-flow congenital vascular malformations originated by John Mulliken [1, 2] is based on the Hamburg classification and lesion flow characteristics as in the International Society for the Study of Vascular Anomalies (ISSVA) classification of 1996 [3, 4]. The details are:

(a) Truncular arterial malformations (AM): aneurysms, coarctation, ectasias, stenosis, and arteriovenous fistulas(AVF)
(b) Extratruncular arteriovenous malformations (AVM): complex combined, regional syndromes

Truncular arterial malformations develop in the late phase of embryonic development, and they have a much better prognosis in terms of recurrence than the extratruncular arteriovenous malformations.

These arterial malformations occur as aneurysms, coarctations and stenosis, or ectasias. The surgical repair applies regular techniques of reconstructive vascular surgery for tangential resection of an aneurysm [5], resection of

the aneurysm and replacement by autologous interposition graft (Fig. 37.1), autologous venous patch graft plastic to treat an arterial stenosis, a coarctation (Fig. 37.2b) or an alloplastic bypass graft to treat several stenoses, or a long-distance stenosis in a coarctation (Fig. 37.2a) [6].

Congenital AVFs of major named vessels are also treated by standard vascular surgery techniques as, e.g., interruption of the venous connection and reconstruction of the arterial defect by an alloplastic interposition graft (Fig. 37.3). AVFs of larger peripheral vessels can be treated by interventional catheter techniques as well as by vascular surgery: ligation and interruption of each AV fistula (Figs. 37.4 and 37.5) [7].

Extratruncular AVMs represent completely different challenges. They are an active lesion, and they have a high tendency to progress and to worsen and to reexpand after treatment. Truncular ones are cured after treatment. Before an indication for treatment of AVMs is worked out, it is mandatory to classify the clinical findings following the Schobinger classification of AVM (Table 37.1). This classification was worked out to assess AVM lesions in different clinical stages and clinical conditions objectively based on the patient's clinical status to select the best-suited time for treatment as a practical guideline [8]. Most (77 %) stage I lesions progress to a higher stage by adulthood. It exists as an increased risk

D.A. Loose
Bereich Angiologie und Gefäßchirurgie,
Facharztklinik Hamburg und Klinik Fleetinsel,
Hamburg, Germany
e-mail: info@prof-loose.de

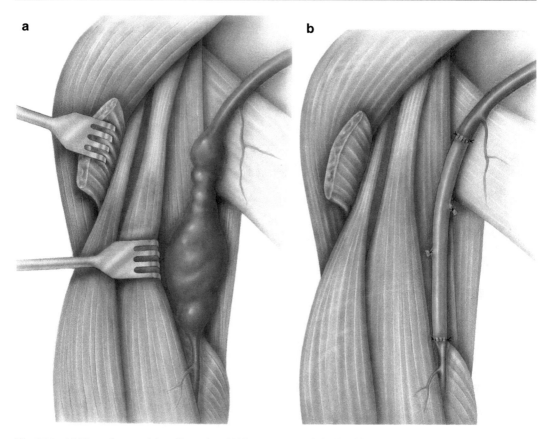

Fig. 37.1 (**a**) Truncular arterial malformation (AM): aneurysm of the brachial/axillary artery. (**b**) Resection of the aneurysm and reconstruction by autologous venous interposition graft

during puberty. Pregnancy does not increase risk of progression for stage I AVMs.

The primary option for treatment of extratruncular AVMs are interventional catheter techniques. These follow best the recommendations given by the arteriographic classification [8] proposed for extratruncular AVM lesions based on the arteriographic findings of the "nidus." Such better management and predicting of the outcome of endovascular treatment is possible.

However, in several cases sole vascular surgery is indicated or more often in combination with interventional treatment [7–9]. Resection plus embolization results in a better control compared to embolization alone. Early intervention for stage I lesions may give improved long-term control.

For example, when localized infiltrating AVMs cannot be treated by direct puncture sclerotherapy or by catheter embolization (Fig. 37.6), the en bloc resection after precise interruption of the afferent and efferent vessels is one option. In cases with secondarily dilated venous plexus by AVM, again the principal vessels (artery and vein) have to be surgically liberated from the fistulous communications precisely (Fig. 37.7). In addition the secondarily dilated veins have to be reduced and/or resected [10, 11].

A combined treatment means first interventional embolization followed by surgical excision of the localized AVM, sometimes together with adjacent tissues (Fig. 37.8) [12].

Infiltrating AVM very often cannot be treated by direct puncture or by catheter embolization

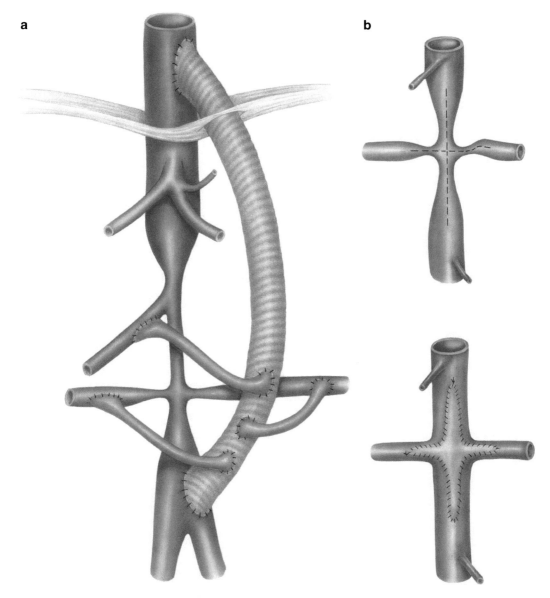

Fig. 37.2 (**a**, **b**) Truncular arterial malformation: stenosis or coarctation of the abdominal aorta. Treatment by (**a**) vascular bypass surgery: alloplastic or autologous venous grafts, (**b**) patch plastic autologous, or alloplastic

techniques [13, 14]. In this situation, the surgical technique of Belov [7] can be adopted: clamping of the infiltrated part of the tissue followed by a continuous Blalock suture and resection of the overcoming part of the AVM (Fig. 37.9). The advantage of this technique is that a cutdown of the infiltrated tissues with dramatic blood loss can be avoided.

A further sophisticated technique can be recommended in cases where the possibilities of interventional treatment have come to an end but leftovers of the nidus or of the infiltrating

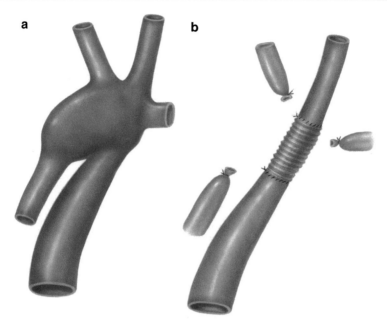

Fig. 37.3 (**a**) Truncular arteriovenous fistula (AVF) of major named vessel; treatment by interruption of the fistulas and (**b**) reconstruction of the arterial side by alloplastic interposition graft

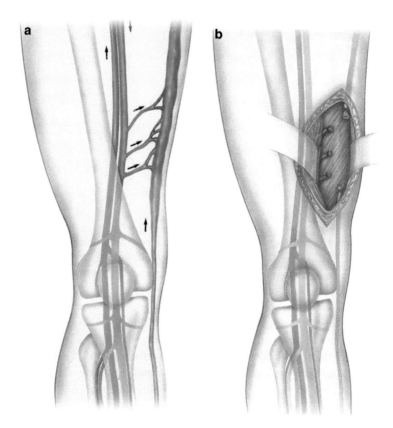

Fig. 37.4 (**a**) Truncular arteriovenous fistulas (AVF) of larger arterial vessels and branches which could not be occluded by interventional catheter techniques sufficiently. (**b**) These residual AVFs can be treated by vascular surgery: ligation and interruption of each arteriovenous fistula

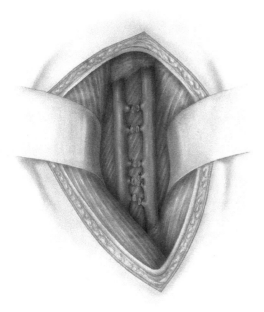

Fig. 37.5 Multiple truncular arteriovenous fistulas (AVF) can be treated by interventional catheter occlusion and/or by ligation by vascular surgery

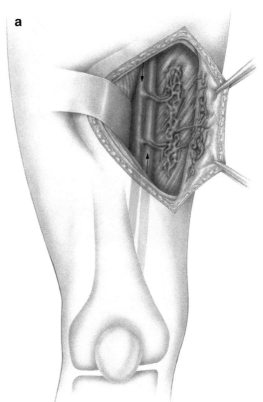

Table 37.1 Schobinger classification of AVM

Stage I (Quiescence): Pink-bluish stain, warmth, and arteriovenous shunting are revealed by Doppler scanning. The arteriovenous malformation mimics a capillary malformation or involuting hemangioma
Stage II (Expansion): Stage I plus enlargement, pulsations, thrill, bruit, and tortuous/tense veins
Stage III (Destruction): Stage II plus dystrophic skin changes, ulceration, bleeding, tissue necrosis. Bony lytic lesions may occur
Stage IV (Decompensation): Stage III plus congestive cardiac failure with increased cardiac output and left ventricle hypertrophy

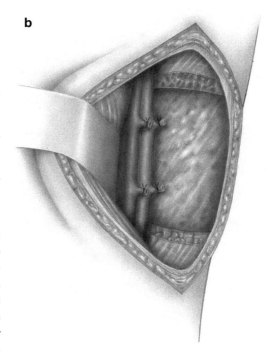

AVM have to be treated in order to avoid an early recurrence. That is the technique according to Loose [15] (Fig. 37.10): (1) identification of tiny AVMs by Doppler ultrasound, (2) clamping of the AVMs under sonographic supervision, (3) surgical closure of tiny AVMs by over-and-over sutures, and (4) Doppler ultrasound control to ensure the complete closure of the specific AVM.

These procedures have to be continued until no more AVM is to be detected by ultrasound [10, 15–20].

Fig. 37.6 (**a**) Extratruncular infiltrating arteriovenous malformation (AVM). (**b**) Treatment by interventional catheter occlusion and/or by vascular surgical ligation of residual AV fistulas and en bloc resection of infiltrated muscle together with superficial veins

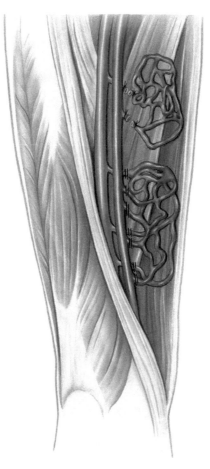

Fig. 37.7 Extratruncular arteriovenous fistulas (AVM) with secondarily dilated venous plexus. Treatment by interventional catheter occlusion of the arteriovenous fistulas and/or vascular surgery and ligation of the residual AV fistulas and resection or extirpation of the secondarily dilated veins

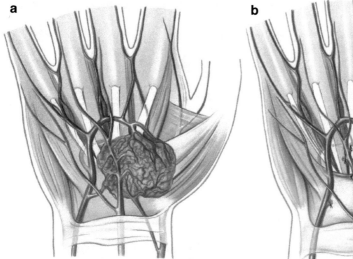
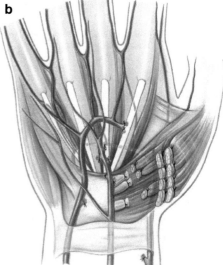

Fig. 37.8 (**a**) Extratruncular infiltrating arteriovenous malformation (AVM) with AV nidus. (**b**) Treatment by interventional catheter embolization and afterwards vascular surgery by en bloc resection of the infiltrated tissues/nidus with partial resection of the adjacent tissues

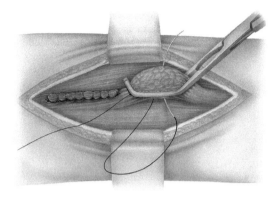

Fig. 37.9 Extratruncular localized infiltrating arteriovenous malformation (AVM): when sclerotherapy or embolization treatment are not possible or not successful, the surgical technique according to Belov [7] is an option: clamping of the infiltrated part of the tissue followed by a continuous Blalock suture and resection of the overcoming part of the AVM

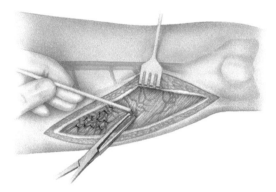

Fig. 37.10 Extratruncular diffuse infiltrating AVM not to be sufficiently treatable by interventional techniques can be treated by the surgical technique according to Loose: before surgery the AVMs are identified by colors. Doppler imaging and precisely marked on the overlying skin. During surgery ultrasonic Doppler mapping of AV fistulas, clamping, and over-and-over sutures of the AV fistulas and directly afterwards ultrasonic control of the complete closure of the AV fistulas. This has to be continued until every AV fistula of the specific region is closed up

References

 1. Mulliken JB, Glowacki J. Hemangiomas and vascular malformations in infants and children: a classification based on endothelial characteristics. Plast Reconstr Surg. 1982;69:412–22.
 2. Enjolras O, Mulliken JB. Vascular tumors and vascular malformations (new issues). Adv Dermatol. 1997;13:375–423.
 3. Mulliken JB. Classification of vascular birthmarks. In: Mulliken JB, AE Y, editors. Vascular birthmarks: hemangiomas and malformations. Philadelphia: WB Saunders; 1988. p. 24–37.
 4. Lee BB, Baumgartner I, Berlien P, Bianchini G, Burrow P, Glovicki P, Huang Y, Laredo J, Loose DA, Markovic J, Mattassi R, Parsi K, Rabe E, Rosenblatt M, Shortell C, Stillo F, Villavicencio L, Zamboni P. Diagnosis and treatment of venous malformations Consensus Document of the International Union of Phlebology (IUP) updated 2013. Int Angiol. 2014. PMID:24566499.
 5. Mattassi R, Loose DA. Treatment of arterial malformations. In: Mattassi R, Loose DA, Vaghi M, editors. Hemangiomas and vascular malformations. Milan: Springer-Italia; 2009. p. 209–13.
 6. Belov S, Loose DA. Surgical treatment of congenital vascular defects. Int Angiol. 1990;9:175–82.
 7. Belov S. Operative- technical peculiarities in operations of congenital vascular defects. In: Balas P, editor. Progress in angiology. Turin: Edizioni Minerva Medica; 1991. p. 379–82.
 8. Lee BB, Baumgartner I, Berlien HP, Bianchini G, Burrows P, Do YS, Ivancev K, Kool LS, Laredo J, Loose DA, Lopez-Gutierrez JC, Mattassi R, Parsi K, Rimon U, Rosenblatt M, Shortell C, Simkin R, Stillo F, Villavicencio L, Yakes W. Consensus document of the International Union of Angiology (IUA)-2013, Current concepts on the management of arteriovenous malformations. Int Angiol. 2013;32(1):9–36.
 9. Loose DA. Combined treatment of congenital vascular defects: indications and tactics. Semin Vasc Surg. 1993;4:260–5.
10. Loose DA. The combined treatment of arteriovenous malformations. In: Mattassi R, Loose DA, Vaghi M, editors. Hemangiomas and vascular malformations. Milan: Springer-Italia; 2009. p. 195–204.
11. Loose DA. Treatment of arteriovenous malformations. In: Mattassi R, Loose DA, Vaghi M, editors. Hemangiomas and vascular malformations. Milan: Springer-Italia; 2009. p. 215–21.
12. Loose DA, Weber J. Indications and tactics for a combined treatment of congenital vascular defects. In: Balas P, editor. Progress in angiology. Turin: Edizioni Minerva Medica; 1991. p. 373–8.
13. Riles TS, Rosen RJ. Peripheral arteriovenous fistulae. In: Rutherford RB, editor. Vascular Surgery. 4th ed. Philadelphia: WB Saunders Company; 1995. p. 1211–7.
14. Lee BB, Bergan JJ. Advanced management of congenital vascular malformations: a multidisciplinary approach. Cardiovasc Surg. 2002;10:523–33.
15. Loose DA. Systematik, radiologische Diagnostik und Therapie vaskulärer Fehlbildungen. In: Hohenleutner U, Landthaler M (Hrsg.) Operative Dermatologie im Kindes- und Jugendalter. Diagnostik und Therapie von Fehl-und Neubildungen. Berlin/Wien: Blackwell; 1997.
16. Jackson JE, Mansfield AO, Allison DJ. Treatment of high-flow vascular malformations aided by flow occlusion techniques. Cardiovasc Intervent Radiol. 1996;19:323–8.
17. Mattassi R, Loose DA, Vaghi M. Surgical techniques in vascular malformations. In: Mattassi R, Loose DA,

Vaghi M, editors. Hemangiomas and Vascular malformations. An atlas of diagnosis and treatment. 2nd ed. Milan: Springer Italia; 2015. p. 249–54.

18. Mattassi R, Loose DA, Vaghi M. Principles of treatment of vascular malformations. In: Mattassi R, Loose DA, Vaghi M, editors. Hemangiomas and vascular malformations. Milan: Springer Italia; 2009. p. 145–51.

19. Weber JH. Interventional therapy in arteriovenous congenital malformations. In: Mattassi R, Loose DA, Vaghi M, editors. Hemangiomas and vascular malformations. Milan: Springer Italia; 2009. p. 153–62.

20. Mattassi R. Surgical treatment of congenital arteriovenous defects. Int Angiol. 1990;9(3):196–202.

Combined Surgical and Endovascular Approaches

38

Byung-Boong Lee, James Laredo,
and Richard Neville

The contemporary management of ever-challenging congenital vascular malformations (CVMs) has been established over a relatively short time period, less than three decades, utilizing both endovascular and surgical therapy [1–4].

The traditional approach to the management of CVMs throughout the last century has long been surgical excision alone based on a minimal understanding of the natural history of CVMs. The excision was often too radical and based on the traditional surgical approach utilized in the treatment of malignant tumors, with a goal of achieving a "cure" and preventing recurrence [5–8].

The collateral damage to the surrounding tissues (e.g., soft tissue and musculoskeletal system) by such extensive surgery was inevitable in addition to the significant intraoperative complications (e.g., massive bleeding) and subsequent

B.-B. Lee, MD, PhD, FACS (✉)
Professor of Surgery and Director,
Center for the Lymphedema and Vascular
Malformations, George Washington University,
Washington, DC, USA

Adjunct Professor of Surgery, Uniformed Services,
University of the Health Sciences, Bethesda,
MD, USA
e-mail: bblee38@gmail.com

J. Laredo, MD • R. Neville, MD
Division of Vascular Surgery, Department of Surgery,
George Washington University Medical Center,
22nd and I Street, NW, Washington, DC, USA
e-mail: bblee@mfa.gwu.edu

morbidity. This aggressive surgical approach, even if a surgical "cure" had been achieved, was associated with significant morbidity and often produced crippling disfigurement and had a profound, negative impact on the patient's quality of life.

Poor surgical outcomes remained the major challenge in the treatment of CVMs throughout the last century and was partly due to the aggressive surgical approach and limited data on the natural history of CVMs. The radical surgical approach, with its inherent significant morbidity and associated complications, was considered the standard and logical approach to the treatment of the entire group of the CVMs, even in the treatment of venous/lymphatic malformations (VM/LM), which seldom become a life-/limb-threatening condition, as which may often be the case in patients with arteriovenous malformations (AVMs) [9–12]. The poor surgical outcomes associated with the long-standing, traditional aggressive surgical approach led to the development of minimally invasive, endovascular treatments.

The development of classification systems for vascular anomalies and CVMs was an important diagnostic advancement to occur in the last century, allowing proper diagnosis and treatment of CVMs. The Hamburg consensus workshop held in Hamburg, Germany, in 1988 and organized by the world experts in the treatment of CVMs opened the door to a new era of contemporary management of CVMs. Soon after the develop-

© Springer-Verlag Berlin Heidelberg 2017
Y.-W. Kim et al. (eds.), *Congenital Vascular Malformations*, DOI 10.1007/978-3-662-46709-1_38

ment of the Hamburg consensus classification, the ISSVA classification of vascular anomalies was established [13–16].

The ISSVA classification system defined both vascular malformations and vascular tumors/hemangiomas as distinct vascular anomalies, taking into account the *hemodynamic* properties of CVMs. The Hamburg classification further defined CVMs based on the *embryologic* origin and the presence of mesenchymal cell characteristics that are found in *extratruncular*-type CVM lesions [17–20].

These two new classification systems based on the etiology, anatomy, embryology, and pathophysiology of CVMs allowed the precise diagnosis of the various malformations. Based on the embryology of each of the different types of CVMs, each malformation was further classified as an extratruncular or truncular lesion.

A "multidisciplinary team approach" emerged based on the new classification systems, the goals of which include the appropriate selection of endovascular and surgical therapy, prevention and control of recurrence, and minimal complications and morbidity [21–24].

This contemporary approach was the result of full utilization and incorporation of newly established *endovascular* treatments in addition to traditional surgical excision. Endovascular therapy has allowed improved diagnosis and management of CVMs [25–28].

Endovascular treatment was initially known for its excellent outcomes in the treatment of "surgically inaccessible" CVM lesions utilizing a variety of embolotherapy and sclerotherapy techniques [25–28]. Endovascular therapy alone, utilizing the currently available embolotherapy and sclerotherapy agents, is *NOT* curative. However, the appropriate selection of endovascular treatments with the appropriate indications has produced excellent outcomes exceeding those observed with traditional surgical excision alone. Hence, endovascular treatment with the various embolo-/sclerotherapies became the treatment of choice as independent

therapy for "surgically inaccessible" lesions, especially in the poor surgical candidate with extensive lesions extending beyond the deep fascia with involvement of muscle, tendon, and bone as diffuse infiltrating extratruncular CVM lesions [29–32].

Furthermore, embolo-/sclerotherapy is considered the first treatment option for all CVM lesions, both "surgically inaccessible" and "surgically accessible" lesions whenever feasible.

Endovascular therapy is utilized in the majority of surgical candidates as adjunctive therapy to improve surgical outcomes and reduce morbidity. Preoperative and postoperative embolo-/sclerotherapy augments the effectiveness of traditional surgical therapy, especially in patients with infiltrating extratruncular CVM lesions. (Fig. 38.1).

Embolization utilizing the various agents (e.g., N-butyl cyanoacrylate (NBCA), coils, particles) is often performed preoperatively in patients with CVM lesions. Preoperative embolization of CVM lesions helps facilitate surgical dissection, minimizes bleeding during subsequent surgical excision, and contributes to lower postoperative complications and morbidity.

The combined treatment approach utilizing both endovascular and surgical therapy allows the treatment of difficult, extensive CVM lesions through a "staged" approach. This often involves limited surgical excision after preoperative embolization, followed by additional sclerotherapy treatment sessions postoperatively (Fig. 38.2).

Traditional open surgical/excisional therapy and endovascular therapy are now fully integrated in the management of the CVMs, as the most effective means to treat all types of CVMs including mixed lesions (e.g., embolo-/sclerotherapy for extratruncular lesion, angioplasty and stent for truncular lesion). This multidisciplinary approach utilizes all of the currently available treatment options to maximize efficacy and minimize risk of complication and morbidity.

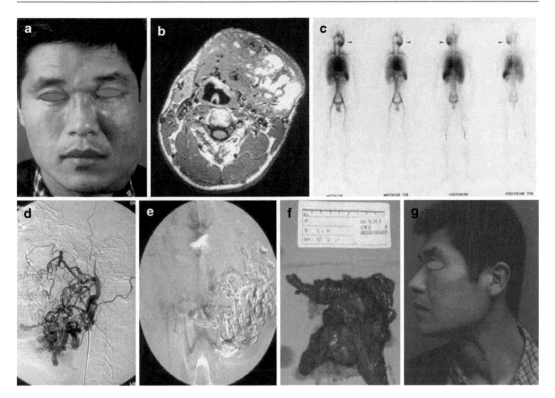

Fig. 38.1 (a–g) New role of endovascular therapy as an adjunct therapy to surgical therapy. As shown in clinical photo (**a**), AV malformation (AVM) lesion in the head and neck region was confirmed as "infiltrating" extratruncular high-flow AVM lesion as shown in MRI (**b**), compatible to duplex ultrasonographic findings. Additional assessment with whole-body blood pool scintigraphy (**c**) has confirmed the lesion located superficially only in the head and neck region with no evidence for further extension. Arteriographic study (**d**) was done as a road map for combined approach to this infiltrating extratruncular lesion; the lesion was filled with N-butyl cyanoacrylate glue as preoperative embolotherapy as shown in (**e**). Whole glue-filled lesions were safely excised in total, as shown in surgical specimen (**f**). The follow-up assessment confirmed no evidence of recurrence with excellent clinical outcome in 5 years shown in (**g**) (Lee and Bergan [22], December 2002)

Identification of the embryological subtype (truncular or extratruncular) of the CVM is essential in order to select the optimal combination of various treatment modalities best suited for each type of CVM.

Assessment of the extent and severity of the CVM lesion and its involvement with the arterial, venous, and lymphatic systems is also important (e.g., confirmation of normal deep vein system for the management of truncular VM lesion in the lower extremity). Individual components of mixed CVM lesions should also be evaluated (e.g., LM).

Not all CVM lesions require treatment. Only symptomatic lesions require treatment and only those associated with significant morbidity where the risk of lesion complication outweighs the risk of treatment. A multidisciplinary treatment approach utilizing combined endovascular and surgical treatment should be undertaken. Low-risk treatment should be the first-line therapy.

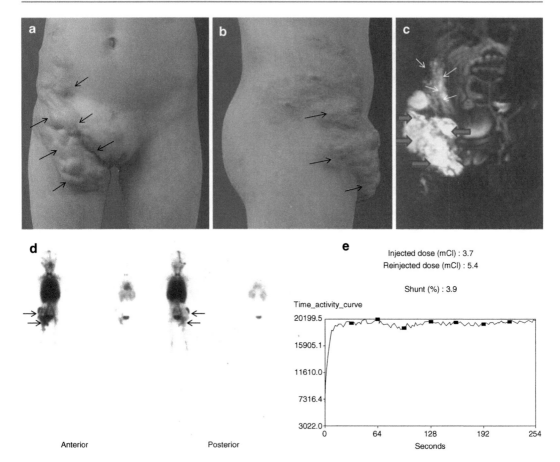

Fig. 38.2 (**a–j**) New role of endovascular therapy through combined approach with surgical therapy. Clinical photos (**a**, **b**) portray large venous malformation (VM) lesions affecting the entire right groin extended to the pubic region, upper thigh, and lower flank (*arrows*). MRI study (**c**) depicts a large superficially located cluster of infiltrating VM lesions (*thick arrows*) as well as another deeply located cluster of the lesions extended into the retroperitoneal space (*thin arrows*). Further assessment with whole-body blood pool scintigraphy (**d**) reveals the magnitude of the entire lesions affecting the right pelvic region as a whole. Transarterial lung perfusion scintigraphy (**e**) also ruled out a hidden risk of AVM involved. Percutaneous direct-puncture phlebography (**f**) demonstrates the outcome of preoperative embolotherapy: VM lesions filled with N-butyl cyanoacrylate (NBCA). Operative finding (**g**) shows an NBCA glue-filled lesion, done preoperatively, which allowed minimal damage to the surrounding tissue, as shown by the surgical specimen (**h**). Clinical photograph (**i**) taken 2 years later shows excellent outcome of combined approach (Lee BB, Villavicencio L: General Considerations. Congenital Vascular Malformations. Fig. 68–7. pp. 1062–3. Section 9. Arteriovenous Anomalies. pp. 1046–1064. *Rutherford's Vascular Surgery*. 7th Edition. Cronenwett JL and Johnston KW, Eds. Saunders Elsevier, Philadelphia, PA, USA. 2010)

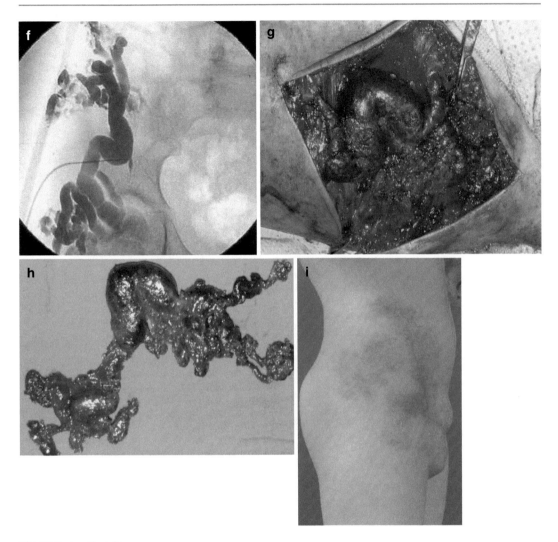

Fig. 38.2 (continued)

Conclusions

Surgical therapy combined with endovascular therapy utilizing a multidisciplinary team approach in the treatment of CVMs can achieve improved long-term treatment results with reduced morbidity and recurrence.

References

1. Lee BB. Advanced management of congenital vascular malformation (CVM). Int Angiol. 2002;21(3):209–13.
2. Lee BB. Critical issues on the management of congenital vascular malformation. Ann Vasc Surg. 2004;18(3):380–92.
3. Lee BB, Baumgartner I, Berlien HP, Bianchini G, Burrows P, Do YS, Ivancev K, Kool LS, Laredo J, Loose DA, Lopez-Gutierrez JC, Mattassi R, Parsi K, Rimon U, Rosenblatt M, Shortell C, Simkin R, Stillo F, Villavicencio L, Yakes W. Consensus Document of the International Union of Angiology (IUA)-2013. Current concept on the management of arterio-venous management. Int Angiol. 2013;32(1):9–36.
4. Lee BB, Baumgartner I, Berlien P, Bianchini G, Burrows P, Gloviczki P, Huang Y, Laredo J, Loose DA, Markovic J, Mattassi R, Parsi K, Rabe E, Rosenblatt M, Shortell C, Stillo F, Vaghi M, Villavicencio L, Zamboni P. Diagnosis and treatment of venous malformations consensus document of the International Union of Phlebology (IUP): updated 2013. Int Angiol. 2015;34(2):97–149.
5. Belov ST, Loose DA. Surgical treatment of congenital vascular defects. Int Angiol. 1990;9(3):175–82.
6. Mattassi R. Experiences in surgical treatment of congenital vascular malformation: changes in diagnosis and surgical tactics in the view of new experiences. In: Belov S, Loose DA, Weber J, editors. Vascular malformations. Reinbek: Einhorn-Presse Verlag GmbH; 1989. p. 202–5.
7. Malan E. Surgical problems in the treatment of congenital arteriovenous fistulae. J Cardiovasc Surg (Torino). 1965;6:251.
8. Lee BB, Laredo J, Kim YW, Neville R. Congenital vascular malformations: general treatment principles. Phlebology. 2007;22(6):258–63.
9. Lee BB, Laredo J. Venous malformation: treatment needs a bird's eye view. Phlebology. 2013;28:62–3.
10. Lee BB. Endovascular management of the Congenital Vascular Malformation (CVM) is not a panacea. Editorial. Damar Cer Derg. 2013;22(1):1–3.
11. Lee BB. Not all venous malformations needed therapy because they are not arteriovenous malformations. Comments Dermatol Surg. 2010;36(3):340–346. Dermatol Surg. 2010;36(3):347.
12. Lee BB. Changing concept on vascular malformation: no longer enigma. Ann Vasc Dis. 2008;1(1):11–9.
13. Belov S. Classification, terminology, and nosology of congenital vascular defects. In: Belov S, Loose DA, Weber J, editors. Vascular malformations. Reinbek: Einhorn-Presse; 1989. p. 25–30.
14. Enjolras O, Wassef M, Chapot R. Introduction: ISSVA classification. In: Color atlas of vascular tumors and vascular malformations. New York: Cambridge University Press; 2007. p. 1–11.
15. Lee BB. New classification of congenital vascular malformations (CVMs). Rev Vasc Med. 2015;3(3):1–5.
16. Lee BB, Antignani PL, Baraldini V, Baumgartner I, Berlien P, Blei F, Carrafiello GP, Grantzow R, Ianniello A, Laredo J, Loose D, Lopez Gutierrez JC, Markovic J, Mattassi R, Parsi K, Rabe E, Roztocil K, Shortell C, Vaghi M. ISVI-IUA consensus document – diagnostic guidelines on vascular anomalies: vascular malformations and hemangiomas. Int Angiol. 2015;34(4):333–74.
17. Belov ST. Anatomopathological classification of congenital vascular defects. Semin Vasc Surg. 1993;6:219–24.
18. Belov ST. Classification of congenital vascular defects. Int Angiol. 1990;9:141–6.
19. Lee BB, Laredo J, Lee TS, Huh S, Neville R. Terminology and classification of congenital vascular malformations. Phlebology. 2007;22(6):249–52.
20. Gloviczki P, Duncan AA, Kalra M, Oderich GS, Ricotta JJ, Bower TC, et al. Vascular malformations: an update. Perspect Vasc Surg Endovasc Ther. 2009;21(2):133–48.
21. Lee BB. Critical role of multidisciplinary team approach in the new field of vascular surgery – endovascular surgery. J Kor Soc Vasc Surg. 2003;19(2):121–3.
22. Lee BB, Bergan JJ. Advanced management of congenital vascular malformations: a multidisciplinary approach. J Cardiovasc Surg. 2002;10(6):523–33.
23. Lee BB. Current concept of venous malformation (VM). Phlebolymphology. 2003;43:197–203.
24. Lee BB, Do YS, Yakes W, Kim DI, Mattassi R, Hyun WS, Byun HS. Management of arterial-venous shunting malformations (AVM) by surgery and embolo-sclerotherapy. A multidisciplinary approach. J Vasc Surg. 2004;3:596–600.
25. Lee BB. New approaches to the treatment of Congenital Vascular Malformations (CVMs) – Single Center Experiences – (editorial review). Eur J Vasc Endovasc Surg. 2005;30(2):184–97.
26. Lee BB, Kim DI, Huh S, Kim HH, Choo IW, Byun HS, Do YS. New experiences with absolute ethanol sclerotherapy in the management of a complex form of congenital venous malformation. J Vasc Surg. 2001;33(4):764–72.
27. Lee BB, Do YS, Byun HS, Choo IW, Kim DI, Huh SH. Advanced management of venous malformation (VM) with ethanol sclerotherapy: mid-term results. J Vasc Surg. 2003;37(3):533–8.

28. Do YS, Yakes WF, Shin SW, Kim DI, Shin BS, Lee BB. Ethanol embolization of arteriovenous malformations: interim results. Radiology. 2005;235(2):674–82.

29. Yamaki T, Nozaki M, Sasaki K. Color duplex-guided sclerotherapy for the treatment of venous malformations. Dermatol Surg. 2000;26(4):323–8.

30. Pascarella L, Bergan JJ, Yamada C, Mekenas L. Venous angiomata: treatment with sclerosant foam. Ann Vasc Surg. 2005;19(4):457–64.

31. O'Donovan JC, Donaldson JS, Morello FP, Pensler JM, Vogelzang RL, Bauer B. Symptomatic hemangiomas and venous malformations in infants, children, and young adults: treatment with percutaneous injection of sodium tetradecyl sulfate. AJR Am J Roentgenol. 1997;169(3):723–9.

32. Cabrera J, Cabrera Jr J, Garcia-Olmedo MA, Redondo P. Treatment of venous malformations with sclerosant in microfoam form. Arch Dermatol. 2003;139(11):1494–6.

Management of Deep Vein Aplasia, Hypoplasia, and Lateral Marginal Vein

39

Raul Mattassi

Anomalies of the venous system in the lower limb are uncommon diseases. They may present in two different forms according to error in the complex vasculogenetic process. A defect in the regression of primitive capillaries brings to an area of dysplastic vessels located in tissues ("extratruncular forms"), while a defect in the morphogenesis of main veins ("truncular forms") may originate deep vein aplasia, hypoplasia, and persistence of embryonal vessels, like marginal and sciatic vein. Truncular defects may combine with extratruncular venous malformations or with lymphatic defects. These combinations are defined as Klippel-Trenaunay syndrome. In a study on 46 cases of Klippel-Trenaunay syndrome, we found a combination of CVM, as reported in Table 39.1.

Aplasia of deep veins is the rarest condition. Inferior caval vein is the result of a complex embryological process in which defects may originate up to 15 different anomalies, including aplasia of the infrarenal or suprarenal caval vein [1]. Incidence of inferior caval vein anomaly is less than 1% but is higher in cardiac malformation [2]. Aplasia of suprarenal cava is characterized by con-

tinuation in azygos/hemiazygos, while infrarenal aplasia has a collateral circulation through pelvic, paravertebral, and superficial abdominal veins. Aplasia of iliac vein, common, external, or bot is mainly monolateral [3] (Fig. 39.1) [1]. Bilateral aplasia of iliac veins is extremely rare [4]. Often those cases have no symptoms, but deep venous thrombosis and pulmonary thromboembolism have been reported [5]. Invasive treatment of those defects, including surgery, is not indicated as collaterals may allow an almost normal life; thrombosis and thromboembolism are treated by anticoagulation. In case or thromboembolism with an occluded iliac or caval vein, differential diagnosis between recent thrombosis and vein aplasia is mandatory, as endovascular recanalization is not indicated nor possible in venous aplasia.

In the lower limbs, deep vein aplasia is mainly limited to a single segment that may be common femoral, superficial femoral, or popliteal vein. Most frequent location is superficial femoral vein, followed by popliteal and common femoral vein. Those defects are compensated by collateral circulation through normal veins, like saphenous or deep femoral vein, by abnormal dilated superficial veins, or by persistent embryonal veins, like marginal or sciatic vein. These collateral systems may combine differently. Cutaneous nevus is common. Limb length discrepancy due to overgrowth of the affected limb is possible but not constant. Combination with extratruncular venous malformations is possible but not constant.

R. Mattassi
Department of Vascular Surgery and Center for Vascular Malformations "Stefan Belov", Clinical Institute Humanitas "Mater Domini" Castellanza, Varese, Italy
e-mail: raulmattassi@gmail.com

© Springer-Verlag Berlin Heidelberg 2017
Y.-W. Kim et al. (eds.), *Congenital Vascular Malformations*, DOI 10.1007/978-3-662-46709-1_39

Treatment of those deep vein aplasia is not possible. Superficial abnormal veins are collaterals of the missing main vessels and should not be removed. Before surgery of venous anomalies in the limb, deep vein aplasia should be excluded by a precise diagnostic process. The recommended tests are duplex scan, performed

Table 39.1 Vascular defects in 46 cases of Klippel-Trenaunay, Castellanza, 2011–2015)

Deep vein aplasia	9 (19%)
Deep vein hypoplasia	9 (19%)
Extratruncular deep infiltrating, dysplastic veins	19 (41%)
Marginal vein	14 (30%)
Superficial dysplastic veins	46 (100%)
Truncular lymphatic defects	13 (28%)

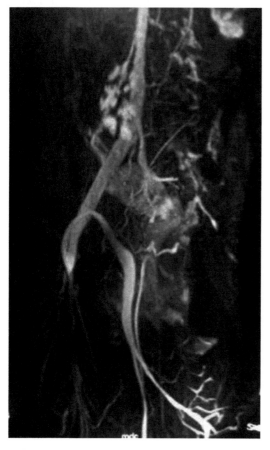

Fig. 39.1 Pelvic angio-MR that demonstrate aplasia of left common and external iliac vein. A suprapubic spontaneous bypass is visible

by an experienced technician in CVM and contrast-enhanced MR or CT.

Hypoplasia of deep veins is much more common than aplasia. The first report of that anomaly was probably due to Stephan Belov which described it in an uncommon location: the internal jugular vein with abnormal dilated submandibular veins connected to external jugular vein. The patient had severe headache and sleep disorders due to face edema on horizontal position [6]. A surgical removal of dilated submandibular veins was performed with immediate disappearance of symptoms. Postoperative control demonstrated dilation to normal size of the hypoplastic jugular vein and normal venous drainage from brain. The possibility of dilation of hypoplastic (congenitally stenotic) veins after removal of superficial dilated and dysplastic vessels was called by Belov "operation of rerouting venous flow." That happens because, after removal of dysplastic veins that has a bypass effect, avoiding blood to flow through deep veins, blood is forced through with a dilating effect [6, 7].

Vein hypoplasia is much more common on the lower limb. Superficial femoral vein is the most frequently involved vessel. This anomaly is often combined with other venous anomalies of the limb, like dilated, dysplastic superficial veins (truncular forms), intra- or extramuscular areas of dysplastic veins (extratruncular defects), or persistence of embryonal vein. Removal of the dysplastic superficial vein is possible in order to normalize vein flow (Fig. 39.2). Crucial is a precise diagnosis in order to distinguish aplasia from hypoplasia, as mentioned above. Intra- or extramuscular extratruncular infiltrating coexisting malformations can be treated surgically or by alcohol sclerosis. Details can be found in Chap. 34.

Marginal vein (MV) is an abnormal vessel, a remnant of an embryonal vein that failed to regress before birth. The vein is sited on the lateral edge of the lower limb and may vary in extension (only at the calf, at the calf and thigh or extended also to the gluteus) and in the connections to the deep venous system (lateral perforants, connections to the saphenous or the

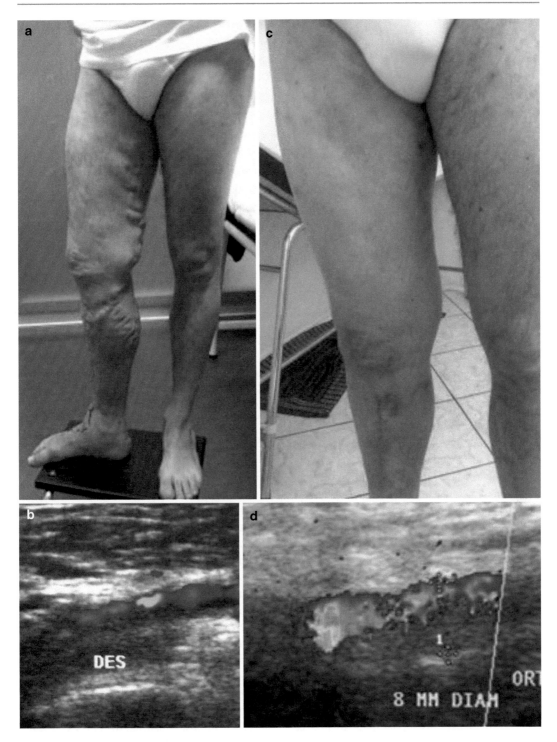

Fig. 39.2 (a) Patient with dilated dysplastic superficial veins of the right limb. (b) Duplex scan that demonstrates a hypoplasia of superficial femoral vein (diameter, 3 mm), (c) after surgical removal by steps of the superficial dysplastic veins, (d) duplex scan after 6 months of the end of the treatment. The vein is now 8 mm width

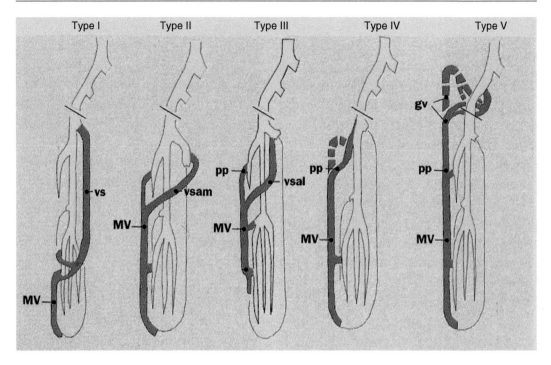

Fig. 39.3 Classification of marginal vein according to Weber. *MV* marginal vein, *cb* anterior arched vein, *vsm* main saphenous vei, *vsam* medial accessory saphenous vein, *mcv* medial crural vein, *pp.* deep perforants, *vsal* lateral accessory saphenous vein, and *gv* gluteal vein (Reproduced with permission from Mattassi [15])

deep femoral system, or connections to the external iliac vein through gluteal veins) (Fig. 39.4 (same as Fig. 13.1)). According to different extension and course, a classification of the VM has been done (Fig. 39.3) [8]. The vein is typically valveless. Beside extension, also morphology may vary, from a size similar to a normal saphenous vein to an extreme dilated vessel. Peculiarity of that vein is the possibility to be connected to the deep system by extreme large and fragile perforants that can easily be damaged during surgery with bleeding [9, 10].

MV may manifest in different ways. In some cases there are no symptoms and the patient may even not be aware of his defect. In other cases, the patient may complain on a sense of limb heaviness by standing, sometimes also with edema. Limb length discrepancy, due to an overgrowth of the affected limb, is possible. An ulcer

is rare. Phlebitis is possible. Recently it has been reported that MV may be the origin of dangerous pulmonary embolism [11]. Sometimes, embolism may happen repeatedly and unrecognized with chronic damage of pulmonary function [12].

A much rarer persistence of embryonal vessel is *sciatic vein*. This valveless vessel is deep sighted in the thigh, often originating by connections with popliteal vein. It follows in part the sciatic nerve and connects through gluteal perforants with the internal iliac vein system. As the vein is valveless, it may create discomfort, like heaviness and even pain in the calf in standing position. As that abnormal vein is less known and not externally visible, diagnostic is often missed. Because of deep thigh intramuscular location, recognition by duplex scan examination requires knowledge and skill. Contrast-enhanced MR or CT is helpful to demonstrate it [13] (Fig. 39.5).

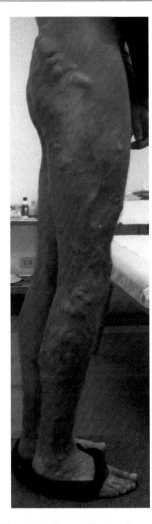

Fig. 39.4 Marginal vein type V according to Weber classification. That patient had an aplasia of external iliac vein (Reproduced with permission from Mattassi [15])

In case of persistent MV, removal of the pathologic vein is recommended, especially if there is limb overgrowth, as this process can be stopped after treatment. However, as in the case of dysplastic superficial veins, also marginal and sciatic vein may be associated to dysplasia of the deep venous system that should be recognized precisely before treatment. Marginal vein should be removed surgically avoiding a closed stripping because large perforants may exist with bleeding risk. Site and size of perforants should be recognized by duplex scan before operation in order to perform selected ligation of those veins, which are often large and fragile [7, 9, 10]. Endovascular procedures, like laser or radiofrequency closure, are also possible [14]. However, marginal vein is often very superficial, and skin damage by laser or radiofrequency application is possible. In case of huge perforants, surgery is preferred by us in order to perform a correct and precise ligation [15]. Good result of surgical treatment of MV is reported [16].

In a very rare condition, a marginal vein may coexist with aplasia of deep venous system and several AV fistulas to the marginal vein itself, creating a flow overloading toward that valveless embryonal vein. That extremely rare condition can be improved by careful skeletonization of the vein and ligation of all incoming fistulas. Results are reduction of stasis in the vein and improvement of symptoms [17].

Sciatic vein is often not the cause of discomfort and treatment is not required. Surgical approach is posterior on the thigh, by opening the muscular fascia and finding out the vein deep between muscles. Removal of a tract of the vein or the simple distal disconnection at popliteal space can be sufficient to eliminate stasis symptoms in the calf.

In conclusion, aplasia and hypoplasia of the veins of the lower limbs are rare congenital diseases that may be well tolerated in some cases, while in others severe discomfort may exist. Surgical treatment is possible in hypoplasia but not in aplasia of main veins. A diagnostic accuracy is requested as differential diagnosis is crucial for treatment strategy. Experienced personnel performing investigations is necessary for good quality result. Marginal and sciatic veins can be removed by surgery if they create discomfort or a limb overgrowth or shortening. Evaluation of the deep system before treatment is mandatory [18, 19].

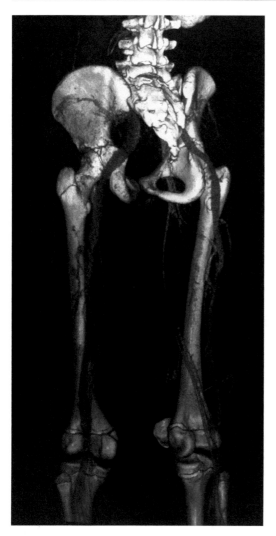

Fig. 39.5 A posterior image of a angio CT scan that demonstrates a bilateral persistent complete sciatic vein

References

1. Chuang VP, Mena CE, Hoskins PA. Congenital anomalies of the inferior vena cava. Review of embryogenesis and presentation of a simplified classification. Br J Radiol. 1974;47(556):206–13.
2. Timmers GJ, Falke TH, Rauwerda JA, Huijgens PC. Deep vein thrombosis as a presenting symptom of congenital interruption of the inferior vena cava. Int J Clin Pract. 1999;53(1):75–6.
3. Kutsal A, Lampros TD, Cobanoglu A. Right iliac vein agenesis, varicosities, and widespread hemangiomas: report of a rare case. Tex Heart Inst J. 1999;26(2):149–51.
4. Onkar D, Onkar P, Mitra K. Isolated bilateral external iliac vein aplasia. Surg Radiol Anat. 2013;35(1):85–7.
5. D'Aloia A, Faggiano P, Fiorina C, Vizzardi E, Bontempi L, Grazioli L, Dei Cas L. Absence of inferior vena cava as a rare cause of deep venous thrombosis complicated by liver and lung embolism. Int J Cardiol. 2003;88(2–3):327–9.
6. Belov ST, Loose DA, Müller E. Angeborene Gefäßfehler (Congenital vascular malformations). Reinbeck: Einhorn Presse Verlag; 1985. p. 148–50.
7. Belov S, Loose DA. Surgical treatment of congenital vascular defects. Int Angiol. 1990;9(3):175–82.
8. JH W. Invasive diagnostics of congenital vascular malformations. In: Mattassi R, Loose DA, Vaghi M, editors. Hemangiomas and vascular malformations. 1st ed. Milan: Springer; 2009. p. 139.
9. Mattassi R. Vaghi M: management of marginal vein: current issues. Phlebology. 2007;22(6):283–6.
10. Mattassi R, Pozzoli W. The marginal vein. Gefässchirurgie. 2014;4(19):311–5.
11. BB L. Marginal vein is not a simple varicose vein: it is a silent killer! review. Damar Cer Derg. 2013;22(1):4–14.
12. Rodríguez-Mañero M, Aguado L, Redondo P. Pulmonary arterial hypertension in patients with slow-flow vascular malformations. Arch Dermatol. 2010;146(12):1347–52.
13. Kenneth J, KJ Jr C, Gloviczki P, Stanson W. Persistent sciatic vein: diagnosis and treatment of a rare condition. J Vasc Surg. 1996;23(3):490–7.
14. King K, Landrigan-Ossar M, Clemens R, Chaudry G, Alomari AI. The use of endovenous laser treatment in toddlers. J Vasc Interv Radiol. 2013 Jun;24(6):855–8.
15. Mattassi R Vascular malformations of the limbs: treatment of venous and arteriovenous malformations. In: Mattassi R, Loose DA, Vaghi M. Hemangiomas and vascular malformations. An atlas of diagnosis and treatment. 2nd Springer, Milan 2015, p. 417–430
16. Kim YW, Lee BB, Cho JH, Do YS, Kim DI, Kim ES. Haemodynamic and clinical assessment of lateral marginal vein excision in patients with a predominantly venous malformation of the lower extremity. Eur J Vasc Endovasc Surg. 2007;33(1):122–7.
17. Belov ST. Congenital agenesia of the deep veins of the lower extremity: surgical treatment. J Cardiovasc Surg. 1972;13:594–8.
18. Lee BB, Laredo J, Kim YW, Neville R. Congenital vascular malformations: general treatment principles. Phlebology. 2007;22(6):258–63.
19. Lee BB, Baumgartner I, Berlien P, Bianchini G, Burrows P, Gloviczki P, Huang Y, Laredo J, Loose DA, Markovic J, Mattassi R, Parsi K, Rabe E, Rosenblatt M, Shortell C, Stillo F, Vaghi M, Villavicencio L, Zamboni P. Diagnosis and treatment of venous malformations consensus document of the International Union of Phlebology (IUP): updated 2013. Int Angiol. 2015;34(2):97–149.

Surgical Treatments for Lymphedema

40

Dong-Ik Kim and Je Hoon Park

Basic Concept of Surgical Treatment of Lymphedema

In the past, surgical excision was the only treatment, if there are secondary changes, without pathophysiological correction. But contemporary therapeutic concept is focused on pathophysiological correction and effective when performed before secondary histological changes. An obstructive factor is that lymphatics is very thin. Thus, development of microsurgery is crucial. Also because various conservative therapeutic options, such as extremity elevation, compressive therapy, complex decongestive therapy, and compressive pump therapy, outweighed the surgery, physicians take account for what surgery to do and when to do.

Historical Background

The first surgical treatment for lymphedema was performed in the name of lymphangioplasty by Handley in 1908 [1]. As the first anatomical

D.-I. Kim (✉)
Vascular Surgery, Samsung Medical Center, Sungkyunkwan University School of Medicine, Seoul, South Korea
e-mail: dongik.kim@samsung.com

J.H. Park
Division of Transplantation and Vascular Surgery, Department of Surgery, International St. Mary's Hospital, Catholic Kwandong University College of Medicine, Incheon, South Korea
e-mail: ceccil@ish.ac.kr

surgery, Kondoleon introduced an operation which removes radical fascia and hypertrophic fat tissue partially, which has been adopted for 50 years. In the same year, Charles introduced complete resection of subcutaneous tissue, and then Thompson and Servell et al. introduced modified operation.

But these operative techniques result in longer hospitalization, slower wound healing, larger operative scar, sensory nerve injury, remnant foot or ankle edema, and cosmetic disadvantages, which are adopted in limited circumstances recently. Brorson [2] and colleagues tried to overcome these demerits by the introduction of liposuction in 1998 (Table 40.1).

Operative techniques which anastomose between lymphatics were developed as a functional surgery for lymphedema in the early period. Recently, operation which anastomoses between lymphatics and vein is the most commonly used method, and operation which anastomoses between lymphatics and venule is performed.

Anatomical Surgery

Surgical strategies are composed of anatomical operation which remove edematous tissue anatomically and functional operation which improve lymphatic flow or reconstruct lymphatics. Anatomical operation consists of direct surgical excision of lymphedema tissue and

Table 40.1 Types of surgical treatment for lymphedema [3, 4]

Category	Operation	Surgeon	Year	References
Anatomical surgery	Direct surgical resection (Charles' operation)	Charles	1912	[5]
	Homans' operation	Homans	1934	[6]
	Staged subcutaneous excision beneath flaps	Miller	1973	[7]
	Liposuction	Illouz	1989	[8]
		Brorson and Svensson	1997	[2]
Functional surgery	FLAP interposition	Gilles	1935	[9]
	Lymphatic bypass	Baumeister and Suida	1990	[10]
	Microsurgery of lymphatics and veins	Yamada	1967	[11]
	Vascularized lymph node transfers	Shim	2015	[12]
Others	Stem cell therapy	Maldonado	2011	[13]
		Shim	2015	[14]

liposuction, and functional surgery consists of flap interposition, lymph-lymph bypass, lymph-vein bypass, lymph-vein or lymph-venule anastomosis, and vascularized lymph node transfer.

Direct Surgical Excision

Indications

These operative techniques recently were not adopted as the first treatment but used in limited circumstances such as recurrent lymphangitis and cellulitis, refractory pain, motor and functional disability due to size and weight of lymphedema tissue, cosmetic purpose, etc. [15].

Surgical Methods

Charles' Operation

This is the operation which is characterized by complete removal of all skin and subcutaneous tissue with preservation of the deep fascia and sole of the foot and sequential performance of split-thickness or full-thickness skin graft from the resected specimen (Fig. 40.1).

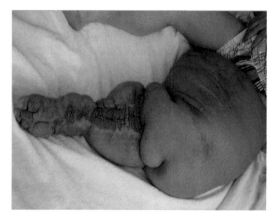

Fig. 40.1 Charles' operation

Homans' Operation

The Homans' operation is a reduction procedure in which the skin is preserved (Fig. 40.2). The procedure is suitable only if the overlying skin is in good condition. An incision is made along the length of the affected part of the limb; anterior and posterior skin flaps are raised, and the lymphedematous subcutaneous tissue is excised down to the deep fascia. The skin flaps are refashioned to size, replaced, and closed using sutures. Each operation typically reduces the limb circumference by one-third, and several operations through separate incisions may be needed to debulk a limb.

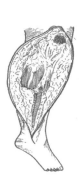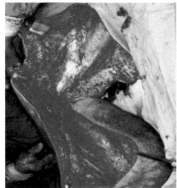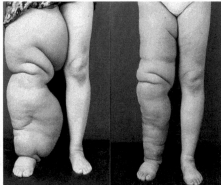

Fig. 40.2 Homans' operation

Usually for a disabling swelling below the knee, an initial medial reduction can be combined with a lateral procedure later.

Sistrunk's Operation and Thompson's Operation

Sistrunk removed skin and soft tissue through an elliptical incision along the medial arm and wide excision of the deep fascia.

Thompson expanded this procedure by embedding the de-epithelialized skin flaps from the entire length of the elliptical incision along the neurovascular bundle. The theory was based on spontaneous lymphangiogenesis from the superficial system to the deep system in order to provide shunting of lymph fluid [16].

Results

Kim et al. [17] reported improving data of eight cases of modified Auchincloss-Homans excision in six refractory patients with conservative treatment. And then they emphasized the beneficial surgical effect of active postoperative physiotherapy via 24 same operations in 20 patients [18].

In 2005, Lee et al. applied various surgical options, such as Auchincloss-Homans excision, lymphovenous bypass, and free lymph nodes transplant surgery, in 26 patients (43 cases) and reported about 50 % effect of functional surgery and 67 % effect in patients with truncular type and 80 % effect in patients with extratruncular type [19].

Also they reported good results of decongestive therapy and/or compression therapy and additional excisional surgery in end stages (stage IV–V) of lymphedema patients (85 %; 28 among 33 cases) [20].

Liposuction

Indications

This surgical concept is based on the prevention of complications caused by direct excision and effective removal of accumulated, hypertrophic subcutaneous fat tissue caused by chronic lymphedema.

Results

Cormier et al. [21] emphasized excisional surgery as the first treatment of lymphedema and especially asserted the usefulness of liposuction in upper extremity disease.

In various studies, the volume reduction rate ranges from 18 to 118 % (mean; 91.1 %), and these studies especially reported a volume reduction rate of more than 100 % in the treatment of upper extremity lymphedema [22–24].

Functional Surgery

Flap Interposition

The basis behind flap interposition is to place functioning lymphatic vessels contained within a segment of vascularized tissue into an affected area to siphon or bypass excess lymph fluid.

In 1935, Gilles and Fraser were the first to treat lower extremity lymphedema by attaching a flap of skin and subcutaneous tissue from the arm to the leg and keeping the arm by the patient's side [9].

Goldsmith et al. reported the use of greater omentum flaps to upper and lower extremity lymphedema. The greater omentum was pedicled off the ipsilateral gastroepiploic vessel and transferred to the extremity via a subcutaneous tunnel. The excess lymph fluid in the extremity was expected to drain into the abdominal lymphatic system through the rich network of lymph vessels in the greater omentum. Thirty-eight percent of lower extremity and 56 % of upper extremity experienced good results in 22 patients [25].

Lymphatic-Lymphatic Bypass

Some investigators have attempted to bypass fibrosed lymphatics by using lymphatic or vein grafts to link distal lymphatics to more proximal lymphatic channels.

Baumeister and Suida [10] attempted to bridge areas of stenosed lymphatic vessels with autologous lymphatic grafts in the upper and lower extremities. For the upper extremity, healthy lymphatic vessels from the medial thigh are harvested as a composite graft and buried in a subcutaneous tunnel between the supraclavicular shoulder region and the upper arm. The lymphatic vessels at either end are microscopically identified and anastomosed to the recipient lymphatics.

Lymphovenous Bypass or Anastomosis and Lymphaticovenular Anastomosis

A lymphovenous shunt was first described by Jacobson in 1962 in a canine model [26] and

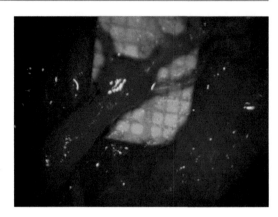

Fig. 40.3 Lymphovenous anastomosis

applied first in clinical trial by Yamada in 1967 [11] but showed poor result until the 1970s.

Since Koshima et al. [27] introduced a supermicrosurgical approach in 1996, there was a new turnover in this procedure. Koshima et al. applied the method using a venule and not a conventional vein as a graft, because distal lymphatics is lesser involved into lymphedema and has lesser venous reflux due to lesser pressure of venule, which result in more good effect. The use of "supermicrosurgery" to anastomose vessels less than 0.8 mm in diameter has recently gained popularity around the world [28–31] (Fig. 40.3).

Vascularized Lymph Node Transfers (VLNT)

Free tissue transfer of lymph nodes has been the most recent development in the treatment of lymphedema. In general, it has been shown that preserving the vascular supply during transfer results in greater improvement in the degree of lymphedema and in lymphatic function [32]. The harvest of vascularized lymph nodes are groin, thoracic, submental, and supraclavicular nodes, with the groin being the most popular [4]. The advantages and disadvantages are presented in Table 40.2.

Outcomes

Since there are a few published high-level studies evaluating the long-term outcomes after surgical treatment of lymphedema, this treatment option remains controversial and is considered experimental in many countries [21].

Summaries of the literature included in the systematic review have been updated through 2014 and are presented in Tables 40.3, 40.4, 40.5, and 40.6 [21, 34].

Table 40.2 Comparison of various recipient sites for vascularized lymph node flap transfer [33]

Recipient site	Potential recipient arteries	Potential recipient veins	Skin paddle required	Advantages	Disadvantages
Upper limb					
Axilla	Subscapular; circumflex scapular; thoracodorsal; lateral thoracic; circumflex humeral	Comitant	No	Concomitant scar contracture release	Scarred bed
Elbow	Inferior ulnar collateral; anterior ulnar recurrent	Comitant; basilic	Yes	Unscarred bed	Less gravity effect
Wrist	Dorsal branch of radial; ulnar	Comitant; cephalic	Yes	Gravity effect	Aesthetic
Lower limb					
Groin	Superficial inferior epigastric; superficial circumflex iliac; deep inferior epigastric	Comitant	No	Concomitant scar contracture release	Scarred bed
Knee	Medial sural; descending genicular	Comitant; great saphenous	Yes	Unscarred bed	Patient positioning; less gravity effect
Ankle	Anterior tibial; posterior tibial	Comitant; greater or lesser saphenous	Yes	Gravity effect	Aesthetic

Table 40.3 Summary of published literature related to excisional procedures for the treatment of lymphedema [34]

Author (year)	Study design	Number of patients	Lymphedema site	Specific surgical procedures	Follow-up time, months	Measurement technique	Volume reduction, %
Kim et al. (2004) [18]	Retrospective	20	Lower extremity	Excision	17.8	Volumeter	16 %
Modolin et al. (2006) [35]	Prospective	17	Penis/scrotum	Excision	72	NR	NR
Lee et al. (2008) [20]	Retrospective	22	Lower extremity	Excision	48	Infrared optometric volumetry and circumference	NR
Salgado et al. (2009) [36]	Prospective	11	Upper extremity	Excision with preservation of perforators	17.8	Circumference	21
Van der Walt et al. (2009) [37]	Retrospective	8	Lower extremity	Modified Charles procedure	27	NR	8.5 kg
Karri et al. (2011) [38]	Retrospective	27	Lower extremity	Charles procedure	48	NR	NR

NR: not reported

Table 40.4 Summary of published literature related to liposuction procedures for the treatment of lymphedema [34]

Author (year)	Study design	Number of patients	Lymphedema site	Specific surgical procedures	Follow-up time, months	Measurement technique	Volume reduction, %
Liu et al. (2005) [39]	Prospective	11	Upper extremity	Liposuction	a	Circumference	a
Bronson et al. (2006) [22]	Prospective	35	Upper extremity	Liposuction	12	Water displacement	103
Qi et al. (2009) [23]	Prospective	11	Upper extremity	Liposuction, myocutaneous flap transfer	26	Circumference	18
Damstra et al. (2009) [24]	Prospective	37	Upper extremity	Suction-assisted lipectomy	12	Water displacement	118
Schaverien et al. (2012) [40]	Prospective	12	Upper extremity	Liposuction	36	Water displacement	123
Granzow et al. (2014) [41]	Retrospective	10	Upper extremity (n = 6), lower extremity (n = 4)	Suction-assisted lipectomy	32	Circumference	111 % (UE), 87 % (LE)

[a]Abstract only available
UE upper extremity, *LE* lower extremity

Table 40.5 Summary of published literature related to tissue transfer procedures for the treatment of lymphedema [34]

Author (year)	Study design	Number of patients	LE site	Specific surgical procedures	Follow-up time, months	Measurement technique	Volume reduction, %
Weiss et al. (2002) [42]	Prospective	12	Upper extremity	ALTT	96	Circumference	22 to 31
Wongtrungkapun (2004) [43]	Prospective	10	Lower extremity	Lymphovenous implantation	4.5	Circumference	3.5 cm at knee, 7.37 cm at 16 cm below knee, 2.75 at metatarsal level
Becker et al. (2006) [44]	Retrospective	24	Upper extremity	Lymph node transplantation	96	Circumference	Reduction to normal (n = 10), some reduction (n = 10), no change (n = 2)
Belcaro et al. (2008) [45]	Retrospective case-control	9	Lower extremity	ALTT (n = 9) vs. control (n = 8)	120	Water displacement	Increase of 13
Hou et al. (2008) [46]	Randomized controlled trial	15	Upper extremity	Autologous bone marrow stromal cell transplantation (n = 15) vs. CDT (n = 35)	12	Circumference	81
Lin et al. (2009) [47]	Retrospective	13	Upper extremity	VLNT	56	Circumference	51
Gharb et al. (2011) [48]	Prospective	21	Upper extremity	VLNT	40	Circumference	NR
Cheng et al. (2012) [49]	Prospective	6	Lower extremity	VLNT	8.7	Circumference	64 % above knee, 64 % below knee, 67 % above ankle
Cheng et al. (2013) [50]	Prospective	10	Upper extremity	VLNT	39	Circumference	40

ALTT autologous lymphatic tissue transplantation, *VLNT* vascularized lymph node transfer, *NR* not reported, *LE* lymphedema, *UE* upper extremity, *LE* lower extremity

Table 40.6 Summary of published literature related to lymphatic reconstructive procedures for the treatment of lymphedema [34]

Author (year)	Study design	Number of patients	LE site	Follow-up time, months	Measurement technique	Volume reduction, %
Koshima et al. (2004) [51]	Retrospective	52	LE	15	Water displacement	42
Matsubara et al. (2006) [52]	Retrospective	9	LE	21–87	Circumference	>5 cm ($n = 6$), 2 cm ($n = 2$), no effect ($n = 3$)
Damstra et al. (2010) [53]	Prospective	10	UE	12	Water displacement	2
Demirtas et al. (2008) [54]	Retrospective	42	LE	12	Circumference	59
Campisi et al. (2010) [28]	Retrospective	1800	UE and LE	120	Water displacement	56 (83 with 67 % reduction)
Chang (2010) [55]	Prospective	20	UE	18	Perometer	35
Maegawa et al. (2010) [56]	Retrospective	111	LE		Circumference	NR
Mihara et al. (2010) [57]	Retrospective	11	LE	23.6	Circumference	92
Narushima et al. (2010) [58]	Prospective	14	UE ($n = 2$), LE ($n = 12$)	809	Circumference	11
Furukawa et al. (2011) [59]	Prospective	9	UE	17	Circumference	>50 in 77.8 % of patients
Yamamoto et al. (2011) [60]	Retrospective	20	LE	8.9	Circumference	11
Auba et al. (2012) [61]	Prospective	12	UE ($n = 7$), LE ($n = 5$)	24	Circumference	1.18 cm circumference
Mihara et al. (2012) [62]	Prospective	6	LE	10	Circumference	NR
Ayestaray et al. (2013) [63]	Prospective	4	Head and neck	12	Circumference	3.7
Boccardo et al. (2013) [64]	Retrospective	23	LE	42	Circumference	80
Chang et al. (2013) [31]	Prospective	100	UE ($n = 89$), LE ($n = 11$)	12 to 36	Perometer	42 (UE), 7 to 42 (LE)

ALTT autologous lymphatic tissue transplantation, *VLNT* vascularized lymph node transfer, *NR* not reported, *LE* lymphedema, *UE* upper extremity, *LE* lower extremity

Summary

Direct surgical excision or liposuction has limited usefulness especially in the patients who are refractory to conservative nonsurgical therapy. Currently a variety of functional surgeries have been developed in concordance to development and improvement of (super)microsurgical techniques; however they have not yet proven their definitive effect. In the future, further high-level studies were needed for the improvement of clinical outcomes.

References

1. Handley WS. Elephantiasis treated by Lymphangioplasty. Proc R Soc Med. 1909;2(Clin Sect):123–5.
2. Brorson H, Svensson H. Complete reduction of lymphoedema of the arm by liposuction after breast cancer. Scand J Plast Reconstr Surg Hand Surg. 1997;31(2):137–43.
3. Baumeister RGH. Lymphedema: Surgical Treatment. In: Cronenwett JL, Johnston KW, editors. Rutherford's Vascular Surgery. Philadelphia: Elsevier; 2014. p. 1028–42.

4. Teng E, Chang DW. Overview of Surgical Techniques. In: Cheng M-H, Chang DW, Patel KM, editors. Principles and Practice of Lymphedema Surgery. Philadelphia: Elsevier; 2016. p. 87–97.

5. Hadamitzky C et al. Surgical procedures in lymphedema management. J Vasc Surg: Venous and Lym Dis. 2014;2(4):461–8.

6. Homans J, Drinker CK, Field M. Elephantiasis and the Clinical Implications of Its Experimental Reproduction in Animals. Ann Surg. 1934;100(4):812–32.

7. Miller TA, Harper J, Longmire Jr WP. The management of lymphedema by staged subcutaneous excision. Surg Gynecol Obstet. 1973;136(4):586–92.

8. Illouz Y-G, Villers YTD. Body Sculpturing by Lipoplasty. New York: Churchill Livingstone; 1989.

9. Gillies H, Fraser FR. Treatment of Lymphoedema by Plastic Operation: (a Preliminary Report). Br Med J. 1935;1(3863):96–8.

10. Baumeister, R.G. and S. Siuda, Treatment of lymphedemas by microsurgical lymphatic grafting: what is proved? Plast Reconstr Surg, 1990. 85(1): p. 64–74; discussion 75–6.

11. Yamashita S, Chang DW, Koshima I. Microsurgical procedures: Lymphovenous anastomosis techniques. In: Cheng M-H, Chang DW, Patel KM, editors. Principles and practice of lymphedema surgery. Edinburgh: Elsevier; 2016. p. 173–9.

12. Shim YK. Experience of lymphedema treated by using free vascularized normal lymph node transfer in 14 cases. International Angiology. 2015;34(Suppl 1):30.

13. Maldonado GE et al. Autologous stem cells for the treatment of post-mastectomy lymphedema: a pilot study. Cytotherapy. 2011;13(10):1249–55.

14. Shim YK. Therapeutic trial of lymphedema using adipocyte derived stem cell grafts with combined therapy. International Angiology. 2015;34(Suppl 1):109.

15. Gloviczki P. Principles of surgical treatment of chronic lymphoedema. Int Angiol. 1999;18(1):42–6.

16. Miller TA. A surgical approach to lymphedema. Am J Surg. 1977;134(2):191–5.

17. Kim DI et al. Excision of subcutaneous tissue and deep muscle fascia for advanced lymphedema. Lymphology. 1998;31(4):190–4.

18. Kim DI et al. Excisional surgery for chronic advanced lymphedema. Surg Today. 2004;34(2):134–7.

19. Lee BB et al. Current concepts in lymphatic malformation. Vasc Endovascular Surg. 2005;39(1):67–81.

20. Lee BB et al. Supplemental surgical treatment to end stage (stage IV-V) of chronic lymphedema. Int Angiol. 2008;27(5):389–95.

21. Cormier JN et al. The surgical treatment of lymphedema: a systematic review of the contemporary literature (2004-2010). Ann Surg Oncol. 2012;19(2):642–51.

22. Brorson H et al. Quality of life following liposuction and conservative treatment of arm lymphedema. Lymphology. 2006;39(1):8–25.

23. Qi F et al. Treatment of upper limb lymphedema with combination of liposuction, myocutaneous flap transfer, and lymph-fascia grafting: a preliminary study. Microsurgery. 2009;29(1):29–34.

24. Damstra RJ et al. Circumferential suction-assisted lipectomy for lymphoedema after surgery for breast cancer. Br J Surg. 2009;96(8):859–64.

25. Goldsmith HS. Long term evaluation of omental transposition for chronic lymphedema. Ann Surg. 1974;180(6):847–9.

26. Jacobson 2nd JH, Suarez EL. Microvascular surgery. Dis Chest. 1962;41:220–4.

27. Koshima, I., et al., Ultrastructural observations of lymphatic vessels in lymphedema in human extremities. Plast Reconstr Surg, 1996. 97(2): p. 397–405; discussion 406–7.

28. Campisi C et al. Microsurgery for lymphedema: clinical research and long-term results. Microsurgery. 2010;30(4):256–60.

29. Koshima I et al. Supramicrosurgical lymphaticovenular anastomosis for the treatment of lymphedema in the extremities. Nihon Geka Gakkai Zasshi. 1999;100(9):551–6.

30. Yamamoto Y et al. Follow-up study of upper limb lymphedema patients treated by microsurgical lymphaticovenous implantation (MLVI) combined with compression therapy. Microsurgery. 2003;23(1):21–6.

31. Chang DW, Suami H, Skoracki R. A prospective analysis of 100 consecutive lymphovenous bypass cases for treatment of extremity lymphedema. Plast Reconstr Surg. 2013;132(5):1305–14.

32. Tobbia D et al. Experimental assessment of autologous lymph node transplantation as treatment of postsurgical lymphedema. Plast Reconstr Surg. 2009;124(3):777–86.

33. Henry SL, Cheng M-H. Recipient site selection in vascularized lymph node flap transfer. In: Cheng M-H, Chang DW, Patel KM, editors. Principles and practice of lymphedema surgery. Edinburgh: Elsevier; 2016. p. 113–21.

34. Cromwel KD, Armer JM, Cormier JN. Evidence-based outcomes. In: Cheng M-H, Chang DW, Patel KM, editors. Microsurgical procedures: Lymphovenous anastomosis techniques. Philadelphia: Elsevier; 2016. p. 191–202.

35. Modolin M, et al. Surgical treatment of lymphedema of the penis and scrotum. Clinics (Sao Paulo). 2006;61(4):289–94.

36. Salgado CJ, et al. Radical reduction of upper extremity lymphedema with preservation of perforators. Ann Plast Surg. 2009;63(3):302–6.

37. van der Walt JC, et al. Modified Charles procedure using negative pressure dressings for primary lymphedema: a functional assessment. Ann Plast Surg. 2009;62(6):669–75.

38. Karri V, et al. Optimizing outcome of charles procedure for chronic lower extremity lymphoedema. Ann Plast Surg. 2011;66(4):393–402.

39. Liu Q, Zhou X, Wei Q. Treatment of upper limb lymphedema after radical mastectomy with liposuction technique and pressure therapy. Zhongguo Xiu Fu Chong Jian Wai Ke Za Zhi. 2005;19(5):344–5.

40. Schaverien MV, et al. Liposuction for chronic lymphoedema of the upper limb: 5 years of experience. J Plast Reconstr Aesthet Surg. 2012;65(7):935–42.

41. Granzow JW, et al. An effective system of surgical treatment of lymphedema. Ann Surg Oncol. 2014;21(4):1189–94.
42. Weiss M, Baumeister RG, Hahn K. Post-therapeutic lymphedema: scintigraphy before and after autologous lymph vessel transplantation: 8 years of long-term follow-up. Clin Nucl Med. 2002;27(11):788–92.
43. Wongtrungkapun R. Microsurgical lymphonodovenous implantation for chronic lymphedema. J Med Assoc Thai. 2004;87(8):877–82.
44. Becker C, et al. Postmastectomy lymphedema: long-term results following microsurgical lymph node transplantation. Ann Surg. 2006;243(3):313–5.
45. Belcaro G, et al. Lymphatic tissue transplant in lymphedema–a minimally invasive, outpatient, surgical method: a 10-year follow-up pilot study. Angiology. 2008;59(1):77–83.
46. Hou C, Wu X, Jin X. Autologous bone marrow stromal cells transplantation for the treatment of secondary arm lymphedema: a prospective controlled study in patients with breast cancer related lymphedema. Jpn J Clin Oncol. 2008;38(10):670–4.
47. Lin CH, et al. Vascularized groin lymph node transfer using the wrist as a recipient site for management of postmastectomy upper extremity lymphedema. Plast Reconstr Surg. 2009;123(4):1265–75.
48. Gharb BB, et al. Vascularized lymph node transfer based on the hilar perforators improves the outcome in upper limb lymphedema. Ann Plast Surg. 2011;67(6):589–93.
49. Cheng MH, et al. A novel approach to the treatment of lower extremity lymphedema by transferring a vascularized submental lymph node flap to the ankle. Gynecol Oncol. 2012;126(1):93–8.
50. Cheng MH, et al. Vascularized groin lymph node flap transfer for postmastectomy upper limb lymphedema: flap anatomy, recipient sites, and outcomes. Plast Reconstr Surg. 2013;131(6):1286–98.
51. Koshima I, et al. Minimal invasive lymphaticovenular anastomosis under local anesthesia for leg lymphedema: is it effective for stage III and IV? Ann Plast Surg. 2004;53(3):261–6.
52. Matsubara S, et al. Long-term results of microscopic lymphatic vessel-isolated vein anastomosis for secondary lymphedema of the lower extremities. Surg Today. 2006;36(10):859–64.
53. Damstra RJ, et al. Lymphatic venous anastomosis (LVA) for treatment of secondary arm lymphedema. A prospective study of 11 LVA procedures in 10 patients with breast cancer related lymphedema and a critical review of the literature. Breast Cancer Res Treat. 2010;113(2):199–206.
54. Demirtas Y, et al. Supermicrosurgical lymphaticovenular anastomosis and lymphaticovenous implantation for treatment of unilateral lower extremity lymphedema. Microsurgery. 2009;29(8):609–18.
55. Chang DW. Lymphaticovenular bypass for lymphedema management in breast cancer patients: a prospective study. Plast Reconstr Surg. 2010;126(3):752–8.
56. Maegawa J, et al. Types of lymphoscintigraphy and indications for lymphaticovenous anastomosis. Microsurgery. 2010;30(6):437–42.
57. Mihara M, et al. Regional diagnosis of lymphoedema and selection of sites for lymphaticovenular anastomosis using elastography. Clin Radiol. 2011;66(8):715–9.
58. Narushima M, et al. The intravascular stenting method for treatment of extremity lymphedema with multiconfiguration lymphaticovenous anastomoses. Plast Reconstr Surg. 2010;125(3):935–43.
59. Furukawa H, et al. Microsurgical lymphaticovenous implantation targeting dermal lymphatic backflow using indocyanine green fluorescence lymphography in the treatment of postmastectomy lymphedema. Plast Reconstr Surg. 2011;127(5):1804–11.
60. Yamamoto T, et al. Lambda-shaped anastomosis with intravascular stenting method for safe and effective lymphaticovenular anastomosis. Plast Reconstr Surg. 2011;127(5):1987–92.
61. Auba C, et al. Lymphaticovenular anastomoses for lymphedema treatment: 18 months postoperative outcomes. Microsurgery. 2012;32(4):261–8.
62. Mihara M, et al. Scarless lymphatic venous anastomosis for latent and early-stage lymphoedema using indocyanine green lymphography and non-invasive instruments for visualising subcutaneous vein. J Plast Reconstr Aesthet Surg. 2012;65(11):1551–8.
63. Ayestaray B, Bekara F, Andreoletti JB. pi-shaped lymphaticovenular anastomosis for head and neck lymphoedema: a preliminary study. J Plast Reconstr Aesthet Surg. 2013;66(2):201–6.
64. Boccardo F, et al. Surgical prevention and treatment of lymphedema after lymph node dissection in patients with cutaneous melanoma. Lymphology. 2013;46(1):20–6.

Ji Hye Hwang

Introduction

Complex decongestive therapy (CDT) (also known as complete decongestive therapy or decongestive lymphatic therapy (DLT)) is now well established as the standard treatment for lymphedema regardless of the etiology (primary or secondary), its site (limb, trunk, or face), or its clinical stage [1]. The best treatment protocol among whole CDT or single therapy (MLD, pneumatic pump, short-stretch bandages, compression garments, and therapeutic exercises) still could not be identified because of heterogeneity in the subject populations, measured outcomes, and follow-up durations in the current studies. Many studies have revealed the short-term and long-term benefits of CDT such as decreasing edema volume and improving quality of life (QOL) in patient with secondary lymphedema on limb [2, 3] or even head/neck area [4].

However, surprisingly, there is no study that reports the effect of CDT in patient with primary lymphedema only. Few studies have reported that patients with primary lymphedema experienced distressful symptoms, functional impairments, and frequent infection [5, 6].

Primary lymphedema can occur in many sites such as leg, arm, face, or genital area. Also, it is common to see patients with bilateral limb or multi-segment, more than one segment affected by lymphedema, e.g., face and arms or arms and leg [7, 8]. The ultimate goals of treatment for patients with primary lymphedema are to improve not only physical impairments of affected limb or area but also QOL and functional disabilities. Especially, the treatment of children with primary lymphedema should be performed with a long-term plan, utilizing CDT.

This chapter will explore the two-phase CDT approach according to involved area especially lower limb and discuss clinical experience on primary lymphedema treatment, comparing it with characteristics of secondary lymphedema.

Complex Decongestive Therapy (CDT) on Limb

General Remarks of Two-Phase CDT [9, 10]

Elements of CDT include manual lymph drainage (MLD), compression therapy, decongestive exercises, basic skin care and education for self-care, and risk reduction. It is performed in two phases. In phase 1, known as the decongestive phase, the patient is treated with all components of CDT on a daily basis until the limb is

J.H. Hwang, MD, PhD
Department of Physical & Rehabilitation Medicine,
Samsung Medical Center, SungKyunKwan University
School of Medicine, Seoul, South Korea
e-mail: jhlee.hwang@samsung.com

decongested. Then, the patient progresses into phase 2 of CDT, self-management phase.

The objectives of CDT are (1) to improve the function of lymphatic vessels, (2) to soften the fibrosclerotic tissues, (3) to reduce increased connective tissues, and (4) to prevent soft tissue infections [8]. The current standard of care for lymphedema is CDT. However, the optimal treatment protocol remains controversial [11]. Recent study reported no significant differences in limb volume between compression garment only and CDT with daily MLD and short-stretch bandaging for arm lymphedema [12].

Phase 1: Decongestive Phase

In this phase, the patient has intensive therapy daily and also is informed about all components of CDT. The end of this first phase is determined by the time when the degree of lymphedema limb volume reduction reaches a plateau. The duration of this phase varies with the severity of the lymphedema and usually averages 2–4 weeks for patients with one limb involved. In extreme patients, this phase may be extended up to 6–8 weeks and can be repeated several times.

MLD is a gentle manual treatment technique, based on basic Vodder strokes – stationary circle, pump, scoop, and rotary designed to reroute the accumulated lymphatic fluid from involved limb/body area to healthy lymphatic and/or venous system. The most common effects of MLD are (1) increase in lymphangiomotoricity, (2) reverse of lymph flow, (3) increase in venous return, (4) soothing, and (5) analgesic effects. MLD is different from other massage techniques in that it has light directional pressure on the superficial lymphatic territories. Another unique characteristic is that the proximal part of affected limb and even contralateral limb is decongested first to treat the more distal part. High-pressure techniques like Swedish muscle massages could damage lymphatic structures including anchoring filaments especially in patient with the early stage of lymphedema. However, for patient with lymphostatic fibrosis, other fibrosis techniques are applied in the target area directly with more intensity and prolonged time than the basic strokes. In this

phase, MLD is applied over 30 min at least once a day, five times a week.

The effects of *compression therapy* are achieved with compression bandages and garments. In decongestive phase, compression therapy is applied using short-stretch bandages (up to 60% elasticity) in combination with proper pads following MLD for all day and night. Short-stretch bandages exert a very low resting pressure to avoid a tourniquet effect and also a high working pressure generated during muscle contraction. To achieve a compression gradient, it is necessary to apply bandages in layers. Bandage techniques that are commonly used are the spiral or figure-of-eight wrapping. The purposes of using special pads with foam materials are not only for protecting bony prominences and making the limb into a cylindrical shape but also for increasing the pressure over the focal fibrotic area. In addition, it is important to educate patient or a family member to make sense of the self-bandaging techniques and skin care [13]. The most significant reduction in volume typically occurs during the first week of treatment [14].

Lymphedematous skin also tends to be dry and may become thickened and scaly. Lymphedema patients are susceptible to infections of the skin and soft tissues. The process of inflammation/infection may not only worsen the swelling and discomfort but can also develop into a serious medical crisis. Therefore, *meticulous care of skin and nail* is essential.

Exercises consist of active, nonresistive, and repetitive protocols, which should be customized by the physician and/or therapist to meet the patient's goals. The stage and type of lymphedema as well as additional comorbidities need to be considered for specific restrictions and limitations of muscle/joint activity. Exercises vary in interstitial tissue pressure, affect lymph propulsion and clearance, and transport fluid and inflammatory proteins from the edematous area [15]. Ideally, decongestive exercises are performed 2–3 times daily for 10–15 minutes Compression garments should be worn during exercise. High-intensity and repetitive activities such as tennis, running, and mountain biking may not be beneficial for the patient during and immediately after phase 1 therapy.

Phase 2: Self-Management Phase

To maintain and more improve the results achieved in phase 1, the patient progresses into phase 2 of CDT. The components in this phase are similar to those in phase 1, but the point that should be emphasized is self-management. The patient assumes a duty like a therapist.

Patients should continue the meticulous skin care and perform simple self-MLD, compression therapy using elastic stocking/garment, and exercises. But it is not easy for patients to self-MLD properly implemented.

Main *compression* in this phase is applied by compression garments during the daytime hours. Patients with limb lymphedema will usually require a compression pressure range of about 30 mmHg for garments for the arm and 40–60 mmHg for garments for the leg, respectively. If a patient's limb is deformed or needs the high degree of compression garment over 50 mmHg, custom-made garments are a better choice. Compression garments should be checked regularly and replaced every 6 months. According to the severity and chronicity of lymphedema, many patients still require short-stretch multilayered bandaging during the night or weekends in this self-management phase. The multilayered short-stretch bandaging is very effective; however, many patients complain about a self-care burden and cosmetic issue with its bulkiness. Less bulky Velcro-band devices such as CircAid® and AutoFit® are recently developed or improved, but still not widely used than bandages in practice. These are applied more easily and allow better movement, and also, a few reports show good results [7].

Exercise is beneficial not only for general health but also for lymphedema itself. Gradual progression is imperative when prescribing exercises. Underwater leg exercises are proven to significantly enhance the effect of CDT [16].

Good patient compliance is indispensable because this phase lasts for a lifetime. Therefore, the physician and/or the lymphedema therapists should educate and check up on the patient regularly to maximize their compliance.

CDT on Genital/Lower Abdominal Area or Face

In the majority of cases, genital lymphedema is combined with leg lymphedema. Because lymph cysts or lymphangioma circumscriptum commonly occurs, daily meticulous skin care with disinfecting agents should be necessary for cellulitis prevention. Parts of MLD including abdominal and genital treatment and genital bandaging must be learned and performed by the patient several times daily. The ready-made or custom-made special foam pads are inserted into the compression pantyhose or bandages for women. For male genital lymphedema, bandaging the penis and scrotum is not easy and often requires cohesive bandages.

Isolated primary head and neck lymphedema is very rare and usually occurs in combination with arm and upper trunk involvement. The majority of facial lymphedema is unilateral. Compared to the secondary head and neck lymphedema after surgery and irradiation, primary patients have little functional problems such as limited mouth opening and neck motion. MLD sequence and compression methods with bandages or special compression garment are similar to the secondary lymphedema patients [17].

Intermittent Pneumatic Compression Pump (IPC)

The use of IPC for lymphedema therapy in decongestive phase and/or self-management phase of CDT or employed as stand-alone therapy is the most controversial issue [18]. Some published reports support the use of IPC [12, 19], but others are not for patients with secondary lymphedema, especially after breast cancer therapy [20]. Major theoretical concerns about using IPC are generation of genital edema and development of a fibrosclerotic ring at the root of the extremity [21]. It should be avoided by careful observation and combined MLD. The American Cancer Society Working Group on the Diagnosis and Management of Lymphedema designated IPC as a potential adjunctive component of CDT. IPC is only effective when combined with low-stretch bandages or stockings to maintain edema reduction. It is still very hard to know whether a particular pressure, cycle, or cuff design is better than others. Still, the most popular pump system is nongraded sequential compression with 3 to 14 chambers. But the guidelines for patient and device selection for incorporating IPC into main therapeutic program continue to evolve. Patient factors include severity of lymphedema, involvement of the trunk or genital area, and the presence of complications that contraindicate the use of simple, classical devices [22]. Recently developed new devices that simulate manual massage and design improvements for area of coverage, ease of use, and sequence/actions may increase the therapeutic effect and patient compliance. By the way, IPC should form part of a long-term therapeutic program for patient with advanced lymphedema, particularly useful in elderly patients, patients in bed, or patients with disabilities.

Special Issues in the Treatment of Primary Lymphedema

Primary lymphedema can occur in many sites such as leg, arm, face, or genital area, but over 90% are leg lymphedema. Also, it is common to see patients with bilateral limb or multi-segment, more than one segment affected by lymphedema, e.g., face and arms or arms and leg. Patients with primary lymphedema are relatively younger compared to those with cancer therapy-related secondary lymphedema. Among those who visited my clinic, over 70% were under the age of 30 and many of them were juvenile patients. Therefore, proper treatment planning, following medical care system model for chronic diseases that require lifetime medical care, is necessary. In addition to edema volume reduction or

maintaining with CDT-based therapy, other therapeutic considerations such as the special shoe prescription including wide-depth shoe or heel lift to correct mild leg length discrepancy are required. When the degree of lymphedema is severe, functional impairment of arm or leg must be assessed regularly.

CDT-Based Therapy Issues of Primary Leg Lymphedema

According to the known epidemiologic data, about one third of leg primary lymphedema patients have bilateral distal leg involvements [8]. MLD sequence and compression therapy with short-stretch bandages for this type are similar to the treatment of chronic venous insufficiency or posttraumatic secondary lymphedema. Proximal parts of the leg do not need to be applied of compression bandages or garments [10].

Primary leg lymphedema patients with involvement of thigh and trunk quadrant usually show extensive leg edema. Its treatment is similar to the treatment for secondary lymphedema [10].

According to long-term observational result in my experience, as similar to the results of other studies on the secondary lymphedema, phase 1 CDT is also found to be effective on reduction of excessive volume of the primary lymphedema patients (Figs. 41.1 and 41.2). However, the amount of volume reduction in edema and long-term maintenance was relatively unsuccessful in primary lymphedema patients compared to that of secondary patients [2, 3, 23]. This might be due to occurrence of tissue change on the involved sites at the time of diagnosis and onset of treatment. Although aggressive CDT-based care with a strict prevention is warranted, especially in the case of children and adolescent patients, it is important to constantly educate them to understand their conditions and to manage themselves on their

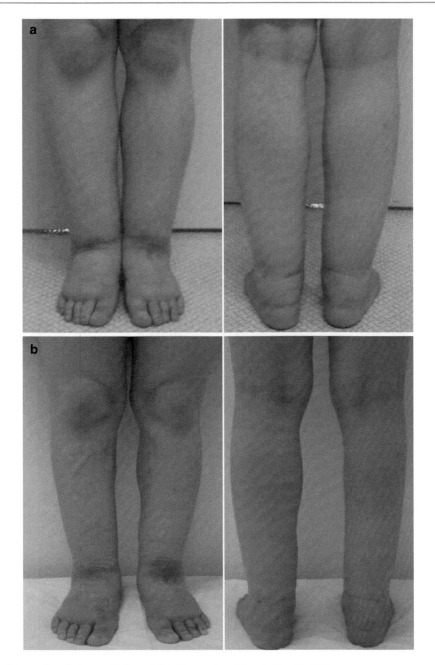

Fig. 41.1 Primary lymphedema of bilateral distal legs before (**a**) and after (**b**) CDT

own. In order to overcome cosmetic and functional problems due to life-long condition, high compliance to CDT is required. Therefore, continuous education paired with professional psychological support must be emphasized above all.

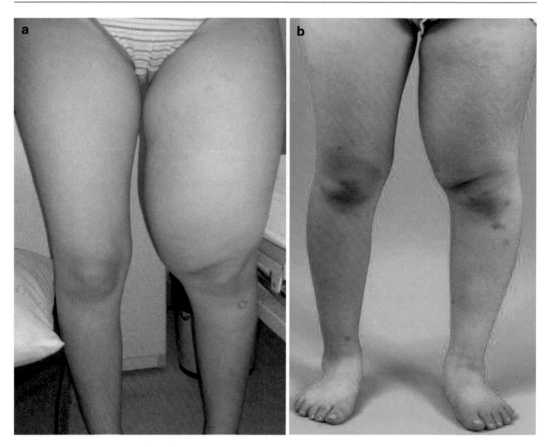

Fig. 41.2 A 15-year-old girl with primary lymphedema of the left leg, mainly thigh involvement before (**a**) and after (**b**) complex decongestive therapy (CDT)

References

1. The diagnosis and treatment of peripheral lymphedema: 2013 consensus document of the international society of lymphology. Lymphology. 2013; 46:1–11.
2. Lasinski BB, TK mK, Squire D, et al. A systematic review of the evidence for complete decongestive therapy in the treatment of lymphedema from 2004 to 2011. PM R. 2012;4:580–601.
3. Kim YB, Hwang JH, Kim TW, et al. Would complex decongestive therapy reveal long-term effect and lymphoscintigraphy predict the outcome of lower-limb lymphedema related to gynecological cancer treatment? Gynecol Oncol. 2012;127:638–42.
4. Smith BG, Hutcheson KA, Little LG, Skoracki RJ, Rosenthal DI, et al. Lymphedema outcomes in patients with head and neck cancer. Otolaryngol Head Neck Surg. 2015;152(2):284–91.
5. Okajima S, Hirota A, Kimura E, et al. Health-related quality of life and associated factors in patients with primary lymphedema. Jpn J Nurs Sci. 2013;10: 202–11.
6. Deng J, Radina E, Fu MR, et al. Self-care status, symptom burden, and reported infections in individuals with lower-extremity primary lymphedema. J Nurs Scholarsh. 2015;47(2):126–34.
7. Lee BB, Andrade M, Antignani PL, et al. Diagnosis and treatment of primary lymphedema consensus document of the international union of phlebology (IUP)-2013. Int Angiol. 2013;32(6):541–60.
8. Connell F, Brice G, Jeffery S, et al. A new classification system for primary lymphatic dysplasias based on phenotype. Clin Genet. 2010;77:438–52.
9. Foldi E, Foldi M. Complete decongestive therapy. In: Lee BB, Bergan J, Rockson SG, editors. Lymphedema; a concise compendium of theory and practice. London: Springer; 2011. p. 220–49.
10. Zuther JE. Lymphedema management: the comprehensive guide for practitioners. 2nd ed. New York: Thieme; 2009.
11. Javid SH, Anderson BO. Mounting evidence against complex decongestive therapy as a first-line treatment for early lymphedema. J Clin Oncol. 2013; 31(30):3737–8.
12. Dayes IS, Whelan TJ, Jullian JA, et al. Randomized trial of decongestive lymphatic therapy for the

treatment of lymphedema in women with breast cancer. J Clin Oncol. 2013;31:3738–63.

13. Schuren J, Mohr K. Pascal's law and the dynamics of compression therapy: a study on healthy volunteers. Int Angiol. 2010;29(5):431–5.

14. Leduc O, Leduc A, Bourgeois P, et al. The physical treatment of upper limb edema. Cancer. 1998;89(12 Suppl American):2835–9.

15. Havas E, Paeviainen T, Vourela J, et al. Lymph flow dynamics in exercising human skeletal muscle as detected by scintigraphy. J Physiol. 1997;504:233–9.

16. Tidhar D, Drouin J, Shimony A. Aqua lymphatic therapy in managing lower extremity lymphedema. J Support Oncol. 2007;5:179–83.

17. Smith BG, Hutcheson KA, Little LG, et al. Lymphedema outcomes in patients with head and neck cancer. Otolaryngology-head and neck surgery. 2015;152(2):284–91.

18. Szolnoky G, Lakatos B, Keskeny T, et al. Intermittent pneumatic compression acts synergistically with manual lymphatic drainage in complex decongestive physiotherapy for breast cancer treatment-related lymphedema. Lymphology. 2009;42:188–94.

19. Haghighat S, Lotfi-Tokaldany M, Yunesian M, Akbari ME, Nazemi F, Weiss J. Comparing two treatment methods for postmastectomy lymphedema: complex decongestive therapy alone and in combination with intermittent pneumatic compression. Lymphology. 2010;43:25–33.

20. Uzkeser H, Karatay S, Erdemci B, Koc M, Senel K. Efficacy of manual lymphatic drainage and intermittent pneumatic compression pump use in the treatment of lymphedema after mastectomy: a randomized controlled trial. Breast Cancer. 2015;22:300–7.

21. Morris RJ. Intermittent pneumatic compression-systems and applications. J Med Eng Technol. 2008;32(3):179–88.

22. Rockson SG. Current concepts and future directions in the diagnosis and management of lymphatic vascular disease. Vasc Med. 2010;15(3):223–31.

23. Lee H, Uhm KE, Hwang JH. Clinical characteristics and long-term outcomes in patients with primary lymphedema. In: Proceedings of 43rd annual meeting of the Korean Academy of Rehabilitation Medicine, Seoul; 2015.

Laser Therapy of Superficial and Deep Capillary Malformation (CM): Principles of Laser Technology

42

Peter Berlien

The difference between laser light and other light sources like intense pulsed light (IPL), LED, and xenon arc lamps is that laser is monochromatic, collimated, and coherent. This means that the tissue interaction is specific and the light distribution is calculable. Generally, one can say in the visible the shorter the wavelength, the more specific the absorption coefficient and, in the near infrared, the longer the wavelength, the more water absorption. Furthermore, the longer the wavelength, the lower the scattering and back scattering; the longer the pulse duration, the more thermal effects. With changing of the biophysical properties of the overlying tissue through compression and/or cooling, one can change the basic absorption of these layers. This allows bedside puncture techniques to make the tissue transparent and bring laser irradiation into deeper tissues. So one has the following application principles:

1. Transcutaneous with/without compression and/or cooling
2. Impression, interstitial, and paravasal application

3. Intraluminal as endovenous, intra-arterial, and intracystic techniques
4. Endoscopic in noncontact, contact, and impression techniques

Principles of Laser Treatment

In principle, the techniques of laser applications in congenital vascular tumors and in vascular malformations are similar, but the aim is different. In tumors, the aim is to induce regression or fibrosis, and in vascular malformations, the aim is to destroy the pathologic vascular structure because there is no spontaneous regression. This means that the parameters for treatment of vascular malformations must be more aggressive than for vascular tumors. But however, in contrast to lymphatic malformations, there is ever a high absorption of the Nd:YAG laser near-infrared radiation in the blood, so the parameters have to be adapted to this absorption.

For superficial small capillaries, the flash lamp-pumped dye laser (FPDL) is the laser of choice; for larger telangiectasias the KTP, Alexandrite, or pulsed Nd:YAG laser; for vessel diameters more than 2 mm or deeper located malformations, the near-infrared lasers as diode with 980 nm or Nd:YAG with 1064 nm; and for

P. Berlien
Wissenschaft und Forschung, Lasermedizin,
Elisabeth Klinik, Berlin, Germany
e-mail: lasermed.elisabeth@pgdiakonie.de

© Springer-Verlag Berlin Heidelberg 2017
Y.-W. Kim et al. (eds.), *Congenital Vascular Malformations*, DOI 10.1007/978-3-662-46709-1_42

315

Table 42.1 The choice of laser types depends on the depth, the thickness, and the kind of malformation

Superficial cutaneous	
Flat findings	Flash lamp-pumped dye laser
Telangiectatic findings	KTP laser
Tuberous findings	Pulsed Nd: YAG
Hyperkeratotic findings	CO$_2$ laser
Intra- and subcutaneous, up to a depth of 1–15 mm	Transcutaneous Nd: YAG (1064) with ice cube cooling
	Bare fiber impression technique
Subcutaneous, voluminous, > depth/ thickness of 10 mm	Nd: YA G (1064/1320) interstitial or intraluminal
Hollow organs, body cavities	Nd: YAG (1064/1320) endoscopic in air/water

In general, the more superficial and the smaller the vessels, the more an indication for short pulse duration; the deeper and the larger the vessel size and the volume, the longer the pulse duration up to exposure

intraluminal application as endovenous, intra-arterial, and endocystic, even additional 1320 nm or 1440 as Nd:YAG or diode laser. The CO$_2$ is only for vaporization of hyperkeratotic tissue (Table 42.1) [1].

Capillary Malformations

With the introduction of the flash lamp-pumped pulsed dye laser (FPDL), port-wine stain (PWS) can be treated in infancy and early childhood. The high-pulse peak power of the pulsed dye laser disrupts the vessels (Fig. 42.1).

Spider vascular lesions can be obliterated by KTP laser directed at the central artery under compression.

Due to the lower erythrocyte concentration in capillary-lymphatic malformations, the basic absorption for the FDL is reduced so the results of dye laser therapy are generally worse than for PWS. However, the ectatic venules in the epidermis are a good indication for the KTP, pulsed Nd:YAG, or chopped cw Nd:YAG with fluid cooling cuvette (Fig. 42.2). So general anesthesia needed for the laser therapy in childhood may also be used for clinical examinations if necessary.

In hyperkeratotic capillary malformation, the KTP laser is mostly not useful due to the high surface absorption. In punctual lesions, a pulsed Nd:YAG laser coagulation is helpful but the popcorn effect due to high energy should be avoided because this can cause bleeding. In disseminated excessive bleeding areas, a homogenous cw Nd:YAG laser coagulation through ultrasound jelly is necessary to avoid carbonization. However, this is followed by scarring. In more hyperkeratotic lesions, CO$_2$ laser vaporization is possible, but even this results in scarring.

If a soft tissue hypertrophy is shown despite the FDL therapy, the growing tissue will be treated in cases of dermal hypertrophy with a double-pulsed Nd:YAG/pulsed dye laser or in cases of more subcutaneous or soft tissue hypertrophy with the transcutaneous ice cube-cooled Nd:YAG laser, as for infantile hemangioma, but with a higher power of 60 W.

The large PWS of the extremities in Klippel-Trenaunay syndrome sometimes needs the same combination of pulsed dye laser, transcutaneous ice cube-cooled Nd:YAG laser, or, in cases with hyperkeratinization, CO$_2$ laser. In Proteus syndrome with patchy PWS of the hands or feet, the effectiveness of pulsed dye laser therapy is limited, just as it is for other mixed capillary lymphatic malformations. However, even here, the treatment of ectatic vessels with pulsed Nd:YAG or KTP laser is possible [6].

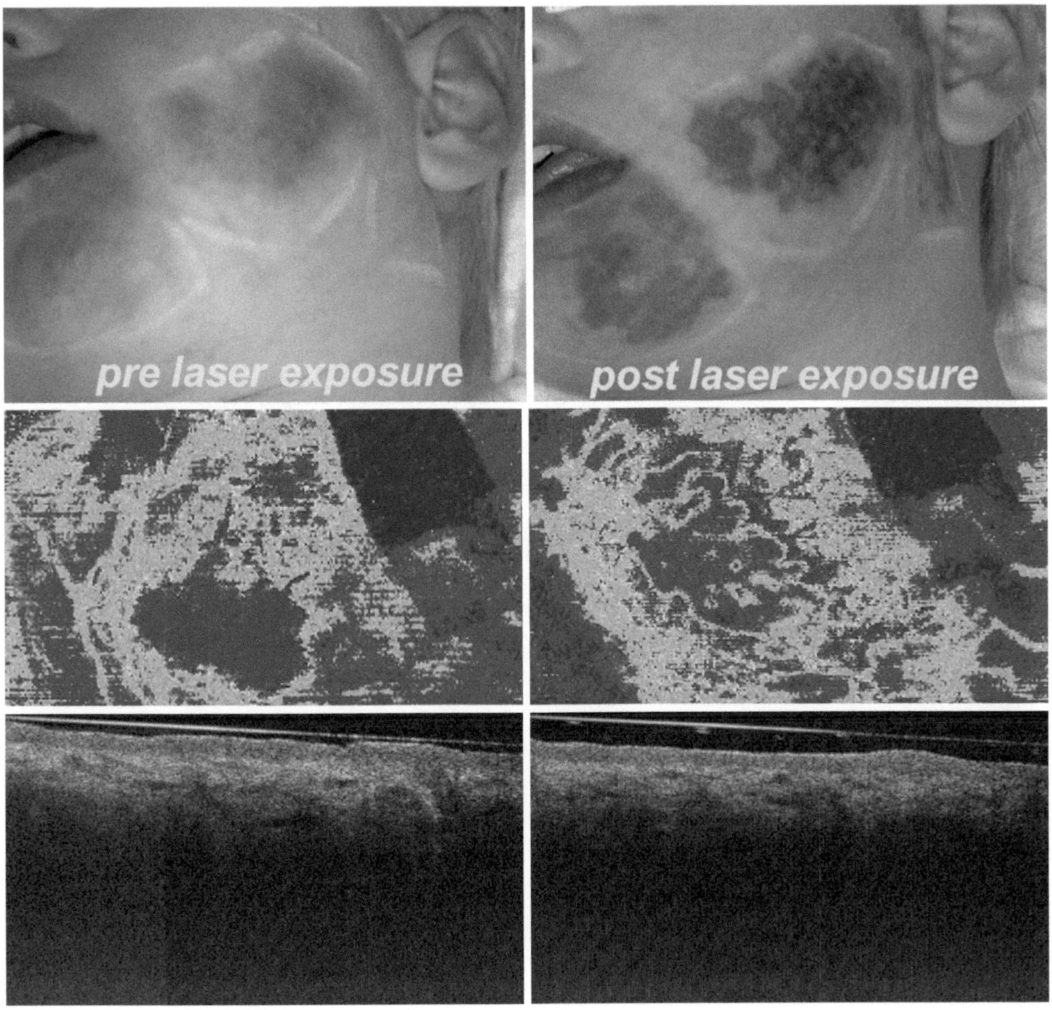

Fig. 42.1 As explained in this chapter, laser treatment of hemangiomas with the principle of FLPDL therapy is the induction of photoacoustic shock waves in small capillaries. This shows the importance of laser Doppler and OCT investigation to detect the vessels' diameters. The figure shows above the clinical picture, in the middle the laser Doppler, and below the OCT. After FPDL it shows the clinical picture the typical gray color, the laser Doppler decreases microcirculation and the OCT occludes vessels

Extratruncular Lymphatic Malformation

Microcystic ("Solid") Lymphatic Malformation "ITT"

If a surgical resection due to the infiltrative growth or other risks is not possible, an interstitial laser coagulation is possible. The biophysical basis is that the thin lymph cyst walls are good transparent for the Nd:YAG laser near-infrared radiation. This means that not only the direct punctured cyst will be irradiated but even also all the surrounding. In contrast to the above or later in venous malformations described, intraluminal techniques here exist as a direct contact of the 600 µ bare fiber with the adjacent tissue. This means that power of more than 5–7 W leads to a carbonization at the fiber end which absorbs all laser energy.

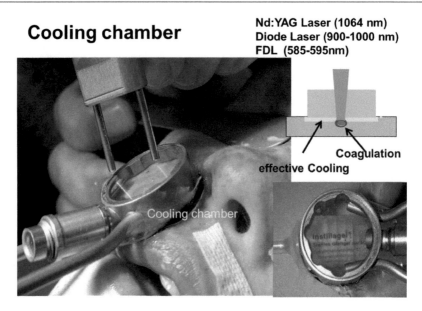

Fig. 42.2 The flexible membrane on the patient side of the fluid cooling cuvette can follow all anatomical contours. This allows complete protection of the skin even in difficult regions

The effect is that vaporization occurs, but no radiation can transmit to the tissue to perform a large volume coagulation. Here an additional sclerotherapy makes no sense and is dangerous.

Mucous Membrane Affection

Palatinal, hypopharyngeal, and/or laryngeal as well as urethral, bladder, and/or intravaginal lymphatic cysts are coagulated with the noncontact method comparable to the methods on laser therapy of hemangiomas. In the oropharynx, a direct coagulation in the near-contact procedure is possible with 15–20 W and chopped mode. The more venous the parts with higher basic absorption, the greater the risk of the popcorn effect or direct vaporization. In a frog egg situation on the larynx, the Werner ice water technique [3] gives you a good overview over the malformation and prevents carbonization of the surface. The power has to be increased to 20–25 W, depending by on the venous component. In the bladder or in the genital tract, the

endoscopic coagulation will be performed under continuous saline rinsing. Even here, the greater the venous component, the greater the risk of popcorn effect. Often they are combined with a chylothorax and chylopericardium and a pleural adhesion and are called Gorham-Stout syndrome (or disappearing bone disease). Here, an endoscopic cw Nd:YAG laser coagulation of the ectatic lymph vessels to reduce the chylous extravasation is possible. This laser application is possible in the treatment of airway, intestinal, intrarectal, and genitourinary tract VM lesions [5]. The treatment is performed with Nd:YAG laser or 1 μ diode laser. The use of the Nd:YAG laser for laryngeal VMs helps to avoid tracheotomy and open surgical resection [7].

Bare Fiber Contact Vaporization

What was described in the previous paragraph has to be avoided and must immediately be induced in the treatment of mucous membrane hyperkeratotic cysts, such as, e.g., enoral or anogenital cysts: with a high power of 30 W and chopped-mode carbonization of the fiber end to prevent uncontrolled deep coagulation and to perform bloodless vaporization. Especially in the mouth, there are mixed venous-lymphatic vesiculas which have a high risk of recurrent bleeding, superinfection, and foetor ex ore. Postoperatively, there is no specific treatment necessary, only continuous rinsing with fluid.

Intraluminal (Intracystic) Technique

Larger cysts were punctured under CCDS [8] control to prevent a direct puncture of interseptal veins and to string several cysts. If the diameter is more than 2 cm, it is helpful to reduce the size by suction of the lymph fluid. In cases of previous hemorrhage, flushing with saline is necessary until the fluid is clear. The kind of puncture cannula depends on the lesion. If possible, 16 or 18 G Teflon vein cannulas are preferred, because this material has no heat conduction risk from the heated tip. In larger lymphangiomas or in anatomically difficult regions where the puncture directions must change, a steel cannula is easier to handle but carries the risk of skin burning by the heated cannula. Because there is a lower basic absorption without erythrocytes, a power of approximately 10 W cw Nd:YAG laser is used [9]. The coagulation is stopped when an extensive color bruit is seen in the CCDS. Near the interseptal veins, the power must be reduced to prevent a vein perforation. If there is no risk of communication with vessels or body cavities, an additional sclerotherapy can be helpful, e.g., with Picibanil [2]. The aim of laser coagulation in this combination is to destroy the lymph cyst's epithelium in order to enhance the effectiveness of the sclerotherapy. The puncture direction must never cross the nerve direction to avoid a direct nerve palsy. But due to the postoperative swelling, an increasing hypesthesia or dysesthesia can occur within the next few days. This is transient and heals without any defects within a few weeks.

Cutaneous/Subcutaneous Malformation

The combination of cutaneous and subcutaneous malformation, also known as the blue rubber bleb nevus syndrome, can be treated like a congenital vascular tumor, with the transcutaneous ice cube-cooled Nd:YAG laser technique. However, here, a higher power of minimum 50–60 W is needed because induction of regression and also direct coagulation is necessary. In cases of intracutaneous lesions, a scar formation in the affected region is not always avoidable.

Soft Tissue Phlebectasias

Because the vessel wall as opposed to the blood is the target, if possible the ectatic vessel will not be punctured, but irradiated paravasally, as with the perforator vein laser coagulation. In cases where a paravasal application is not possible, but only an intraluminal application similar to the truncular procedure, the fiber tip has to be rinsed with saline solution to prevent carbonization followed by perforation. If there is no direct drainage over larger veins, an additional sclerotherapy can be performed. Postoperatively, a compression bandage is obligatory for 24 h. Localized intravascular coagulopathy (LIC) is not a contraindication for this technique because a thrombus formation can be avoided with this procedure.

Glomuvenous Malformation ("Glomangioma")

Due to the similar morphology with the infantile hemangioma, an effective therapy for multiple glomangiomas (glomangiomatosis) is treatment with Nd:YAG laser with continuous surface cooling. In solitary lesions, the interstitial puncture technique is used as for microcystic lymphangioma.

Arterial Malformations

In general the pure truncular AV malformation is successfully treated with embolization [10]. However, in some cases, the peripheral smaller vessels remain and are an indication for laser therapy. Depending on the size and origin, the pulsed dye laser, the KTP laser, the pulsed Nd:YAG laser, or the cw Nd:YAG laser chopped with the fluid cooling chamber are used. For fistulas which are not treated by embolization, a paravasal or intraluminal Nd:YAG laser coagulation is performed [9]. The surrounding pathological vessels are treated in the same session with high-power transcutaneous ice cube-cooled Nd:YAG laser. Depending on the size of the lesion, multiple punctures with the afterloading technique and several sessions are necessary. For extensive lesions, interstitial Nd:YAG laser coagulation may help by obliterating all microfistulas in order to collapse the arteriovenous malformation permanently, or collateral vessels can develop very slowly.

Besides the case of the capillary malformations described earlier, the most important malformation for laser therapy is the hamartous AV malformation ("angioma racemosum"). Here an interstitial laser therapy or a transcutaneous ice cube-cooled Nd:YAG laser therapy is needed. Mucous membrane bleeding is directly coagulated because here scar formation is not a concern.

Rendu-Osler-Weber Syndrome (Hereditary Hemorrhagic Telangiectasia)

For gastrointestinal bleeding spots endoscopically, the argon beamer electrofulguration is easier to handle than side fire laser fiber.

However, for all other manifestations, Nd:YAG laser therapy is the treatment of choice. For nasal or enoral spots, including tongue mucous membrane, cw Nd:YAG laser with 600 μ bare fiber in near contact with 12–15 W at 300–400 ms in the repetition mode. Higher power can induce vaporization with opening of the central shunt artery, and longer exposure times can cause a popcorn effect with massive bleeding. If acute bleeding has occurred, one has to remove the blood with continuous saline rinsing during lasering (Fig. 42.3). Here, the power must increase to 20–25 W and cw mode. Another option is to compress the bleeding vessel with the Hopf/Jovanovic glass spatula during lasering. Here, even with 20–25 W, the exposure time has to be reduced to prevent carbonization under the glass spatula. For skin lesions including the face, finger, or subungual areas, the pulsed Nd:YAG laser with intermittent ice cube cooling is the first choice. The parameters vary depending on the laser system, mainly between 50 and 100 J/cm^2. For micro AV shunts, CCDS-guided interstitial coagulation with 5 W and in cw mode is necessary. In larger AV shunts with life-threatening bleeding on the face, additional arterial embolization is indicated [4].

So from the standpoint of the lesions, generally one can say the smaller the vessels like capillaries, the shorter the wavelength and the pulse duration and the larger the diameter, the longer the wavelength and longer exposure time. Due to these biophysical rules, one can say the more extratruncular malformation, the more a laser indication and the more truncular, the more surgical and other intraluminal techniques.

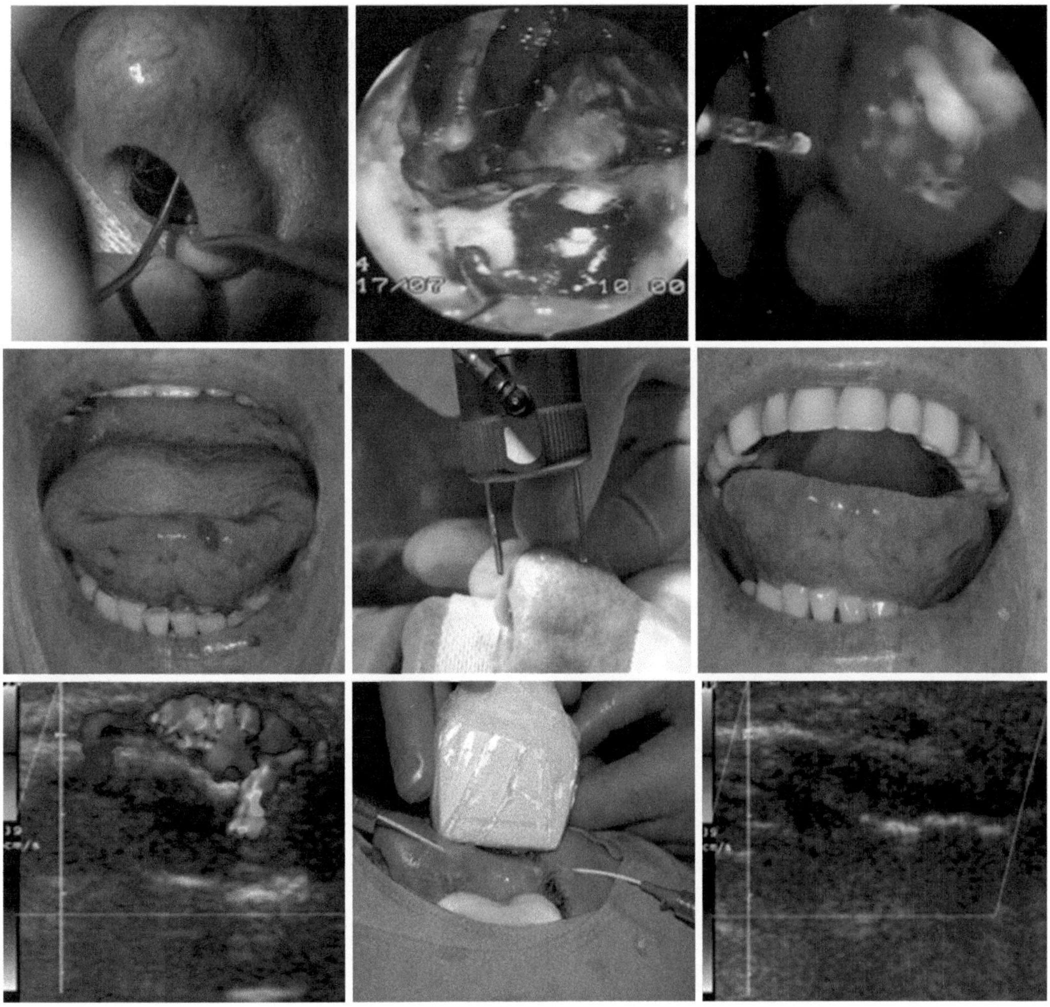

Fig. 42.3 The glass spatula compression or rinsing of the blood is necessary during cw Nd:YAG – or NIR diode laser – coagulation of bleeding Osler spots to prevent vaporization and septum perforation (*above*). *Middle*: Besides nasal bleeding, there are often the same malformations on the skin and mucosal membranes. Here, direct pulsed Nd:YAG over KTP laser coagulation is indicated. *Below*: As an AV malformation of the Osler's disease in the same way of AV fistulas in organs like the liver and lung, one can find AV fistulas in soft tissue. Here an interstitial laser coagulation of a not for embolization-suitable fistula

References

1. Berlien HP, Waldschmidt J, Müller G. Laser treatment of cutaneous and deep vessel anomalies. In: Waidelich W, editor. Laser optoelectronics in medicine. Berlin/Heidelberg/New York: Springer; 1988. p. 526–8.
2. Berlien HP. Laser treatment of vascular malformations. In: Mattassi R, Loose DA, Vaghi M, editors. Hemangiomas and vascular malformations. Milan/Berlin/Heidelberg/New York: Springer; 2015. p. 291–305.
3. Eivazi B, Wiegand S, Teymoortash A, Neff A, Werner JA. Laser treatment of mucosal venous malformations of the upper aerodigestive tract in 50 patients. Lasers Med Sci 2010;25(4):571–6. Epub 2010 Mar 9.
4. Menefee MG, Flessa HC, Glueck HI, Hogg S. Hereditary hemorrhagic telangiectasia (Osler-Weber-Rendu disease): an electron microscopy study of the vascular lesions before and after therapy with hormones. Arch Otolaryngol. 1985;101:246–51.
5. Philipp CM, Poetke M, Berlien HP. Vascular tumors and malformations of the pelvic and genital region-classification and laser treatment. Med Laser Appl. 2008;24:27–51.

6. Poetke M, Philipp C, Großewinkelmann A, et al. Die Behandlung von Naevi flammei bei Säuglingen und Kleinkindern mit dem blitzlampengepumpten Farbstofflaser. Monatsschr Kinderheilkd. 2001; 32:405–15.

7. Scherer K, Waner M. Nd:YAG lasers (1,064 nm) in the treatment of venous malformations of the face and neck: challenges and benefits. Lasers Med Sci 2007;22(2):119–26. Epub 2007 Feb 22.

8. Urban P, Philipp CM, Poetke M, Berlien HP. Value of colour coded duplex sonography in the assessment of haemangiomas and vascular malformations. Medical Laser Application. 2005;20(4):267–78.

9. Urban P, Poetke M, Müller U, Philipp C, Berlien H-P. Interstitial Nd:YAG Laser treatment of vascular malformations controlled by color coded duplex sonography (CCDS). Med Laser Appl. 2011;26:85.

10. Yakes WE. Alcohol embolotherapy of vascular malformation. Sem Interv Radiol. 1989;6:146–61.

Conservative/Medical Treatment of CVM

43

Iris Baumgartner and Byung-Boong Lee

Patients with congenital vascular malformations (CVM) span a wide variety of manifestations. The complexity of CVM often requires difficult and, sometimes, invasive treatment. Conservative and medical management is focused on prevention of symptoms and complications.

Conservative Treatment

For the majority of patients with CVM, the most important conservative treatment by far is compression therapy. Adequate compressive treatment can minimize symptoms and possibly prevents complications. Specifics of compression therapy do not differ from those for chronic venous insufficiency or lymphedema [1].

Conservative approaches also include proper skin, local wound-, bleeding or ulcer care, and compression therapy with elastic garment and/or bandage. Lifestyle modification and appropriate physical therapy including special orthopedic footwear would improve daily life and limb function.

A considerable number of patients with CVM report signs of anxiety, depression, and somatic or psychological distress if specifically prompted [2]. The need for psychological support especially for a visible deformity should not be underestimated. Treating physicians should be aware of the psychological impact that a CVM can have and should offer appropriate support.

Factors known to trigger progression include elevation of systemic vascular growth factors such as are seen with generalized growth, during and after puberty/menarche or pregnancy and following tissue trauma including surgery. Patients with early-stage AVM therefore should be counseled to minimize these risks, by avoiding the use of estrogen-containing contraceptives [3].

I. Baumgartner, MD (✉)
Clinical and Interventional Angiology, Swiss
Cardiovascular Center, University Hospital Bern,
Bern, Switzerland
e-mail: iris.bgtn@gmail.com

B.-B. Lee, MD, PhD, FACS (✉)
Professor of Surgery and Director, Center for the
Lymphedema and Vascular Malformations,
George Washington University, Washington,
DC, USA

Adjunct Professor of Surgery, Uniformed Services,
University of the Health Sciences, Bethesda,
MD, USA
e-mail: bblee38@gmail.com

Medical Treatment

There is currently no medical option to cure CVM. Medical therapies can be roughly divided at controlling cellular proliferation/abnormal growth, and others are aimed at avoiding hemostatic complications (bleeding, thrombosis) and general medical consequences (infection, anemia, pain).

Venous Malformations

Venous malformations (VMs) are associated with an increased risk for thrombosis as well as bleeding [4]. In extensive venous malformations, ectatic vessels can lead to stasis with activation of the coagulation cascade, and several studies have been able to demonstrate this localized intravascular coagulopathy (LIC) [5, 6]. A large skin surface and/or muscle involvement by the VM represents strong predictable criteria for coagulation disorders associated with VM showing strong positive statistical correlation. This is not only true for large VMs but also for multifocal VMs. Laboratory assessments show low levels of fibrinogen and elevated D-dimers. Severity of LIC seems to be related to the extent of the malformation [7].

LIC rarely results in serious complications, but it can be aggravated by different stimuli such as surgery, endovascular therapy, or trauma, resulting in disseminated intravascular coagulopathy (DIC). It is especially important to bear this in mind in the perioperative management of patients with CVM, and diligent prophylaxis with low molecular weight heparin (LMWH) is recommended [1].

It seems reasonable to assume that large malformed draining veins, such as the marginal vein which is frequently ectatic and typically valveless, can be a source of pulmonary embolism [8]. Elimination of such veins should be considered in patients who have suffered a pulmonary embolism. In general, any extensive VM should be assumed to be a risk factor for venous thromboembolism, and prophylactic measures should be contemplated in any situation with increased risk.

Patients with VM frequently suffer from painful episodes of local thrombosis within the malformed veins. These can often be successfully treated – minimizing intensity and duration of pain – with short courses of LMWH similar to the treatment of superficial vein thrombosis in patients without vascular malformations [1]. Extensive, multifocal, infiltrating, painful VMs should be treated with weight-adjusted dose (100 U/kg/day) of LMWH. Based on available data, LMWH treatment should be continued for 20 days. However, the introduction and duration of anticoagulation therapy should be based on

clinical and hematological grounds and to be reevaluated regularly for each patient and each VM. It has been proposed to initiate prophylactic therapy with weight-adjusted (100 U/kg/day) subcutaneous LMWH 10 days before and to continue 10–20 days after any surgical procedure (including abovementioned minimally invasive procedures).

In patients who experience such episodes very frequently and in whom this treatment has proven beneficial, self-administration of LMWH at the onset of symptoms should be discussed. With the increasingly widespread use of novel oral anticoagulants, an alternative to treat superficial thrombosis might be emerging, although at this point, there is very little experience in this setting, and the use of these agents is off-label. Depending on the site of the malformation, recurrent bleeding can cause chronic anemia. It is often not possible to completely eliminate the lesion to prevent bleeding. Anemia in these patients should be treated the same as chronic anemia by other causes. This might require iron replacement therapy or even regular red blood cell transfusions [9].

Lymphatic Malformations

Malformations with a lymphatic component carry a risk of infection. These patients need to be aware of this risk and instructed on how to act appropriately to prevent infection, how to recognize early signs, and when to seek medical attention or, in select cases, initiate self-medication. Preventive measures include good skin care and treatment of possible sources of infection. When an infection occurs, prompt treatment with an appropriate anti-infective agent is important. Choice of the specific antibiotic does not differ from similar infections in patients without vascular malformations. If infections are recurring, patients should be given the option to initiate treatment themselves at the first sign of infection. In patients with frequent infections, a long-term antibiotic prophylaxis should be considered. Two recent studies performed by the "Prophylactic Antibiotics for the Treatment of Cellulitis at Home" (PATCH) group have clearly confirmed the efficacy of antimicrobial prophylaxis.

Penicillin remains the drug of choice. Treatment options in patients with penicillin allergy are limited by the rising prevalence of macrolide resistance among group A streptococci [10].

Arteriovenous Malformations

Doxycycline has been used to treat patients with brain AVMs, where it may be associated with a reduced rate of bleeding. It is a matrix metalloproteinase inhibitor with mild antiangiogenesis effects. Clinically, it usually does not lead to any significant change.

Thalidomide has also been used to treat symptomatic AVMs. In the experience of physicians at Children's Hospital Boston, the drug led to significant improvement in swelling and pain, especially for patients with AVM associated with PTEN hamartoma syndrome. Unfortunately, the AVM usually does not diminish with this medication.

Avastin/bevacizumab has been used to treat several patients with HHT and has shown a significant reduction in epistaxis as well as arteriovenous shunting. Unfortunately it can also lead to bleeding.

Sirolimus has been shown to be highly effective in shrinking the painful hamartomas in PTEN hamartoma syndrome. Unfortunately, the lesions recur when the drug is stopped, and the AVM does not regress on this medication [3, 11–15].

Drugs in CVM

Thalidomide

Thalidomide has been shown to reduce bleeding in patients with hereditary hemorrhagic telangiectasia, possibly by promoting vessel maturation [16]. The drug is also known by his antiangiogenic effect by suppression of endothelial growth factor. Several reports about positive effects of thalidomide in the treatment of gastrointestinal bleeding due to vascular malformations have been published [17]. Combination of thalidomide (100 mg daily) and interferon (6 million units 3 times a week) has also been used in extensive CVM with acceptable results [14]. Main side effect of thalidomide is peripheral neuropathy (about 20%) [18]. Other side effects are somnolence, constipation, macular rash, and neutropenia. In conclusion, the real utility of this drug in CVM is to be demonstrated. Moreover, beside some reports of effect in gastrointestinal bleeding, no significant data exist about real effect in other VM, LM, or AVM.

Sildenafil

Sildenafil is a drug that selectively inhibits phosphodiesterase-5, preventing the breakdown of cyclic guanosine monophosphate. Inhibition of phosphodiesterase-5 decreases the contractility of vascular smooth muscle, producing vasodilation.

Some positive effect of this drug on complex lymphatic malformations has been reported [19, 20]. The effect has been explained by smooth muscle relaxation in cysts, induced by sildenafil that could facilitate cyst relaxation or emptying of them. However, a randomized study is necessary to recognize the real effectiveness of that drug.

Sirolimus

Sirolimus known also as rapamycin is a macrolide produced by the bacteria *Streptomyces hygroscopicus*, discovered by Brazilian researchers in the pacific island Rapa Nui. Sirolimus (also known as rapamycin) is potent to control many cellular processes involved in growth, but seems to be particularly important for vascular growth. It was originally developed as an antifungal agent, but his target changed when it was demonstrated an immunosuppressive and antiproliferative effect. The drug has been used to prevent kidney transplant rejection and to improve coronary stenting by developing sirolimus-eluting stents. Further studies demonstrate an anticancer effect by inhibition of angiogenesis. The drug has been used with good results in tumors [21]. Recently, some reports indicate a possible positive effect in the treatment of CVM, mainly of the lymphatic variety [22, 23]. A recent phase

II clinical trial on different types of vascular malformations, mainly lymphatic, but also venous and kaposiform hemangioendothelioma treated with sirolimus (62 cases, at a dosage of 0.8 mg/ m^2 per dose, twice daily), were reported at the 20th International Workshop of International Society for the Study of Vascular Anomalies (ISSVA), held in Melbourne, Australia, in 2014. Eighty-two percent had partial response, 5% were stable, and in 12% a progression of the disease was noticed [24]. Specifically, some lymphatic malformations (LMs) and blue rubber bleb nevus syndrome (BRBNS) can be treated quite successfully with sirolimus [25].

Sirolimus toxicity is reported (interstitial pneumonitis and decreased glucose tolerance), but it has not been recognized in these preliminary reports. Further investigations are necessary to assess the real efficacy of this drug.

Estrogen and Progesterone

Estrogen and progesterone have been widely investigated mainly to treat gastrointestinal bleeding because of gut vascular malformations. Interest in this therapy was based on the observation that epistaxis in HHT improved in pregnancy and worsened after menopause.

Some data, based only on anecdotal basis, showed reasonable results. However, a multicenter, randomized study failed to demonstrate advantage on placebo [26].

Octreotide

Octreotide is a somatostatin analogue which has been used for the treatment of gastrointestinal bleeding due to CVM. The drug may have an antiangiogenic effect, beside some gastrointestinal effects, like reduction of gastrin and pepsin and also reduction of duodenal and splanchnic blood flow. Some published series demonstrate a reasonable reduction of transfusions after that therapy (dosage in children, 4–8 μg/kg; in adults, from 100 μg subcutaneously two times per day to 500 μg subcutaneously two times per day) [27].

This drug can be considered as a reasonable adjunctive treatment for gastrointestinal bleeding due to CVM or as the only treatment if other more aggressive possibilities are excluded. No data exist about the usefulness of octreotide in CVM sited outside the gastrointestinal tract.

References

1. Lee BB, Baumgartner I, Berlien P, Bianchini G, Burrows P, Gloviczki P, Huang Y, Laredo J, Loose DA, Markovic J, Mattassi R, Parsi K, Rabe E, Rosenblatt M, Shortell C, Stillo F, Vaghi M, Villavicencio L, Zamboni P. Diagnosis and treatment of venous malformations consensus document of the international union of phlebology (IUP): updated 2013. Int Angiol. 2015;34(2):97–149.
2. Fahrni JO, Cho E-YN, Engelberger RP, Baumgartner I, von Känel R. Quality of life in patients with congenital vascular malformations. J Vasc Surg Venous Lym Dis. 2014;2:46–51.
3. Lee BB, Baumgartner I, Berlien HP, Bianchini G, Burrows P, Do YS, Ivancev K, Kool LS, Laredo J, Loose DA, Lopez-Gutierrez JC, Mattassi R, Parsi K, Rimon U, Rosenblatt M, Shortell C, Simkin R, Stillo F, Villavicencio L, Yakes W. Consensus document of the international union of angiology (IUA) – 2013 Current concepts on the management of arteriovenous malformations. Int Angiol. 2013;32(1):9–36.
4. Oduber CE, van Beers EJ, Bresser P, van der Horst CM, Meijers JC, Gerdes VE. Venous thromboembolism and prothrombotic parameters in Klippel-Trenaunay syndrome. Neth J Med. 2013;71(5):246–52.
5. Dompmartin A, Acher A, Thibon P, Tourbach S, Hermans C, Deneys V, Pocock B, Lequerrec A, Labbé D, Barrellier MT, Vanwijck R, Vikkula M, Boon L. Association of localized intravascular coagulopathy with venous malformations. Arch Dermatol. 2008;144(7):873–7.
6. Mazoyer E, Enjolras O, Laurian C, Houdart E, Drouet L. Coagulation abnormalities associated with extensive venous malformations of the limbs: differentiation from Kasabach-Merritt syndrome. Clin Lab Haematol. 2002;24(4):243–51.
7. Mazoyer E, Enjolras O, Bisdorff A, Perdu J, Wassef M, Drouet L. Coagulation disorders in patients with venous malformation of the limbs and trunk: a case series of 118 patients. Arch Dermatol. 2008;144(7):861–7.
8. Mattassi R, Vaghi M. Management of the marginal vein: current issues. Phlebology. 2007;22(6):283–6.
9. Lee BB, Laredo J: Chapter 7. Coagulation issue in venous malformation and its management. pp 93–127. Clinical handbook of management of antithrombotic & thrombolytic therapy. GHR Rao, E. Kalodiki, WA Leong, J Fareed (eds). 2014, Kontentworx, New Delhi

10. Chlebicki MP, Oh CC. Recurrent cellulitis: risk factors, etiology, pathogenesis and treatment. Curr Infect Dis Rep. 2014;16(9):422–32.

11. Iacobas I, Burrows PE, Adams DM, Sutton VR, Hollier LH, Chintagumpala MM. Oral rapamycin in the treatment of patients with hamartoma syndromes and PTEN mutation. Pediatr Blood Cancer. 2011;57:321–3.

12. Dupuis-Girod S, Ginon I, Saurin JC, Marion D, Guillot E, Decullier E. Bevacizumab in patients with hereditary hemorrhagic telangiectasia and severe hepatic vascular malformations and high cardiac output. JAMA. 2012;307:948–55.

13. Burrows PE, Mulliken JB, Fishman SJ, Klement GL, Folkman J. Pharmacological treatment of a diffuse arteriovenous malformation of the upper extremity in a child. J Craniofac Surg. 2009;20(Suppl 1): 597–602.

14. Adam Z, Pour L, Krejčí M, Pourová E, Synek O, Zahradová L, Navrátil M, Mechl M, Nebeský T, Neubauer J, Feit J, Vokurková J, Král Z, Bednařík O, Slampa P, Dolezalová H, Hájek R, Mayer J. Successful treatment of angiomatosis with thalidomide and interferon alpha. A description of five cases and overview of treatment of angiomatosis and proliferating hemangiomas. Vnitr Lek. 2010;56(8):810–23.

15. Bauditz J, Lochs H. Angiogenesis and vascular malformations: antiangiogenic drugs for treatment of gastrointestinal bleeding. World J Gastroenterol. 2007;13:5979–84.

16. Lebrin F, Srun S, Raymond K, Martin S, van den Brink S, Freitas C, Bréant C, Mathivet T, Larrivée B, Thomas JL, Arthur HM, Westermann CJ, Disch F, Mager JJ, Snijder RJ, Eichmann A, Mummery CL. Thalidomide stimulates vessel maturation and reduces epistaxis in individuals with hereditary hemorrhagic telangiectasia. Nat Med. 2010;16(4):420–8.

17. Tan HH, Ge ZZ, Chen HM, Gao YJ. Successful treatment with thalidomide for a patient with recurrent gastrointestinal bleeding due to angiodysplasia diagnosed by capsule endoscopy. J Dig Dis. 2013;14(3):153–5.

18. Molloy FM, Floeter MK, Syed NA, Sandbrink F, Culcea E, Steinberg SM, Dahut W, Pluda J, Kruger EA, Reed E, Figg WD. Thalidomide neuropathy in patients treated for metastatic prostate cancer. Muscle Nerve. 2001;24:1050–7.

19. Swetman GL, Berk DR, Vasanawala SS, Feinstein JA, Lane AT, Bruckner AL. Sildenafil for severe lymphatic malformations. N Engl J Med. 2012;366(4):384–6.

20. Danial C, Tichy AL, Tariq U, Swetman GL, Khuu P, Leung TH, Benjamin L, Teng J, Vasanawala SS, Lane AT. An open-label study to evaluate sildenafil for the treatment of lymphatic malformations. J Am Acad Dermatol. 2014;22(14):01119.

21. Guba M, von Breitenbuch P, Steinbauer M, Koehl G, Flegel S, Hornung M, Bruns CJ, Zuelke C, Farkas S, Anthuber M, Jauch KW, Geissler EK. Rapamycin inhibits primary and metastatic tumor growth by antiangiogenesis: involvement of vascular endothelial growth factor. Nat Med. 2002;8(2):128–35.

22. Hammill AM, Wentzel M, Gupta A, Nelson S, Lucky A, Elluru R, Dasgupta R, Azizkhan RG, Adams DM. Sirolimus for the treatment of complicated vascular anomalies in children. Pediatr Blood Cancer. 2011;57(6):1018–24.

23. Reinglas J, Ramphal R, Bromwich M. The successful management of diffuse lymphangiomatosis using sirolimus: a case report. Laryngoscope. 2011;121(9):1851–4.

24. Adams D, Hammill A, Trenor C. Phase II clinical trial of Sirolimus for the treatment of complicated vascular anomalies; initial results. Proceedings 20th international workshop on vascular anomales, Melbourne, 2014, p. 20–1.

25. Yuksekkaya H, Ozbek O, Keser M, Toy H. Blue rubber bleb nevus syndrome: successful treatment with sirolimus. Pediatrics. 2012;129(4):e1080–4.

26. Junquera F, Feu F, Papo M, Videla S, Armengol JR, Bordas JM, Saperas E, Piqué JM, Malagelada JR. A multicenter, randomized, clinical trial of hormonal therapy in the prevention of rebleeding from gastrointestinal angiodysplasia. Gastroenterology. 2001;121:1073–9.

27. Nardone G, Rocco A, Balzano T, Budillon G. The efficacy of octreotide therapy in chronic bleeding due to vascular abnormalities of the gastrointestinal tract. Aliment Pharmacol Ther. 1999;13:1429–36.

Multidisciplinary Team Approach for Patients with Congenital Vascular Malformation (CVM): Experience at Samsung Medical Center

44

Young-Wook Kim, Young Soo Do, Dong Ik Kim, and Byung-Boong Lee

Samsung Medical Center (SMC) has been a tertiary referral center in Seoul, South Korea, for the last 20 years. Since the early 1990s, led by a vascular surgeon, Dr. B.B. Lee who founded vascular malformation clinic at SMC, a multidisciplinary team was created for serving patients with congenital vascular malformation (CVM) [1, 2]. This dedicated team for the treatment of CVM started to see patients with CVM together once a month

Y.-W. Kim (✉)
Sungkyunkwan University, School of Medicine, Samsung Medical Center, Seoul, South Korea
e-mail: young52.kim@samsung.com; ywkim52@gmail.com

Y.S. Do
Interventional Radiology, Sungkyunkwan University, School of Medicine, Samsung Medical Center, Seoul, South Korea
e-mail: ys.do@samsung.com

D.I. Kim
Department of Surgery, Samsung Medical Center and Sungkyunkwan University, School of Medicine, Seoul, South Korea

B.-B. Lee, MD, PhD, FACS (✉)
Professor of Surgery and Director, Center for the Lymphedema and Vascular Malformations, George Washington University, Washington, DC, USA

Adjunct Professor of Surgery, Uniformed Services, University of the Health Sciences, Bethesda, MD, USA
e-mail: bblee38@gmail.com

sharing valuable data and knowledge and create a patient database following the Hamburg classification of CVM since its inception.

We would like to describe the rationales for the multidisciplinary approach for the patients with CVM [3, 4]. CVM is embryological defects of the vascular system and often affects more than one vascular system (capillary, arterial, venous, and/or lymphatic systems). This disorder manifests a varying array of characteristics and behaviors in its clinical course.

CVM lesions affect various anatomic sites or organs, and the timing of clinical presentation ranges from newborn to the elderly usually at the onset of overt symptomatic presentation. The presenting clinical features of CVM may be of the primary lesion or of its secondary complications. Furthermore, their clinical course is dynamic with time passage and unpredictable.

For treatment of CVM, curative surgical removal is uncommon and carries a high rate of recurrence and morbidities. Accordingly, it has been challenging for a given expert in one specialty to cope with all of the various complications that are presented, alone.

As described in previous chapters, treatment of CVM patients is challenging. Treatment of CVM usually aims at symptomatic, functional, cosmetic improvements and/or with minimal rates of recurrence or complication after the treatment of CVM lesion. It starts from an accurate assessment of the CVM lesion, choosing an optimal therapeutic strategy and preparing to cope with the expected complications related to treatment.

Proper and thorough assessment of CVM prior to the treatment is of utmost importance. This includes an accurate identification of the extent, the depth, and the type of the CVM lesions and organ or adjacent tissue involvement.

An accurate assessment of subtype of CVM entails identifying all components of the CVM lesion with the consideration for all of the "evolution potential" in the embryonic vascular tissue.

Selection of an optimal treatment strategy starts with choosing patients who are right candidate with proper indication(s) to conventional surgical and/or an interventional treatment on the basis of the risk-benefit analysis.

The role of a multidisciplinary team includes performing a pretreatment assessment to confirm the indication, choosing the treatment strategy, executing a treatment protocol using various treatment options (endovascular, surgical, laser, medical, or combined), scheduling appropriate periodic follow-up (particularly in pediatric patients with higher risk of development of deformity, disfigurement, or psychiatric trauma due to CVM), and performing clinical as well as basic research endeavors.

Early detection of CVM lesion with potential of life-threatening complications (e.g., CVM adjacent to the air way) or prevention of late development of major complications (e.g., major disfigurement, deformity, or dysfunction) is another important role for the multidisciplinary team.

Multidisciplinary team consists of vascular specialists in the field of vascular surgery and interventional radiology, pediatric orthopedic surgeons, pediatric surgeons, plastic surgeons, oral and dental surgeons, rehabilitation specialists, designated anesthesiologists, cardiologists, pathologists, dermatologists, nuclear medicine specialists, specialized nurses, and trained vascular ultrasonographers, (RVTs) data managers.

Through our extensive experience over the past 20 years with the multidisciplinary approach for patients with CVM, we think we have achieved improved results in all aspects of patient

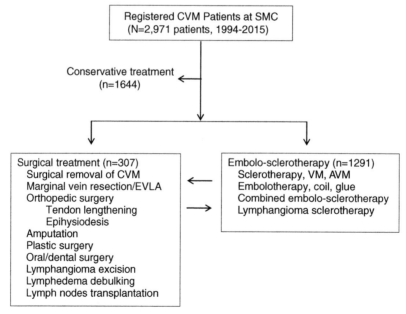

Registered CVM patients were included but capillary malformation (CM) patient who underwent laser therapy only were not included in this data.

Fig. 44.1 Management of CVM patients* at SMC during the past 20 years

care by extending treatment indications, using diversified therapeutic tools, and more efficiently coping with the complications related to CVM treatment. Above all, it affords us the opportunity to make a more reasonable decision in establishing treatment strategy.

Figure 44.1 shows our management of CVM patients at SMC during the past 20 years.

We think our future task includes developing a new embolic or sclerosing agents with less toxicity and higher efficiency, new therapeutic modality to ablate CVM lesion (e.g., laser, thermal ablation, photodynamic therapy), continued research to understand the biologic properties of the embryonic tissue, screening of the patients with higher "evolution potential" using biologic marker or specific imaging study, and to develop an inhibitor of the progression or evolution of CVM lesion. Among them, clinical research

work based on careful observations of CVM patients is also very important job for us.

References

1. Lee BB, Bergan JJ. Advanced management of congenital vascular malformations: a multidisciplinary approach. J Cardiovascular Surgery. 2002;10(6): 523–33.
2. Lee BB. Critical role of multidisciplinary team approach in the new field of vascular surgery – endovascular surgery. J Kor Soc Vasc Surg. 2003;19(2):121–3.
3. Lee BB, Do YS, Yakes W, Kim DI, Mattassi R, Hyun WS, Byun HS. Management of arterial-venous shunting malformations (AVM) by surgery and embolosclerotherapy. A multidisciplinary approach. J Vasc Surg. 2004;3:596–600.
4. Lee BB. New approaches to the treatment of congenital vascular malformations (CVMs) – single center experiences – (Editorial Review). Eur J Vasc Endovasc Surg. 2005;30(2):184–97.

Young-Wook Kim and Raul Mattassi

Introduction

Congenital vascular malformation (CVM) affecting lower extremity (LE) can cause bone and/or joint abnormality which can cause joint pain, early development of osteoarthritis, joint contracture, bone deformity, or limb length discrepancy (LLD) particularly in patients of growing age. Congenital vascular bone syndrome (CVBS) is defined as LLD due to an abnormal bone growth in patients with CVM [1].

Development of LLD attributes either overgrowth or undergrowth of the affected limb. In clinical practice, congenital vascular bone syndrome (CVBS) was often diagnosed by the presence of lower limb length discrepancy ≥ 2 cm in CVM patients.

Prevalence

The prevalence of CVBS is not exactly known among patients with CVM affecting lower extremity. It can be found in all types of CVM.

Y.-W. Kim, MD, PhD (✉)
Sungkyunkwan University, School of Medicine, Vascular Surgery, Samsung Medical Center, Seoul, South Korea
e-mail: young52.kim@samsung.com; ywkim52@gmail.com

R. Mattassi, MD (✉)
Vascular Malformation Center, "Stefan Belov"
Istituto Clinico Humanitas "Mater Domini",
Castellanza (Varese), Italy
e-mail: raulmattassi@gmail.com

According to Mattassi and Vaghi's report, the prevalence of long bone overgrowth was reported in 19 % and undergrowth in 7 % in venous-dominant CVM patients. In AVM patients, the prevalence was, respectively, overgrowth in 49 % and undergrowth in 4 % [1].

Though AVM more frequently coexist with CVBS compared to other types of CVM, CVBS is most prevalent in patients with venous type CVM because patients with venous type CVM outnumber AVM patients.

According to Samsung Medical Center (SMC) data, we found 71 (5.8%) patients with CVBS among 1215 registered patients with CVM affecting lower extremity during the past 21 years (from 1994 to 2015). Table 45.1 shows relative frequencies of CVBS according to the types of CVM. Over half of the CVBS patients were found in venous-predominant CVM patients, whereas CVBS most frequently found in patients with AV malformation, particularly microshunting (extratruncal) type arteriovenous malformation (AVM) (40%).

Pathophysiology of CVBS

There have been case reports of limb length discrepancy in patients with CVM patients since the nineteenth century. Among them, Klippel and Trenaunay described cases of CVM patients with limb elongation, skin nevus, and varicose veins in 1900 [2]. And Parkes Weber (R, R) also described

Table 45.1 Frequency of congenital vascular bone syndrome (CVBS) among patients with congenital vascular malformation (CVM) affecting lower extremity (1994–2015 at SMC)

Type of CVM	No (%) of patients	CVBS* patients	
		No (%)	Frequency (%) according to type of CVM
Venous malformation	728 (60%)	38 (53.5%)	5.2%
AV malformation	138 (11.3%)	14 (19.7%)	10%
Microshunting	10 (0.8%)	4 (5.6%)	40%
Macrofistula	128 (10.5%)	10 (14.1%)	7.8%
Lymphatic-dominant malformation	349 (28.7%)	19 (26.8%)	5.4%

CVM congenital vascular malformation, *CVBS* congenital vascular bone syndrome which was diagnosed when limb length discrepancy (LLD) $\geq$ 2 cm present on lower extremity bone spot scanogram, *AV* arteriovenous

cases of CVM patients showing limb hypertrophy and clinical signs of arteriovenous (AV) fistula [3, 4].

The above-described conditions (Klippel and Trenaunay syndromes and Parkes Weber syndrome) have been well known for causes of limb overgrowth and hypertrophy. However, the pathology of the limb overgrowth has not been well explained so far.

To explain the overgrowth in limb length in patients with CVM in lower extremity, various hypotheses have been proposed including increased vascularity of the growth plate of long bone, increased intramedullary small vessels, high oxygen tension, and elevated temperature [5].

A possible relationship of CVM with bone undergrowth was also noticed. Servelle and Trinquecoste [6] described two cases of CVM patients with limb undergrowth with phleboliths and hamartomas in 1948, and Martorell [7] reported a case of arm shortening with severe bone destruction in 1949.

In 1986, Belov et al. [8] described undergrowth of bone ascribed to the blood flow reduction in a limb.

To explain the undergrowth of long bone in patients with CVMs, mechanical or hemodynamic cause is proposed. Mechanical cause means a pressure effect on the metaphysis of long bone [9], and hemodynamic cause means decreased perfusion to the bone which can occur in an AVM lesion owing to steal phenomenon [10].

In the past, there were many animal studies attempting to explain the causes of CVBS. An overgrowth of long bones was observed in animal

study by ligation of deep veins. The authors concluded that the cause of an overgrowth of the long bone may be venous stasis rather than hyperemia in the growth plate [11]. Other authors performed angiography after deep vein ligation and noticed the development of multiple small AV shunts [12, 13].

Based on these experiments, it was stated that bone hypertrophy was always induced only by AV shunts either large (macrofistula) or small (microfistula) arteriovenous fistula.

The effect of AV shunts on osteoblasts is controversial whether bone growth may be induced by high oxygen tension or by hypoxia secondary to a steal phenomenon. Recently, relations between the bone vasculature, bone growth, and molecules with both angiogenic and osteogenic activity are revealed. It revealed that vascular endothelial growth factor (VEGF) can act directly on osteoblasts [14, 15].

Other known factors that influence skeletal development are fibroblast growth factor (FGF), transforming growth factor (TGF), bone morphogenetic protein (BMP), insulin-like growth factor (IGF), and platelet-derived growth factor (PDGF) [16]. The role of these molecules in the development of CVBS needs to be investigated.

Clinical Features

We found that CVBS can develop in all types of CVM patients. It is frequently associated with clinical features of other types of CVM such as port-wine stain; nevus; varicosity; limb hypertrophy; intermittent episodes of leg pain, leg heaviness, joint pain, or joint contracture; pathologic long bone fracture; lateral scoliosis of the spine; etc.

It can cause not only physical deformity but also functional and psychosocial problems.

Risk Factors for Development of CVBS in CVM Patients

Predicting development of LLD is important in pediatric patients with CVM affecting lower extremity. Kim et al. attempted to determine risk factors for LLD in patients with CVM [17]. A retrospective analysis was conducted for 361 patients (153 (42%) males and 208 (57%) females, mean age of 20 ± 14 years (range, 1–62)) who underwent MRI assessment of a CVM lesion and measured LLD using lower extremity scanogram. The risk factor analysis for LLD >2 cm was performed with test variables of age, gender, type, extent and depth of CVM, and the deep vein agenesis or hypoplasia of the affected limb. The types of CVMs included 215 VM (60%), 43 AVM (12%), 46 LM (13%), and 57 (16%) combined VLM. On the lower extremity scanogram, 26 patients (7%) had an LLD of >2 cm due to overgrowth ($n = 20$) or undergrowth ($n = 6$) of the affected limbs. On a multivariate analysis, whole leg CVM lesion was identified as a single independent risk factor for LLD ($P = 0.004$; OR, 6.512, 95% CI, 1.788–23.713). And overgrowth was significantly ($P = 0.022$) more common in female than in male patients.

Diagnosis of CVBS

The presence of LLD can be assessed with the patient in standing position on a flat floor by observing symmetry of gluteal and popliteal folds of both legs. Femur lengths can be compared by observing for inequality of knee height in supine position with hips and knees flexed with feet flat on examining table (Galeazzi test). However, inequality can be caused in patients with congenital hip dislocation. In addition to the LLD, pelvic tilting, spine scoliosis, or leg or foot deformities can be seen.

Clinical access usually includes studies for the type and extent of CVM; location and extent of bone involvement, particularly intraosseous CVM; amount of limb length discrepancy (LLD); and presence of secondary bone or joint abnormality.

LLD of the lower extremity is a common orthopedic condition. According to an old study of 1000 US Army recruits, two-thirds of this population showed to have limb length discrepancies up to 2 cm [18].

Many investigations [19–21] examining the effects of LLD have shown that minor length discrepancies are usually inconsequential, while greater discrepancies may result in gait problems, scoliosis and pelvic tilting, consequent low back pain and knee contracture, in addition to the dissatisfaction with appearance.

"Two-cm threshold of LLD" has been often used by the orthopedic surgeons since a single publication by Gross in 1978 [22]. Vitale MA et al. [23] reported that patients with a limb length discrepancy of 2 cm or below generally fared better than patients with larger discrepancies, but no discrete cutoff could be identified within this group.

Table 45.2 shows results of diagnostic assessment in 71 patients with CVBS in Samsung Medical Center. In the diagnosis of CVBS, it is important to demonstrate the type, extent, and depth of CVM lesion, coexisting vascular anomaly such as deep vein hypoplasia or aplasia, and involvement of joint or bone. We summarized diagnostic workup for patients with CVBS in Table 45.3.

To determine LLD, lower extremity scanogram, CT scan/digital localization image, and microdose digital scan can be used. The lower extremity scanogram was developed to minimize

Table 45.2 Clinical features of congenital vascular bone syndrome (*n*= 71 patients, 1994 ~2015 at SMC)

	Number (%)	
	LLD > 2 cm (due to overgrowth): *n* = 63 (89%)	LLD > 2 cm (due to undergrowth): *n* = 8 (11%)
Type of CVM		
Venous-dominant malformation	34 (54)	4 (50)
Arteriovenous malformation	13 (21)	1 (12.5)
Lymphatic-dominant malformation	16 (25)	3 (37.5)
Age at initial presentation (year of age)	Mean 1 year (0~17)	Mean 3 years (0~8)
Male/female	30:33	7:1
Extent of CVM in the leg		
Whole leg	49 (67)	5 (62.5)
Upper leg	3 (5)	2 (25)
Lower leg	11 (17)	1 (12.5)
Coexisting lesion		
Port-wine skin lesion	42 (67)	2 (25)
Marginal vein	17 (27)	2 (25)
Limb hypertrophy	35 (56)	–
Limb hypotrophy	–	2 (25)
Depth of CVM involvement		
Skin	43 (68)	2 (25)
Subcutaneous tissue	61 (97)	5 (62.5)
Muscle	39 (62)	6 (75)
Bone	8 (13)	3 (37.5)
Knee joint	6 (9)	1 (12.5)
Femoropopliteal vein		
Intact	51 (81)	7 (87.5)
Aplasia	8 (13)	0
Hypoplasia	3 (5)	1 (12.5)
Phlebectasia	1 (2)	0
LLD (mean cm, range)	3.3 cm (2~12.1)	4.7 cm (2~9.5)

CVM congenital vascular malformation, *VM* venous malformation, *AVM* arteriovenous malformation, *LM* lymphatic malformation, *LLD* limb length discrepancy, congenital vascular bone syndrome was defined as presence of CVM with lower limb LLD > 2 cm due to overgrowth or undergrowth, *LLD* limb length discrepancy

measurement error due to magnification of the peripherally located subject by the X-ray projection angle. A lower extremity scanogram in which the X-ray tube is centered precisely over the hip, knee, and ankle joints and three successive exposures of the lower extremity centered over the three joints are performed. LLD can be determined by the sum of length discrepancies in the three segments. Figure 45.1 shows diagnostic work up used for patients with CVBS.

Although scanography is known as the most accurate radiographic technique for measurement of LLD, problems with interpretation can result from calculation or measurement errors in patients with significant limb length inequalities or hip or knee joint contracture.

Table 45.3 Diagnostic workup of patients with congenital vascular bone syndrome (CVBS)

	Examinations
Type and extent of CVM	Ultrasonography MRI Whole-body blood pool scintigraphy (WBBPS) Catheter arteriography; CT angiography (for AVM) Lymphoscintigraphy (for LM)
Deep vein aplasia or hypoplasia	Ultrasonography (iliac and femoral veins) Whole-body blood pool scintigraphy (WBBPS) Ascending venography or percutaneous direct puncture venography
Bone structure and extent of the bone involvement; secondary bone or joint abnormality	Plain X-ray MRI
Limb length discrepancy (LLD)	Spot scanogram
Interosseous CVM lesion	Contrast-enhanced MRI angiography

CVM congenital vascular malformation, *LM* lymphatic malformation

Instead of using the scanogram, some authors recommend full-length standing anteroposterior radiography to determine LLD.

Management of CVBS

Generally, fairly straightforward guidelines expressed in terms of the magnitude of the predicted discrepancy can be used to choose from among the major treatment categories (Table 45.4).

There are two main treatment strategies for patients with CVBS. The first strategy is treatment of CVM to prevent further progression of LLD, and the second strategy is aiming to correct LLD with orthopedic procedures. If the patient is in age of still growing and CVBS is evident, the treatment should be targeted to the CVM lesion first. If intraosseous CVM (AV fistulas, venous or lymphatic) exist, these lesions should be target for treatment. The detailed treatment procedure for CVM lesion is described in other chapters.

Correction of LLD can be achieved once the cause of CVBS is eradicated in the growing age. Many orthopedic surgical techniques have been used to correct LLD, which include epiphysiodesis, leg shortening, and leg lengthening.

Subischial leg length is used as the length of the lower limb. It is measured by subtracting sitting height from standing height. The lower limb grows more than the trunk and the growth cycle in the lower limb is predictable. After birth, not only does the overall rate of growth vary at different ages, the rate at which various segments of the body grow also differs [24].

By predicting the time of the completion of leg growth taking into consideration of patient age and bone age, orthopedic surgeons attempt to stop an expected growth of the one leg by epiphysiodesis. For example, temporary epiphysiodesis is an orthopedic procedure to correct LLD by deterring from long bone growth of one leg by compression of growth plate with rigid stapling or percutaneous placement of transphyseal screws at the growth plate. When the staples or screws are removed, it is known that normal bone growth resumes. Figure 45.2 show an example of epiphysiodesis for a patient with LLD due to AVM affecting the lower leg and foot.

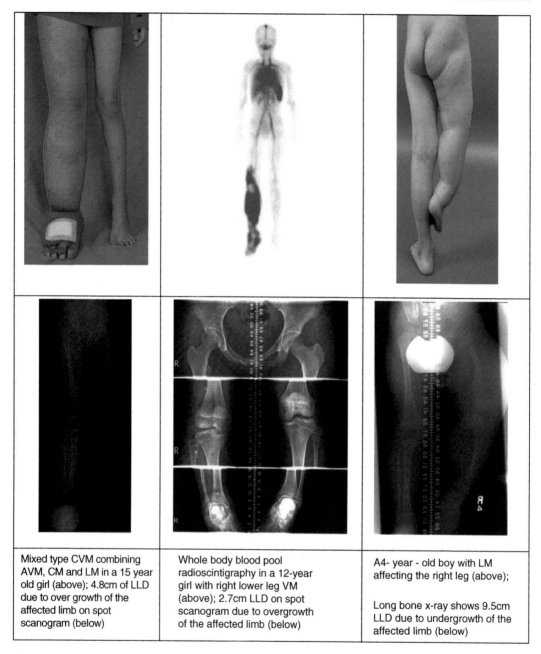

| Mixed type CVM combining AVM, CM and LM in a 15 year old girl (above); 4.8cm of LLD due to over growth of the affected limb on spot scanogram (below) | Whole body blood pool radioscintigraphy in a 12-year girl with right lower leg VM (above); 2.7cm LLD on spot scanogram due to overgrowth of the affected limb (below) | A4- year - old boy with LM affecting the right leg (above); Long bone x-ray shows 9.5cm LLD due to undergrowth of the affected limb (below) |

Fig. 45.1 Congenital vascular bone syndrome (CVBS) in various types of CVM patients. Mixed type CVM combining AVM, CM, and LM in a 15-year-old girl (*Left, top*); 4.8 cm of LLD due to overgrowth of the affected limb on long bone X-ray (*left, bottom*). Whole-body blood pool radioscintigraphy in a 12-year-old girl with right lower leg VM (*middle, top*); 2.7 cm LLD on spot scanogram due to overgrowth of the affected limb (*middle, bottom*). A 4-year-old boy with LM affecting the right leg (*right, top*); long bone X-ray shows 9.5 cm LLD due to undergrowth of the affected limb (*right, bottom*)

There are many other forms of orthopedic procedure to correct LLD. It is beyond the scope of this chapter. In patients with completed long bone growth, a correction of CVM is not benefi-

Table 45.4 General guideline for treatment of patients with LLD

Limb length discrepancy (cm)	Recommended treatment
0–2	No treatment
2–6	Orthotic use, epiphysiodesis, skeletal shortening
6–20	Limb reconstruction (limb lengthening with or without adjunctive procedures)
>20	Prosthetic fitting (with or without surgical optimization)

Weintstein and Flynn [25]

cial in correction of LLD. Therefore, exact timing of epiphysiodesis before completion of long bone growth is critical to correct LLD.

In cases of LLD due to limb undergrowth, bone-lengthening procedure is an attractive treatment option; however, it may be difficult to achieve because the dysplastic bone of the affected limb is often too fragile to perform bone surgery.

In summary, CVBS is a rare form of CVM affecting lower extremity. Considering the difficulty of treatment of CVM, it is more challenging to treat CVBS. However, multidisciplinary approaches by vascular specialist, pediatric orthopedic surgeons, and rehabilitation specialist can make physical and functional improvement in selective patients with CVBS.

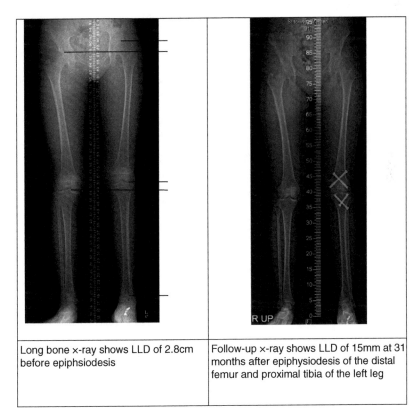

Long bone x-ray shows LLD of 2.8cm before epiphsiodesis	Follow-up x-ray shows LLD of 15mm at 31 months after epiphysiodesis of the distal femur and proximal tibia of the left leg

Fig. 45.2 Temporary epiphysiodesis to correct limb length discrepancy in a patient with CVBS due to left lower leg and foot AVM. Long bone X-ray shows LLD of 2.8 cm before epiphysiodesis. Follow-up X-ray shows LLD of 15 mm at 31 months after epiphysiodesis of the distal femur and proximal tibia of the left leg

References

1. Mattassi R, Vaghi M. Vascular bone syndrome--angio-osteodystrophy: current concepts. Phlebology/Venous Forum R Soc Med. 2007;22(6):287–90.
2. Klippel M, Trenaunay P. Du naevus variqueux et osteo-hypertrophique. Arch Gen Med. 1900;3:641–72.
3. Weber FP. Haemangiectasic hypertrophies of the foot and lower extremity Congenital or acquired. Presse Med. 1908;15:261–6.
4. Weber FP. Haemagiectasis hypertrophy of limbs. Congenital phlebarteriectasis and so called congenital 'varicose veins'. Br J Child Dis. 1918;15:13–7.
5. Kelly PJ, Janes JM, Peterson LFA. The effect of arterio-venous fistulae on the vascular pattern of the femora of immature dogs, a microangiographic study. J Bone Joint Surg Am. 1959;41:1101–8.
6. Servelle M, Trinquecoste P. Des angiomes veineux (about venous angiomas). Arch Mal Couer. 1948;41:436–8.
7. Martorell F. Hemangiomatosis braquial osteolı'tica. Angiologia. 1949;1:219.
8. Belov St, Loose DA, Mu¨ller E. Angeborene Gefa¨Xfehler (Congenital vascular defects). Reinbeck: Einhorn Presse Verlag. 1986:35–37.
9. Janes JM, Musgrove JE. Effect of arteriovenous fistula on growth of bone; an experimental study. Surg Clin North Am. 1950;30(4):1191–200.
10. Mattassi R. Differential diagnosis in congenital vascular-bone syndromes. Semin Vasc Surg. 1993;6(4):233–44.
11. Servelle M. Stase veineuse et croissance osseuse (venous stasis and bone growth). Bull Acad Natl Med. 1948;132:471–4.
12. Soltesz L. Contribution of clinical and experimental studies of the hypertrophy of the extremities in congenital arteriovenous fistulae. J Cardiovasc Surg (Torino). 1965;260
13. Brookes M, Singh M. Venous shunt in bone after ligation of the femoral vein. Surg Gynecol Obstet. 1972;135(1):85–8.
14. Zelzer E, McLean W, Ng YS, et al. Skeletal defects in VEGF(120/120) mice reveal multiple roles for VEGF in skeletogenesis. Development. 2002;129(8):1893–904.
15. Deckers MM, van Bezooijen RL, van der Horst G, et al. Bone morphogenetic proteins stimulate angiogenesis through osteoblast-derived vascular endothelial growth factor A. Endocrinology. 2002;143(4):1545–53.
16. Carano RA, Filvaroff EH. Angiogenesis and bone repair. Drug Discov Today. 2003;8(21):980–9.
17. Kim YW, Lee SH, Kim DI, Do YS, Lee BB. Risk factors for leg length discrepancy in patients with congenital vascular malformation. J Vasc Surg. 2006;44(3):545–53.
18. Rush WA, Steiner HA. A study of lower extremity length inequality. Am J Roentgenol Radium Ther. 1946;56(5):616–23.
19. Gofton JP. Persistent low back pain and leg length disparity. J Rheumatol. 1985;12(4):747–50.
20. Grundy PF, Roberts CJ. Does unequal leg length cause back pain? A case-control study. Lancet (London, England). 1984;2(8397):256–8.
21. Soukka A, Alaranta H, Tallroth K, Heliovaara M. Leg-length inequality in people of working age. The association between mild inequality and low-back pain is questionable. Spine. 1991;16(4):429–31.
22. Gross RH. Leg length discrepancy: how much is too much? Orthopedics. 1978;1(4):307–10.
23. Vitale MA, Choe JC, Sesko AM, et al. The effect of limb length discrepancy on health-related quality of life: is the '2 cm rule' appropriate? J Pediatr Orthop Part B. 2006;15(1):1–5.
24. DiMeglio A, Canavese F, Charles YP. Growth and adolescent idiopathic scoliosis: when and how much? J Pediatr Orthop. 2011;31(1 Suppl):S28–36.
25. Weintstein SL, Flynn JM. Lovell and Winter's pediatric orthopedics. 7th ed. Philadelphia: Wolter Kluwer. Lippincott Williams and Wilkins; 2014. p. 1341–87.

Patricia E. Burrows

AV Malformation (AVM)

The mechanisms for development and progression of AVM are incompletely understood, but have been most thoroughly studied in patients with familial AVM, especially hereditary hemorrhagic telangiectasia [HHT], known to be caused by mutations in endoglin, ALK1, and SMAD4, receptors for the transforming growth factor [TGF] beta superfamily. AVMs and similar vascular lesions have been created in animal models by creating mutations in ALK1, endoglin, and Notch in mice and zebra fish [4–6]. While the animal models do not exactly replicate human disease, it has been possible to study the development of AVMs and observe the effects of various interventions including drug treatment. In addition, studies of the molecular milieu of resected cerebral AVMs have shown inflammatory markers, and matrix metalloproteinases are increased in cerebral AVMs [7, 8]. Histochemical study of resected vascular malformations has also shown increased receptors to growth hormone and follicle-stimulating hormone [FSH] but not estrogen or androgens [9, 10]. Endothelial progenitor cells [EPCs] are also increased in higher stage AVMs, possibly in response to ischemia [11].

Antiangiogenesis treatment for human AVMs has been based partly on findings in the animal models and human AVM tissue studies and partly on anecdotal observations.

Bevacizumab, which is an antibody to vascular endothelial growth factor [VEGF], was first used in patients with lung cancer who coincidentally had HHT. Initially, a patient with liver failure and cardiac overload due to hepatic AVM received treatment with bevacizumab and was found to have dramatic reduction in cardiac output and improvement in hepatic function. Subsequently, there have been some small clinical trials showing efficacy in epistaxis, GI bleeding, hepatic failure, and cardiac overload in patients with HHT [12–15]. Complications of the drug have been relatively infrequent, and it has been noted that patients with HHT require lower doses to achieve a result than patients with cancer [16].

Thalidomide, which is a beta FGF antagonist, has been used anecdotally in patients with sporadic AVM and more recently in patients with HHT who have GI bleeding and epistaxis [17]. Lenalidomide, an analog of thalidomide, has also been found to be effective in anecdotal cases of GI bleeding in HHT. Both drugs have been used successfully for epithelial hemangioendothelioma. Both drugs are teratogenic, and complications include peripheral neuropathy, somnolence, thrombosis, cytopenias, and pseudotumor cerebri.

Matrix metalloproteinase [MMP] inhibitors, such as doxycycline, minocycline, and marimastat, have been tried in patients with sporadic

P.E. Burrows, MD
Medical College of Wisconsin,
Children's Hospital of Wisconsin,
Milwaukee, WI, USA
e-mail: PBurrows@chw.org

AVM, including brain AVMs. This approach is supported by findings of upregulation of MMPs 2 and 9 in brain AVMs and peripheral vascular malformations. In vitro and animal studies have shown that doxycycline and minocycline change the proteomic expression of endothelial cells and, in some cases, reverse the AVMs in animal models. In the brain AVM trial, there was a trend, not statistically significant, suggesting that MMP inhibition might reduce the risk of bleeding from cerebral AVMs [18]. A 3-year-old child with AVM of the forearm, resulting in significant progress of bone destruction and not responding to embolization, was treated with marimastat, a broad-spectrum MMP inhibitor with dramatic dose-related sustained response [19]. She has been taking this medication for 17 years without side effects. Unfortunately, this drug is not FDA approved and has not been available for compassionate use. Several centers prescribe doxycycline or minocycline to AVM patients, but as yet there is no conclusive data supporting its effectiveness. Tetracyclines are known to cause dental discoloration when administered chronically to children under 8 years of age. In addition, MMP inhibitors can cause allergic reactions, gastrointestinal distress, tendinopathies, and pseudotumor cerebri.

Cox-2 inhibitors [nonsteroidal anti-inflammatory drugs] have a mild antiangiogenic effect and are helpful in controlling pain in patients with AVM.

Venous Malformations (VM) and Lymphatic Malformations (LM)

Sirolimus [rapamycin] is an MTOR inhibitor that has been shown to be effective in reducing mass and symptoms related to the hamartomas in patients with PTEN mutations [3] and is also effective in decreasing symptoms and fluid leakage in patients with diffuse lymphatic malformations [1–2] [20–22].

Early studies also show benefit using sirolimus in patients with extensive venous malformations,

including those with blue rubber bleb nevus syndrome [23]. A novel animal model showed that endothelial cells with TIE2 mutation, injected into mice, form vascular lesions resembling human venous malformations. Treatment of the cells and the mice with rapamycin resulted in decreased growth of the vascular lesions, by suppression of AKT. Patients with severely symptomatic venous malformations also improved. It has been noted that the response may require several months of treatment, but treated patients have shown significant improvement in pain, bleeding, lesion size, function, and coagulopathy. Unfortunately, symptoms recur quickly after discontinuation of treatment, but then improve on resuming treatment.

Presently, no benefit has been shown in patients with sporadic AVM treated with sirolimus. Octreotide, a somatostatin analog, has been used in a small series of patients with angioectasias of the bowel [24].

Sildenafil appeared to be effective in a few patients with lymphatic malformation, but subsequent trials did not show a benefit. A larger clinical trial is underway.

Antiestrogen drugs such as tamoxifen and raloxifene have been studied in patients with HHT with possible improvement of epistaxis.

At the time of this writing, the only active clinical trial for drug treatment of patients with AVM with is a European multicenter trial using sirolimus.

Summary

Early studies support the effectiveness of pharmacotherapy for certain vascular malformations, especially extensive lymphatic malformations [rapamycin], hamartomas associated with PTEN mutation [rapamycin], and AVMs associated with ALK1 and ENG mutations [bevacizumab, thalidomide]. As we learn more about the molecular pathways involved in development and progression of vascular malformations, it is likely that new pharmacologic approaches will be identified (Figs. 46.1 and 46.2).

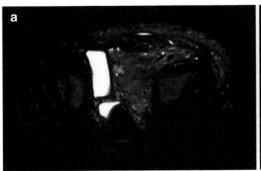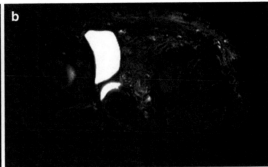

Fig. 46.1 Rapamycin treatment of symptomatic LM in 3-year-old patient with CLOVES syndrome. Patient had bulky overgrowth and leakage from lymphatic vesicles associated with cellulitis. (**a**) Axial STIR of pelvis shows overgrowth and microcystic LM with displacement of bladder. (**b**) After 2 years of rapamycin, the fluid leakage and cellulitis had resolved. MRI shows mild improvement in the bulkiness and fluid content of the LM

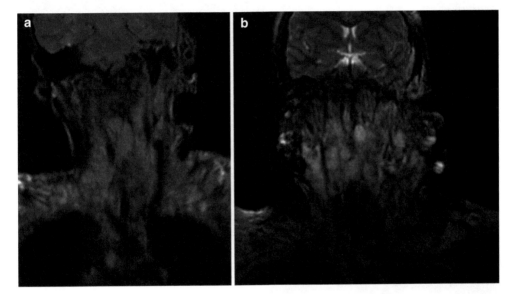

Fig. 46.2 Diffuse VM of the neck, face, airway, scalp, thoracic inlet, and shoulder, presenting with airway obstruction at 4 years of age. VM grew aggressively over childhood and early adulthood. Patient did not do well on rapamycin due to poor compliance. This case shows the need for biological treatment. (**a**) Coronal T2-weighted image at 4 years of age showing the extensive VM. Patient was treated with tracheostomy, extensive percutaneous embolization, and partial resection. Patient did not tolerate ethanol. Treatment continued twice a year after initial hospitalization. (**b**) Five years after presentation, VM still present. Treated with laser therapy, partial resection, and additional sclerotherapy using STS foam. Decannulated.

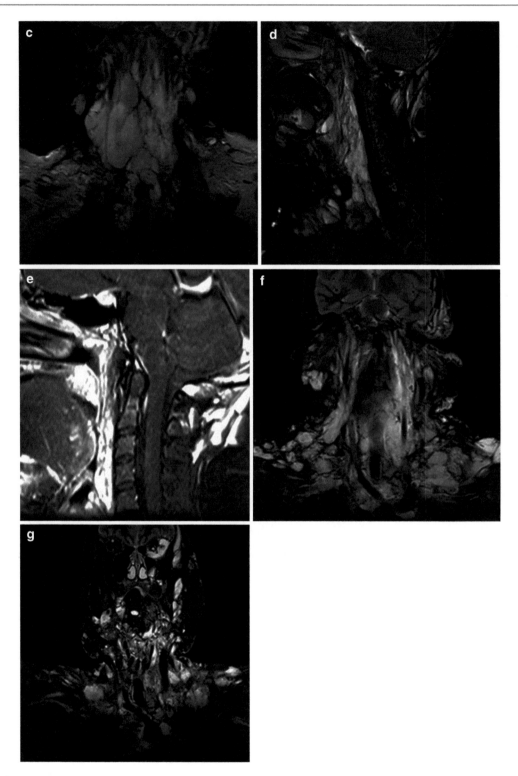

Fig. 46.2 (continued) (**c, d**) Six years after presentation, increased growth of VM. Emergency tracheostomy, started new series of sclerotherapy with foam and bleomycin. (**e**) Improved airway after three sessions of foam and bleomycin. (**f**) Eight years after presentation, increase growth of supraclavicular VM. (**g**) 14 years after presentation, after a trial of rapamycin with continued biannual sclerotherapy with foam and bleomycin. Improved but still having pain and tracheostomy dependence

References

1. Blatt J, McLean TW, Castellino SM, Burkhart CN. A review of contemporary options for medical management of hemangiomas, other vascular tumors, and vascular malformations. Pharmacol Ther. 2013;139(3): 327–33.
2. Margolin JF, Soni HM, Pimpalwar S. Medical therapy for pediatric vascular anomalies. Semin Plast Surg. 2014;28(2):79–86.
3. Iacobas I, Burrows PE, Adams DM, Sutton VR, Hollier LH, Chintagumpala MM. Oral rapamycin in the treatment of patients with hamartoma syndromes and PTEN mutation. Pediatr Blood Cancer. 2011; 57(2):321–3.
4. Murphy PA, Kim TN, Lu G, Bollen AW, Schaffer CB, Wang RA. Notch4 normalization reduces blood vessel size in arteriovenous malformations. Sci Transl Med. 2012;4(117):117ra8.
5. Tual-Chalot S, Oh SP, Arthur HM. Mouse models of hereditary hemorrhagic telangiectasia: recent advances and future challenges. Front Genet. 2015;6:25.
6. Walcott BP. BMP signaling modulation attenuates cerebral arteriovenous malformation formation in a vertebrate model. J Cereb Blood Flow Metab. 2014; 34(10):1688–94.
7. Mouchtouris N, Jabbour PM, Starke RM, Hasan DM, Zanaty M, Theofanis T, et al. Biology of cerebral arteriovenous malformations with a focus on inflammation. J Cereb Blood Flow Metab. 2015;35(2):167–75.
8. Rangel-Castilla L, Russin JJ, Martinez-Del-Campo E, Soriano-Baron H, Spetzler RF, Nakaji P. Molecular and cellular biology of cerebral arteriovenous malformations: a review of current concepts and future trends in treatment. Neurosurg Focus. 2014;37(3):E1.
9. Kulungowski AM, Hassanein AH, Nose V, Fishman SJ, Mulliken JB, Upton J, et al. Expression of androgen, estrogen, progesterone, and growth hormone receptors in vascular malformations. Plast Reconstr Surg. 2012;129(6):919e–24e.
10. Maclellan RA, Vivero MP, Purcell P, Kozakewich HP, DiVasta AD, Mulliken JB, et al. Expression of follicle-stimulating hormone receptor in vascular anomalies. Plast Reconstr Surg. 2014;133(3):344e–51e.
11. Lu L, Bischoff J, Mulliken JB, Bielenberg DR, Fishman SJ, Greene AK. Increased endothelial progenitor cells and vasculogenic factors in higher-staged arteriovenous malformations. Plast Reconstr Surg. 2011;128(4):260e–9e.
12. Dupuis-Girod S, Ginon I, Saurin JC, Marion D, Guillot E, Decullier E, et al. Bevacizumab in patients with hereditary hemorrhagic telangiectasia and severe hepatic vascular malformations and high cardiac output. Jama. 2012;307(9):948–55.
13. Kanellopoulou T, Alexopoulou A. Bevacizumab in the treatment of hereditary hemorrhagic telangiectasia. Expert Opin Biol Ther. 2013;13(9):1315–23.
14. Lupu A, Stefanescu C, Treton X, Attar A, Corcos O, Bouhnik Y. Bevacizumab as rescue treatment for severe recurrent gastrointestinal bleeding in hereditary hemorrhagic telangiectasia. J Clin Gastroenterol. 2013;47(3):256–7.
15. Young LH, Henderson KJ, White RI, Garcia-Tsao G. Bevacizumab: finding its niche in the treatment of heart failure secondary to liver vascular malformations in hereditary hemorrhagic telangiectasia. Hepatology. 2013;58(1):442–5.
16. Azzopardi N, Dupuis-Girod S, Ternant D, Fargeton AE, Ginon I, Faure F, et al. Dose – response relationship of bevacizumab in hereditary hemorrhagic telangiectasia. MAbs. 2015;7(3):630–7.
17. Lebrin F, Srun S, Raymond K, Martin S, van den Brink S, Freitas C, et al. Thalidomide stimulates vessel maturation and reduces epistaxis in individuals with hereditary hemorrhagic telangiectasia. Nat Med. 2010;16(4):420–8.
18. Frenzel T, Lee CZ, Kim H, Quinnine NJ, Hashimoto T, Lawton MT, et al. Feasibility of minocycline and doxycycline use as potential vasculostatic therapy for brain vascular malformations: pilot study of adverse events and tolerance. Cerebrovasc Dis. 2008;25(1-2):157–63.
19. Burrows PE, Mulliken JB, Fishman SJ, Klement GL, Folkman J. Pharmacological treatment of a diffuse arteriovenous malformation of the upper extremity in a child. J Craniofac Surg. 2009;20(Suppl 1):597–602.
20. Hammill AM, Wentzel M, Gupta A, Nelson S, Lucky A, Elluru R, et al. Sirolimus for the treatment of complicated vascular anomalies in children. Pediatr Blood Cancer. 2011;57(6):1018–24.
21. Lackner H, Karastaneva A, Schwinger W, Benesch M, Sovinz P, Seidel M, et al. Sirolimus for the treatment of children with various complicated vascular anomalies. Eur J Pediatr. 2015;174(12):1579–84.
22. Trenor 3rd CC. Sirolimus for refractory vascular anomalies. Pediatr Blood Cancer. 2011;57(6):904–5.
23. Boscolo E, Limaye N, Huang L, Kang KT, Soblet J, Uebelhoer M, et al. Rapamycin improves TIE2-mutated venous malformation in murine model and human subjects. J Clin Invest. 2015;125(9):3491–504.
24. Brown C, Subramanian V, Wilcox CM, Peter S. Somatostatin analogues in the treatment of recurrent bleeding from gastrointestinal vascular malformations: an overview and systematic review of prospective observational studies. Dig Dis Sci. 2010;55(8):2129–34.

Pelvic Arteriovenous Malformation (AVM)

47

Young-Wook Kim, Young Soo Do, Dong-Ik Kim, and Byung-Boong Lee

Arteriovenous malformations (AVMs) can affect any part of the human body containing blood vessels. Traumatic arteriovenous fistula in the uterus secondary to pelvic surgery, dilatation and curettage, or trauma is not described in this chapter.

Pelvic AVM lesions can affect the pelvic wall and pelvic organs and they have a specific clinical importance particularly in female patients.

As described in previous chapters, AVM lesions characteristically have a potential to evolve over time from quiescent lesion to lesion with active arteriovenous shunting which results in venous hypertension, feeding artery and draining vein enlargement, and even as a late complication. Evolution of AVM lesion is often stimulated by trauma (e.g., blunt trauma, surgery of the AVM lesion) or hormonal change (e.g., puberty, pregnancy, or use of contraceptive agent). Clinically, it is more common to encounter female patients with pelvic AVMs during the period of puberty or pregnancy compared to male patients. Among 3066 CVM patients registered in our CVM clinic at Samsung Medical Center (SMC) in Seoul, South Korea, we found that pelvic AVM comprised of 0.7% of all CVM patients and 4.2% of all AVM patients.

Y.-W. Kim (✉) • D.-I. Kim
Department of Vascular Surgery, Samsung Medical Center, Sungkyunkwan University School of Medicine, Seoul, South Korea
e-mail: young52.kim@samsung.com; ywkim52@gmail.com

Y.S. Do
Department of Radiology, Samsung Medical Center, Sungkyunkwan University School of Medicine, Seoul, South Korea

B.-B. Lee, MD, PhD, FACS (✉)
Professor of Surgery and Director, Center for the Lymphedema and Vascular Malformations, George Washington University, Washington, DC, USA

Adjunct Professor of Surgery, Uniformed Services, University of the Health Sciences, Bethesda, MD, USA
e-mail: bblee38@gmail.com

Clinical Manifestations

Symptoms of pelvic AVM range from asymptomatic or mild pelvic discomfort to significant vaginal or rectal bleeding or event to congestive cardiac failure (Table 47.1).

In other previous case series, pelvic AVM patients presented with sciatic pain, hydronephrosis, or gynecologic problems in female patients [1–3].

Diagnosis of Pelvic AVM

Many AVM lesions are detected with ultrasonography (US). With duplex US, AVM can be easily detected showing abnormal high-velocity flow in

© Springer-Verlag Berlin Heidelberg 2017
Y.-W. Kim et al. (eds.), *Congenital Vascular Malformations*, DOI 10.1007/978-3-662-46709-1_47

the venous channels and dilated arterial and venous vascular components. MRI findings include presence of vascular flow voids within

Table 47.1 Demonstrates demographic and clinical features of patients with pelvic AVM (*n*=21)

Features	No (%)
Age at the initial presentation	36 ± 15(16~70)
Gender (male)	13 (62%)
Chief complaint	
Occasionally detected without symptom	8 (38%)
Pelvic pain or discomfort	7 (33%)
Vaginal bleeding	4 (19%)
Gross hematuria	3 (14%)
Repeated abortion	1 (5%)
Symptoms due to pelvic nerve compression	1 (5%)

the effected tissues. MR angiography (MRA), best performed as a time-resolved contrast-enhanced three-dimensional acquisition, can demonstrate the extent and vascular anatomy of AVM lesions [4].

Compared to the AVM lesion at the other parts of the body, pelvic AVM is more likely to be overlooked due to its deep location and quiescent nature of the lesion in an early stage of the AVM. In our experiences, most patients with pelvic AVM were referred to specialized center after being occasionally detected on imaging study (e.g., ultrasound, contrast-enhanced CT, MRI).

In the diagnosis of pelvic AVM, abdominal-pelvic CT angiography is the diagnostic tool of choice. Figure 47.1 shows CT angiogram of patients with pelvic AVM.

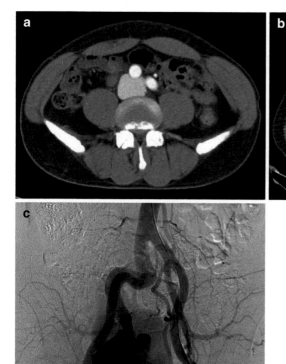

Fig. 47.1 A 49-year-old asymptomatic female with pelvic AVM. (**a**), (**b**) Contrast-enhanced axial CT images show multiple fine feeding arteries from the iliac artery and enlarged draining vein. (**c**) Catheter arteriogram shows multiple fine feeding arteries from both internal iliac arteries and enlarged early draining vein

Angiographic Anatomy

Catheter angiography is usually performed to attain more detailed anatomic and hemodynamic features of the AVM lesions not for a diagnostic confirm. Typically, AVM consists of feeding arteries, nidus (a complex vascular networks connecting feeding arteries with draining veins) of AVM, and dilated drainage veins. As time passes, feeding artery, nidus, and draining veins became enlarged, tortuous, and massive in size resulting in not easy to identify them among all dilated blood vessels.

Pelvic AVMs can be supplied by all arteries in the pelvis including the internal iliac arteries as well as the median sacral and inferior mesenteric arteries [5, 6].

AVM lesions may drain into a single draining vein, often, internal and external iliac, pudendal, or obturator veins or into multiple veins.

Small feeding arteries (or arterioles) or draining veins can be identified on catheter angiograms which cannot be identified on CT angiograms. With these anatomic information, we can determine the target vessels (nidus of AVM) of endovascular treatment. Therefore, catheter arteriography has more important role in treatment of AVM than patients with other types of congenital vascular malformation (CVM).

Treatment of Pelvic AVM

For the treatment of AVM lesion, surgery of endovascular occlusion of the feeding artery of AVM is not used anymore in current practice. There are several reasons not to recommend feeding artery occlusion the treatment of AVM. Feeding artery occlusion only leaving untreated AVM lesions may lead distal organ or tissue ischemia, aggravation of AVM lesions stimulated by local ischemia, and abolishing endovascular access route for future endovascular treatment.

Currently, various procedures were introduced for treatment of AVM lesion. Characteristically, AVM lesion has high flow rate. When we inject certain type of sclerosing agent into the AVM lesion, it passes rapidly through the target lesion.

Therefore, we cannot achieve sclerosis of the AVM lesion. If too large amount of sclerosing agent are used, its side effect will be problem. To overcome this obstacle, Jackson et al. used intravenous balloon occlusion to decrease the blood velocity in AVM lesions [7].

Houbballah et al. [8] reported embolization of the internal iliac vein (draining vein of pelvic AVMs) with Ethibloc or Horsley's bone wax via a percutaneous puncture while clamping the infrarenal aorta and the iliac arteries. After embolization, the internal iliac vein was ligated to prevent pulmonary embolism by the migration of the embolic agent. After then, arterial flow was restored.

Choi et al. [9] reported a patient with pelvic AVM with multiple feeding arteries from the left internal iliac artery draining to the external iliac vein. They used stent graft in the external iliac vein to occlude multiple draining veins before injection of the sclerosing agent into the feeding artery.

Various kinds of embolic materials have been used to treat AVM lesions including metal coils, rapidly polymerizing acrylic adhesives (e.g., NBCA or isobutyl cyanoacrylate [IBCA]), polyvinyl alcohol foam particles (Ivalon), detachable silicon balloons, and ethylene-vinyl alcohol copolymers (Onyx) [5, 10–13].

When embolic material is delivered into AVM lesion via catheter, it forms casts of multiple small vessels on contact with ionic material such as blood.

Relatively high clinical and radiological recurrence has been reported after embolization alone with those materials [5, 14].

As described before, AVM lesions originated from undifferentiated mesenchymal cells having an evolutional potential by certain stimulus. Incomplete embolization of the AVM carries potential risk of recurrence or aggravation of the AVM lesion. Through the arteriographic examinations of AVM lesion, we found that many of AVM lesions have multiple feeding arteries and a single draining vein (see Chap. 10) [15].

On the ground of above-described anatomical and biologic characteristics of AVM lesions, we currently use combined therapy using embolization (embolization of the draining vein with coils or wire) and sclerotherapy (ablation of arteriovenous fistulae and nidus with high-concentration ethanol) with obtaining better treatment results than before.

The concept of our treatment strategy is to convert the high-flow AVM lesion to lower flow condition with embolization of the dilated draining veins as the first stage and then use sclerosing agent to ablate remaining AVMs lesions as the second stage. As embolic materials, we usually use coils or wire depending on the size of the vascular cavity to be embolized. As sclerosing agent, we often use high concentration ethanol. By reducing flow velocity in the AVM lesion with embolization, interacting time of the sclerosing agent with AVM lesions can be increased while reducing the amount of the sclerosing agent.

We believe that the combination of ethanol sclerotherapy and embolization (embolotherapy) is a more efficacious treatment for patients with pelvic AVMs.

Regarding the technical issues of embolotherapy, AVM nidus can be assessed transarterially using microcatheter, transvenous or percutaneous approach, or combined approach. Figure 47.2 shows schematic drawing of the access routes to a dilated draining vein during endovascular therapy of pelvic AVM [6].

Ethanol injection is known to cause pulmonary hypertension secondary to precapillary arterial spasm and hemodynamic changes. According to our study, hemodynamic changes after ethanol injection are more likely due to bolus injection than the total volume of ethanol used. To reduce hemodynamic complications, the minimum therapeutic amount (<0.14 mL/kg body weight) of 100% ethanol is recommended when bolus injection is required. As complications of high-concentration ethanol, hemoglobinuria secondary to hemolysis, pelvic nerve damage (usually transient), and hematuria due to urinary bladder wall damage can occur. We have experienced one patient with massive hematuria requiring partial cystectomy after embolosclerotherapy of pelvic AVM.

In summary, pelvic AVM is a rare form of CVM with potential risk of serious complications such as bleeding, compression of surrounding tissue, and cardiac failure.

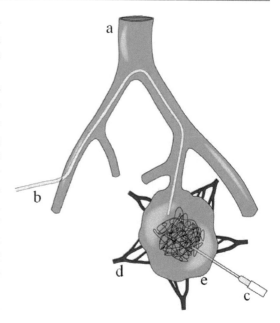

Fig. 47.2 Schematic drawing of access routes to a dilated draining vein during the embolosclerotherapy of the pelvic arteriovenous malformation. (*a*) Inferior vena cava, (*b*) transvenous catheter, (*c*) percutaneous needle, (*d*) feeding arterioles, (*e*) dilated draining vein of pelvic AVM. (YS Do et al. *J Vasc Surg* 2012;55:465–71

For a successful treatment of pelvic AVM, it is required understanding anatomic and biologic characteristics of AVM lesion. In our experience, and combined embolization and sclerotherapy is an effective treatment option with an acceptable risk for complications for patients with pelvic AVMs.

References

1. Vos LD, Bom EP, Vroegindeweij D, Tielbeek AV. Congenital pelvic arteriovenous malformation: a rare cause of sciatica. Clin Neurol Neurosurg. 1995;97(3):229–32. PubMed PMID: 7586854. Epub 1995/08/01. eng.
2. Kelly J, Alvarez RD, Roland PY. Arteriovenous malformation presenting as a complex pelvic mass with ureteral obstruction. A case report. J Reprod Med. 1998;43(10):916–8. PubMed PMID: 9800678. Epub 1998/11/04. eng.
3. Beller U, Rosen RJ, Beckman EM, Markoff G, Berenstein A. Congenital arteriovenous malformation of the female pelvis: a gynecologic perspective. Am J Obstet Gynecol. 1988;159(5):1153–60. PubMed PMID: 3189450. Epub 1988/11/01. eng.

4. Burrows PE. Vascular malformations involving the female pelvis. Semin Intervent Radiol. 2008;25(4):347–60. PubMed PMID: 21326576.Pubmed Central PMCID: PMC3036526. Epub 2008/12/01. eng.

5. Jacobowitz GR, Rosen RJ, Rockman CB, Nalbandian M, Hofstee DJ, Fioole B, et al. Transcatheter embolization of complex pelvic vascular malformations: results and long-term follow-up. J Vasc Surg. 2001;33(1):51–5. PubMed PMID: 11137923. Epub 2001/01/04 eng.

6. Do YS, Kim YW, Park KB, Kim DI, Park HS, Cho SK, et al. Endovascular treatment combined with embolosclerotherapy for pelvic arteriovenous malformations. J Vasc Surg. 2012;55(2):465–71. PubMed PMID: 22051867. Epub 2011/11/05. eng.

7. Jackson JE, Mansfield AO, Allison DJ. Treatment of high-flow vascular malformations by venous embolization aided by flow occlusion techniques. Cardiovasc Intervent Radiol. 1996;19(5):323–8. PubMed PMID: 8781152. Epub 1996/09/01. eng.

8. Houbballah R, Mallios A, Poussier B, Soury P, Fukui S, Gigou F, et al. A new therapeutic approach to congenital pelvic arteriovenous malformations. Ann Vasc Surg. 2010;24(8):1102–9. PubMed PMID: 21035702. Epub 2010/11/03. eng.

9. Choi SY, Do YS, Lee d Y, Lee KH, Won JY. Treatment of a pelvic arteriovenous malformation by stent graft placement combined with sclerotherapy. J Vasc Surg. 2010;51(4):1006–9. PubMed PMID: 20347698. Epub 2010/03/30. eng.

10. Pritchard DA, Maloney JD, Bernatz PE, Symmonds RE, Stanson AW. Surgical treatment of congenital pelvic arteriovenous malformation. Mayo Clin Proc. 1978;53(9):607–11. PubMed PMID: 682689. Epub 1978/09/01. eng.

11. Kaufman SL, Kumar AA, Roland JM, Harrington DP, Barth KH, Haller Jr JA, et al. Transcatheter embolization in the management of congenital arteriovenous malformations. Radiology. 1980;137(1 Pt 1):21–9. PubMed PMID: 7422847. Epub 1980/10/01. eng.

12. Arat A, Cil BE, Vargel I, Turkbey B, Canyigit M, Peynircioglu B, et al. Embolization of high-flow craniofacial vascular malformations with onyx. AJNR Am J Neuroradiol. 2007;28(7):1409–14. PubMed PMID: 17698554. Epub 2007/08/19. eng.

13. Murakami K, Yamada T, Kumano R, Nakajima Y. Pelvic arteriovenous malformation treated by transarterial glue embolisation combining proximal balloon occlusion and devascularisation of multiple feeding arteries. BMJ case Rep. 2014;2014. PubMed PMID: 24907213. Epub 2014/06/08. eng.

14. Palmaz JC, Newton TH, Reuter SR, Bookstein JJ. Particulate intraarterial embolization in pelvic arteriovenous malformations. AJR Am J Roentgenol. 1981;137(1):117–22. PubMed PMID: 6787861. Epub 1981/07/01. eng.

15. Cho SK, Do YS, Shin SW, Kim DI, Kim YW, Park KB, et al. Arteriovenous malformations of the body and extremities: analysis of therapeutic outcomes and approaches according to a modified angiographic classification. J Endovasc Ther: Off J Int Soc Endovasc Spec. 2006;13(4):527–38. PubMed PMID: 16928170. Epub 2006/08/25. eng.

Treatment Strategy on Chylolymphatic/Lymphatic Reflux

48

Cristóbal Miguel Papendieck
and Miguel Angel Amore

Introduction: Historical Background

Through the seventeenth century, the whole concept of chyle circulation was finally accepted since the lacteal vessels or chyliferous vessels were found by G. Aselli in 1622. Following the discovery of the direction of chylous flow, from intestine to cisterna chyli and then to thoracic duct into the blood circulation by J. Pecquet in 1651, chyloreflux has been well documented: chylous reflux (1670), chylous ascites (1685), and chylothorax (1689). But modern concept of lymphatic circulation has been established barely half century ago, essential for the vertebrates to maintain normal life together with the chyle lymph [8, 9].

Definition

Chyle is a milky fluid formed in intestinal lacteals as a part of normal fatty acid metabolism. It is transported first through the lymphatics to reach thoracic duct before entering the venous circulation. Chyle is rich with triglycerides, long-chain aminoacids, lipoproteins, and related vitamins besides white blood cells, especially T lymphocytes. Therefore, chylorrhea will deplete serum levels of protein, lymphocytes, and fat-soluble vitamins, resulting in immune dysfunction through loss of immunoglobulins and lymphocytes besides a metabolic acidosis by the electrolyte imbalances. The term "chylous reflux" represents the abnormal direction of the chyle flow, either backward (backflow) or forward through other directions (diverted flow), thus appearing in various conditions of chylorrhea (chyle leakage through fistulas (lymphangiectasia), capillary microcystic malformations (lymphangiomatosis) or through mesothelium (pleura, peritoneum) or epithelia (intestine mucosa, skin), or as a collection in cavities [1]. Most commonly chyle leakage is into the peritoneal cavity (chylous ascites) or pleural space (chyloperitoneum). But the leakage also results in chyluria (chyle in the urine), chyloptysis (chyle in the sputum), chylopericardium, or cutaneous chyle leakage.

C.M. Papendieck, MD, PhD, FACS (✉)
Angiopediatria, Universidad del Salvador (USAL),
Buenos Aires, Argentina
e-mail: cmpapendieck@angiopediatria.com.ar

M.A. Amore, MD, FACS (✉)
Phlebology and Lymphology Unit, Cardiovascular Surgery Division, Central Military Hospital, Buenos Aires, Argentina

III Chair of Anatomy, Buenos Aires University, Buenos Aires, Argentina
e-mail: mamore@fmed.uba.ar,
miguelangelamore@hotmail.com

© Springer-Verlag Berlin Heidelberg 2017
Y.-W. Kim et al. (eds.), *Congenital Vascular Malformations*, DOI 10.1007/978-3-662-46709-1_48

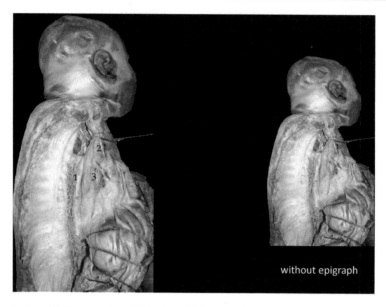

Fig. 48.1 Thoracic duct. (*1*) Thoracic duct. (*2*) Trachea. (*3*) Esophagus

Thoracic Duct

Normal chyle circulation starts in the chyliferous vessels, from the ileum/jejunum, toward (Pecquet)cisterna chyli and then to thoracic duct, ending at the venous circulation through the left jugular–subclavian venous junction.

Thoracic ductis a part of main lymphatic collector system. It transports between 2and 4 liters of systemic lymph plus chyle daily. It is formed by the union of two lumbar, right and left, lymph trunks and gastrointestinal lymph trunk at the level of the lumbar vertebrae I and II. This dilated ampulla, resulting from this union, is named to (Pecquet) cisterna chyli. The chyle joins with the interstitial systemic lymph at this level so that chyle is no longer milky white but turns into an opalescent color.

The thoracic duct ascends at posterior mediastinum and at cervical level end at the posterior wall of the left jugular subclavian venous junction directly or indirectly through interposed lymph nodes [2–4] (Fig.48.1).

Adverse Effects of Anomalous Lymph/Chyle Circulation

Obstruction or direct trauma to the lymphatic vessels by various etiologies will cause chylous leaks into the pleural or peritoneal cavity, known as chylothorax and chyloascites. Chylothorax has a high morbidity, often presenting as a pleural effusion, and diagnosis can be made by analysis of fluid from pleurocentesis.

Chyle leakage can occur in the prenatal as well as postnatal, pediatric, and adult populations with age-related etiological correlation. In adults, chyle leaks are more commonly related to malignancy.

Pleural effusion of the lymph in prenatal age may cause pulmonary hypoplasia, while postnatal pleural effusion may precipitate respiratory failure, the same as chylous ascites [10–12].

Chyle-lymph collections or their external leakage will cause the malnutrition due to hypoproteinemia.

Chyle backflow through the lymphatic vessels in the interstitial tissue is a frequent cause of primary lymphedema.

Bronchopulmonary lymph/chylous effusion always causes some degree of respiratory failure (e.g., lymphangioleiomyomatosis). It may present malnutrition if it occurs at the intestinal mucous level as in the case of primary intestinal lymphangiectasia (Waldmann disease) [1, 5, 7, 13].

Furthermore, percutaneous or transmucosal leaks cause a severe psychosocial disability, as it occurs at the genital or perineal level (Figs. 48.2 and 48.3).

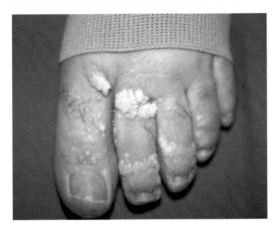

Fig. 48.2 Primary lymphedema and chylous reflux in foot

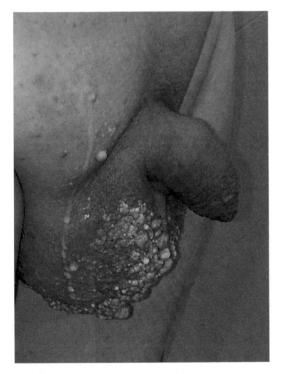

Fig. 48.3 Genital chylous fistulas

Lymph reflux or chyloreflux to the urinary tract is known as chyluria although rarely diagnosed in pediatrics.

Lymph or chyle lymphcysts at the mesentery, greater omentum, retroperitoneum, bone tissue, or cystic lymphangiomas-hygromas in other locations have the meaning of benign expansive tumor, and it can be clinically significant in

mediastinum or bones (phantom bone disease: Gorham Stout syndrome, or associated with angiosarcoma: Gorham Stout Haferkamp, a malignant disease) [14].

A disease with microcystic lymph or chyle lymph, such as lymphangiomatosis, is an oncological risk [15].

Lymph leakage through intestinal mucus means exudative enteropathy. It can be local, regional, or systemic, and the severity of the disease depends on its extension. Chyle leak to the intestinal lumen means the presence of a single or multiple fistula.

The normal chyle formation, and its simultaneous leak at the intestinal lumen (Waldmann disease), is a result of intestinal lymphangiectasia. It may occur moreover in Hennekam syndrome, with segmentary lymphangiomatosis. Chylous ascites or other chyleleaks (chylothorax) can be present in this syndrome.

Primary lymphedema due to chylous reflux means a retrograde hypertension of the involved network at the interstitial lymphatic system (Figs. 48.4 and 48.5).

All mentioned syndromes are an expression of the lymphangiodysplasia.

Treatments

Medical Management

Before the consideration of specific treatment, general treatment strategy for chylous reflux/chylorrhea should be based on dietary regimen to reduce the fatty acid metabolism with appropriate modification of enteral nutrition with either nonfat or low-fat diet and medium chain triglycerides. Also, total parenteral nutrition with bowel rest may be considered as an additional option for chyle leaks when indicated. If such nutritional measures alone are not sufficient, additional medical or surgical interventions should be considered.

Octreotide (Sandostatin, Novartis Pharmaceuticals) is a long-acting somatostatin analogue that inhibits many hormones (including growth, glucagon, and insulin), decreasing intestinal and pancreatic secretion, thus reducing intestinal motility [6, 11, 17]. It has been known for the

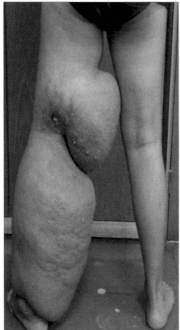
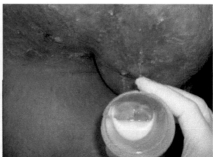

Fig. 48.4 Primary lymphedema and chylous reflux. Chylous fistula

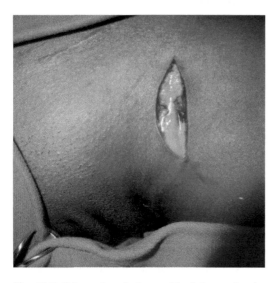

Surgical Management

Drainage of accumulated chylous fluid is an adjunctive management to surgical treatment. Thoracentesis and paracentesis can relieve symptoms of respiratory failure, but tube thoracostomy is often indicated to obtain continuous drainage.

But for persistent leakage after two attempts at drainage, definitive surgery is generally mandated [30–32], and drainage procedures as primary treatment should be abandoned in favor of surgery especially for cutaneous chyle reflux caused by lymphangiomyomatosis [33, 34].

The cutaneous manifestation of chyle reflux in the external genitalia, thigh, or trunk can be managed first with various sclerosing agents directly injecting to precipitate obliterative lymphangitis: tetracycline, doxycycline, alcohol, OK-432, and bleomycin [35, 36].

But, cutaneous lesions in the groin area have a high rate of recurrence so that combined therapy with excision and laser or sclerotherapy is often mandated. The leaking lymphatic ducts, identified after the ingestion of a fatty meal, can be ligated, oversewn, clipped, or excised.

Fig. 48.5 Primary lymphedema with chylous reflux by transnodal pathway. Inguinal incision

efficacy in managing primary or secondary chylothorax and chylous ascites [26, 27], including in newborns [28]. It has also been effective in traumatic thoracic duct trauma-related chyle leak [29].

Sirolimus (rapamycin, Wyeth Pharmaceuticals) was also reported to be effective in the cases of lymphangioleiomyomatosis [16].

The excision of lymphatic malformation lesion is often the most ideal way to relieve the symptoms caused by cutaneous chylorrhea including the skin, bowel, thorax, and abdomen [37]. However, percutaneous drainage tubes inserted postoperatively accompany the risk of converting an internally draining system into an externally draining system so that close monitoring of the drainage amount is warranted to prevent worsening the malnutrition with high volume chyle loss.

The ideal surgical solution is to reconstruct damaged lymphatics with microsurgical techniques to restore "physiological" lymphatic flow by microsurgical anastomoses between lymphatics and veins bypassing disrupted or malformed lymphatics. The most common surgical approaches are lymphatico-venous anastomoses and lymphatico-veno-lymphatic anastomoses with variable long-term patency rates [38].

Chylothorax

Chylothorax is caused by various injuries to the lymph vessels often as iatrogenic injury during cardiac, pulmonary, esophageal, or head and neck surgery, or direct trauma to thoracic duct. Chylothorax may also result from congenital defects: lymphatic malformations, lymphangiectasia, lymphangioleiomyomatosis, and lymphatic obstruction caused by congenital anomalies or hypoplasia of lymphatic vessels. But it also develops as a consequence of malignancy or infections (e.g., tuberculosis) [26, 39–41].

Chest tube drainage is often implemented first as an adjunct treatment to improve respiratory dysfunction, but definitive therapy will be generally needed to follow with various indications. Videoscope-assisted thoracoscopy (VATS) is a safe and effective technique to allow necessary intervention to manage chylous leakage based on the amount and location of output of the chylous leak [42].

Pleural abrasion and pleurodesis with talc or other agents are effective when output is less than 500 mL/day [43]. Fibrin glue can be used when no focal drainage point can be determined [44].

With diffuse drainage, partial pleurectomy is another option to resolve symptoms [45].

However, the ligation of the thoracic duct is often indicated for high-output chylous drainage exceeding 1 L/day, either by VATS or thoracotomy. Alternatively, coil embolization of the thoracic duct may be performed through the cannulation of the cisterna chyli. The Denver pleuroperitoneal shunt has also been used for extreme cases of chylothorax [46].

Nevertheless, congenital chylothorax secondary to lymphatic aplasia, hypoplasia, fibrosis, and superior vena caval obstruction remains a clinical challenge.

Primary/idiopathic chylothorax found during prenatal age can be managed with a prenatal pleural puncture followed by pleuro-amniotic shunting to reduce the risk of the pulmonary hypoplasia.

In the newborn with chylothorax, following a diagnostic puncture intermittent drainage might be needed for the symptomatic improvement though often difficult for an extended period of time.

Therefore, primary chyle leak to pleura, peritoneum, or pericardium, due to dysplasia of the chyle circuit, requires a lymphovenous bypass (e.g., video-assisted thoracic surgery). If the leak is secondary to the surgery (e.g., cardiovascular surgery for the coartaction of the aorta or tricuspid atresia, Fontan operation), the collection must be drained first, and if it persists, a ligation of the thoracic duct or its bypass to the venous system (e.g., azygos vein) should be considered in addition to the pleurodesis with talc and the use of octreotide [18–20].

Chylous Ascites

Chylous ascites is also indicated for percutaneous embolization of retroperitoneal lymphatics which is preferred as the first-line therapy for symptomatic chylous ascites.

The treatment of chylo-lymph collections in the peritoneum requires various combinations of the treatment, following the diagnostic puncture, with intermittent drainage by serial paracentesis,

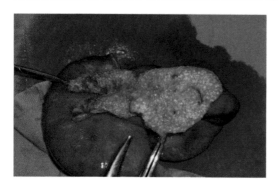

Fig. 48.6 Waldmann disease in children. Ileum segment resected

a specific diet with MCT, and octreotide per indication.

But if it persists, it requires surgical intervention as indicated for chylothorax. A complementary option is a peritoneal–venous shunt (e.g., Degni and Le Veen bypass valves and Denver Shunt), shunting the fluid from the peritoneal cavity to the internal or external jugular vein [47]. However, complications include electrolyte imbalance, subclavian vein thrombosis, wound infection, peritonitis, and various extent of coagulopathy including disseminated intravascular coagulation [48].

Therefore, they shouldn't be used before age of 7 years, and the possible coagulation alteration should be controlled judiciously. They could give only interim temporary solution but do not solve the pathology itself [21].

For retrograde chyle flow caused by thoracic duct obstruction may be managed by a thoracic duct to azygos vein anastomosis to control the backflow lymphedema using the consensus protocol of the International Society of Lymphology (ISL) and International Lymphedema Framework (ILF), as the guidelines including specific diets and octreotide [22, 23].

In the event of chylo reflux to intestine such as in Waldmann disease, the study with videocapsule is indicated as well as the eventual resection of the pathological ileum jejunum segment. Eventually associated chylothorax, chyloperitoneum, and primary lymphedema have the same indications, as already mentioned [1, 13, 24, 25] (Fig. 48.6).

Finally, in view of effective control [49, 50] of recurrent chylothorax after neck surgery with

percutaneous thoracic duct, embolization has been reported to be but has not been proven as primary treatment for the chylorrhea;selective embolization of the reflux point/s and, otherwise, of the thoracic duct can be considered to control the chylous reflux as a new option depending upon the types of lymphatic malformation with different anatomy.

References

1. Papendieck CM. Lymphatic dysplasias in pediatrics. Int Angiol. 1999;18:6–9.
2. Amore M, Tapia L, Mercado D, Pattarone G. Lymphedema: A general outline of its anatomical base. J Reconstr Microsurg. 2015;32:2–9.
3. Kubik S. Atlas fotográfico en color de anatomía humana con sus aplicaciones clínicas. Torax. Barcelona: Ed. Labor; 1969.
4. Rouviere. H. Anatomie des lymphatiques de l homme. Paris: Masson; 1932.
5. Sahn SA. The pathophysiology of pleural effusion. Annu Rev Med. 1990;41:7–13.
6. Yang YS, Ma GC, Shih JC, et al. Experimental treatment of bilateral fetal chylothorax usingintra utero pleurodesis. Ultrasound Obstet Gynecol. 2012;39:56–62.
7. Mc Grath EE, Blades Z, Anderson PB. Chylothorax. aetiology, diagnosis and therapeutic options. Respir Med. 2010;104:1–8.
8. Servelle M. Les chylifères. Paris: Expansion scientifique francaise; 1981.
9. Dieter R, Dieter Jr R, Dieter III R. Venous and lymphatic diseases. New York: Ed. McGraw-Hill; 2011.
10. Soto-Martinez M, Massie J. Chylothorax. diagnosis and management in children. Pediatr Respir Rev. 2009;10:199–207.
11. Bellini C, Eergaz M, Radicioni M, et al. Congenital fetal and neonatal visceral chylous effusions: neonatal chylothorax and chylous ascites revisited. A multicentric retrospective. Lymphology. 2012;45(31):91–102.
12. Vignes S, Beilanger J. Primary Intestinal Lymphangiectasia(Waldmann's disease). OrphanetJ Rare Dis. 2008;3:5.
13. Gorham WL, Stout PH. Massive osteolysis (acute spontaneous absorption of bone, phantom bone disease, disappearing bone disease). Bond Joint Surg. 1955;37A:985–1004.
14. Papendieck CM. Sindrome de Gorham Stout Haferkamp cpn reflujo de quilo. Rev Argent Cir. 2000; 79(1–2):7–10.
15. Chachaj A, Drozdz K, Chabowski H, et al. Chyloperitoneum, chylothorax and lower extremity lymphedema in woman with sporadic lymphangioleiomyomatosis: successfully treated with sirolimus. a case report. Lymphology. 2012;45:53–7.
16. Ergaz Z, Bar-Oz B, Yatsiv I, et al. Congenital chylothorax. Clinical course and prognostic significance. Pediatr Pulmonol. 2009;44:806–11.

17. Rosa CM, Campisis C, Boccardo F, et al. Chylopericardium. A case report demonstrating utility of lymphography combined with 3D computed tomography for corrective surgical treatment using VATS. Lymphology. 2014;47:40–4.
18. Bellini C, Boccardo F, Campisis C, et al. Congenital pulmonary lymphangiectasia. OrphanetJ Rare Dis. 1990;30:43.
19. Kreutzer G, Galindez H, Bono H. An operation for the correction of tricuspid atresia. JCardiovasc Surg. 1973;66(3):613–21.
20. Gleysteen JJ, Hussey CV, Heckman MG. The cause of coagulopathy after peritoneovenous shunt for malignant ascites. Arch Surg. 1990;125(4):474–7.
21. International Society of Lymphology. The diagnosis and treatment of peripheral lymphedema: 2013 Consensus Document of the International Society of Lymphology. Lymphology. 2013;46:1–11.
22. Lee BB, Andrade M, Antignani PL, Boccardo F, Bunke N, Campisi C, et al. Diagnosis and treatment of primary lymphedema. Consensus document of the International Union of Phlebology (IUP) -2013. Int Angiol. 2013;32(6):541–74.
23. Campisi C, Bellini C, Campisi C, et al. Microsurgery for Lymphedema. Clinical research and long-term results. Microsurgery. 2010;30(4):256–60.
24. Olszewski WL. The treatment of lymphedema of the extremities with microsurgical lymphovenous anastomosis. Int Angiol. 1988;7:312–21.
25. Chen E, Itkin M. Thoracic duct embolization for chylous leaks. Semin Intervent Radiol. 2011;28:63–74.

Medical Management

26. Soto-Martinez M, Massie J. Chylothorax: diagnosis and management in children. Paediatr Respir Rev. 2009;10(4):199–207.
27. Ferrandiere M, Hazouard E, Guicheteau V, et al. Chylous ascites following radical nephrectomy: efficiency ofoctreotide as treatment of a ruptured thoracic duct. Intensive Care Med. 2000;26(4):484–5.
28. Bulbul A, Unsur EK. Octreotide as a treatment of congenital chylothorax. Pediatr Pulmonol. 2010;45(6): 628. author reply 9–30
29. Rosing DK, Smith BR, Konyalian V, Putnam B. Penetrating traumatic thoracic duct injury treated successfully with octreotide therapy. J Trauma. 2009; 67(1):E20–1.

Surgical Management

30. Campisi C, Eretta C, Pertile D, Da Rin E, Campisi C, et al. Microsurgery for treatment of peripheral lymphedema: long-term outcome and future perspective. Microsurgery. 2007;27(4):333–8.
31. Wheeler AD, Tobias JD. Tension chylothorax in two pediatric patients. Paediatr Anaesth. 2007;17(5):488–91.

32. Marts BC, Naunheim KS, Fiore AC, Pennington DG. Conservative versus surgical management of chylothorax. Am J Surg. 1992;164:532–4.
33. Lim ST, Ngan H, Wong KK, Ong GB. Leakage of lymph through scrotal skin. J Urol. 1981;125(6): 889–90.
34. Sales F, Trepo E, Brondello S, Lemaitre P, Bourgeois P. Chylorrhea after axillary lymph node dissection. Eur J Surg Oncol. 2007;33(8):1042–3.
35. Alomari AI, Karian VE, Lord DJ, Padua HM, Burrows PE. Percutaneous sclerotherapy for lymphatic malformations: a retrospective analysis of patient-evaluated improvement. J Vasc Interv Radiol. 2006;17:1639–48.
36. Dasgupta R, Adams AD, Elluru R, Wentzel MS, Azizkhan RG. Noninterventional treatment of selected head and neck lymphatic malformations. J Pediatr Surg. 2008;43(5):869–73.
37. Kim NR, Lee SK, Suh YL. Primary intestinal lymphangiectasia treated by segmental resections of small bowel. J Pediatr Surg. 2009;44(10):e13–7.
38. Narushima M, Mihara M, Yamamoto Y, Lida T, Koshima I, et al. The intravascular stenting method for treatment of extremity lymphedema with multiconfiguration lymphaticovenous anastomoses. Plast Reconstr Surg. 2010;125(3):935–43.
39. McGrath EE, Blades Z, Anderson PB. Chylothorax: aetiology, diagnosis and therapeutic options. Respir Med. 2010;104(1):1–8.

Chylothorax

40. Teichgraber UK, Nibbe L, Gebauer B, Wagner HJ. Inadvertent puncture of the thoracic duct during attempted central venous catheter placement. Cardiovasc Intervent Radiol. 2003;26(6):569–71.
41. Fishman SJ, Burrows PE, Upton J, Hendren WH. Life-threatening anomalies of the thoracic duct: anatomic delineation dictates management. J Pediatr Surg. 2001;36(8):1269–72.
42. Maldonado F, Cartin-Ceba R, Hawkins FJ, Ryu JH. Medical and surgical management of chylothorax and associated outcomes. Am J Med Sci. 2010;339(4): 314–8.
43. Paul S, Altorki NK, Port JL, Stiles BM, Lee PC. Surgical management of chylothorax. Thorac Cardiovasc Surg. 2009;57(4):226–8.
44. Nguyen D. Successful management of postoperative chylothorax with fibrin glue in a premature neonate. Can J Surg. 1994;37(2):158–60. Review
45. Barret DS. Pleurectomy for chylothorax associated with intestinal lymphangiectasia. Thorax. 1987;42: 557–8.
46. Podevin G, Levard G, Larroquet M, Gruner M. Pleuroperitoneal shunt in the management chylothorax caused by thoracic lymphatic dysplasia. J Pediatr Surg. 1999;34:1420–2.
47. Roehr CC, Jung A, Proquitte H, Blankenstein O, Hammer H, et al. Somatostatin or octreotide as treatment options for chylothorax in young children: a systematic review. Intensive Care Med. 2006;32:650–7.

Chylous Ascites

48. Kobayashi T, Kishimoto T, Kamata S, Otsuka M, Miyazaki M, et al. Rapamycin, a specific inhibitor of the mammalian target of rapamycin, suppresses lymphangiogenesis and lymphatic metastasis. Cancer Sci. 2007;98(5):726–33.
49. Patel N, Lewandowski RJ, Bove M, Nemcek Jr AA, Salem R. Thoracic duct embolization: a new treatment for massive leak after neck dissection. Laryngoscope. 2008;118(4):680–3.
50. Repko BM, Scorza LB, Mahraj RP. Recurrent chylothorax after neck surgery: percutaneous thoracic duct embolization as primary treatment. Otolaryngol Head Neck Surg. 2009;141(3):426–7.

Cristóbal Miguel Papendicek
and Miguel Angel Amore

Abbreviation

AV   Arterial venous
CVMs   Congenital vascular malformations
ISSVA   International Society for the Study of Vascular Anomalies

Introduction

The classification of vascular anomalies by J. B. Mulliken in 1989 and the CVM identification according to ISSVA–Hamburg (truncular and extratruncular CVM) and ISSVA (1996) (low- and fast-flow CVMs) have enabled the unification of criteria or basic consensus on the diagnostic methodology and therapeutic technical principles.

In the last years, interventional radiology has been more accurately involved as part of the

C.M. Papendicek, MD PhD FACS (✉)
Angiopediatria, Universidad del Salvador (USAL), Buenos Aires, Argentina
e-mail: cmpapendieck@angiopediatria.com.ar

M.A. Amore, MD FACS (✉)
Phlebology and Lymphology Unit,
Cardiovascular Surgery Division,
Central Military Hospital,
Buenos Aires, Argentina
e-mail: mamore@fmed.uba.ar

III Chair of Anatomy, Buenos Aires University,
Buenos Aires, Argentina
e-mail: miguelangelamore@hotmail.com

diagnosis and eventual therapeutic procedure and progressively to the systemic (e.g., propranolol, sildenafil) and local (timolol, bleomycin, and others) pharmacology, which has given a new orientation to many therapeutic aspects, some of them, unsuspected.

CVMs are observed and diagnosed more and more accurately in infants and in some cases in prenatal age. In fact, they are congenital, either diagnosed or not at birth [1–4].

Non-congenital malformations are not taken into consideration in this chapter.

Epidemiology

There is no epidemiologic data referred to the vascular anomaly frequency. It is believed that 3% of the population has some type of angioma. Eighty percent are hemangiomas.

Moreover, it is estimated that there are 70 million patients worldwide that suffer from a lymphatic system malformation. At least 12 malformations or dysplasia in this system are known, apart from hypoplasia, hyperplasia, and aplasia, which are this precisely, and not dysplasia.

From 70 million patients who present this problem, in most of them, it is expressed as primary lymphedema. The congenital, early, and late lymphedema is so far a name for its diagnosis or clinical identification. From the whole primary lymphedema, 80% are degrees 0–I; therefore, they are not diagnosed or treated in infants.

© Springer-Verlag Berlin Heidelberg 2017
Y.-W. Kim et al. (eds.), *Congenital Vascular Malformations*, DOI 10.1007/978-3-662-46709-1_49

Twenty-four millions approximately are degrees II and III.

Truncular venous malformations may present primary and secondary lymphedema. These are expressed as large angiodysplasia syndromes with combined vascular malformations [5–7].

General Therapeutic Analysis

The use of anticoagulant (e.g., heparin of low molecular weight) and antithrombotic therapy (e.g., acetylsalicylic acid) and other drugs such as immunomodulatory (e.g., interferon alpha-2b) has enabled, in some cases, survival or its course without serious complications in pediatric patients. Chronicity of some of the treatments encouraged the search of new supplementary or substitute alternatives (e.g., sclerotherapy, embolization, the use of endoluminal laser or radiofrequency) [8].

It is important to relate the pathology with its extension and location. A CVM in the mediastinum, encephalon, genitals, hands, and feet does not present the same clinical relevance as if it also presented involvement of areas (e.g., pericardium, peritoneum, pleura, etc.). In this last case, pleuro-amniotic shunting is a therapeutic indication.

In large angiodysplasia syndromes or combined vascular malformations, the biochronogram is different if the CVM is primary, single, or combined or if it is simply an associated pathology. Examples of these include overgrowth syndromes such as Klippel-Trenaunay, CLOVES, Proteus, and Gorham-Stout-Haferkamp syndromes and primary or secondary lymphedema due to venous hypertension in truncular venous malformations, the latter possibly the most frequent cause of nonparasitic secondary lymphedema in infants [5, 9].

The Klippel-Trenaunay syndrome with hypertrophy exists, as originally described, but it also exists with segmental body hypotrophy. This allows us to think that the vascular cause for overgrowth is not just one. But the CVM effect does generally mean a life course with overgrowth; this should be foreseen. Contrary to this, overgrowth may be induced or provoked, with therapeutic reasons, to attenuate or avoid growth discrepancy [10, 11].

Other CVMs, as the macro-arteriovenous fistula, deserve a special consideration on its hemodynamic and central meaning. These, especially in the neonatal period, are pathologies with an early systemic risk.

In the newborn, all the fast-flow pathologies, or those space-occupying pathologies with low flow, require an early treatment. The diameter of a malformation may probably determine a therapeutic attitude.

The CVMs' large diameter or volume represents the surgical indication, as well as the presence of multiple micro-AV fistulas.

Multicystic or macrocystic lesions expose the newborn to the Kasabach-Merritt syndrome, with all its implications and the abovementioned treatment.

Pharmacological sclerotherapy is an alternative, but not the only one, especially if the use of bleomycin is considered. This procedure has been used with good results in the cavernous angiomas. In the same way, systemic sildenafil as well as Picibanil, OK432, has been used in lymphangiomas/cystic hygromas [3, 4, 8].

Some CVMs already occur in the newborn with chylo collections or systemic lymph in pleura and/or peritoneal cavity; this may imply a pulmonary hypoplasia. Cystic formations in spaces such as the mediastinum, or at the axilo-cervical level, may have the same meaning; furthermore, this is a reason to perform prenatal surgery and/or premature labor through a non-natural route [6, 7].

Some syndromes, such as the abovementioned Waldmann disease, or lymphangioleiomyomatosis and its actual benefit with the use of rapamycin deserve special considerations. This drug is also used in the Bean syndrome.

Venous-lymphatic CVMs may also be treated with sildenafil, especially if they are large or multicenter.

Greater omentum lymphangiomatosis is surgical, while in the mesentery, in principle, it responds with medical treatment.

Gorham-Stout syndrome requires early treatment with rapamycin and the repair of bone

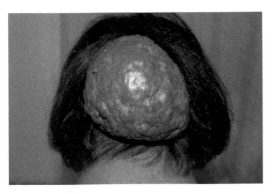

Fig. 49.1 Occipital vascular hamartoma in a child

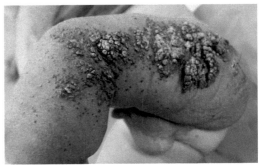

Fig. 49.3 Klippel-Trenaunay-Servelle syndrome, lower limb

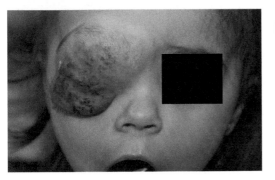

Fig. 49.2 Cavernous angioma cavernoso cara. Orbit

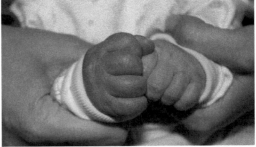

Fig. 49.4 Klippel-Trenaunay-Weber syndrome. Osteohypertrophic nevus in a hand of a newborn

lesions, especially the spine and head/femoral neck (phantom bone disease or bone disappearing syndrome). In the Haferkamp variety, with expected angiosarcoma, the only treatment is the early broad resective surgery. The same attitude should be considered in Maffucci syndrome in acral lesions with hamartomas, apart from their medical treatment [12] (Fig. 49.1).

AV CVMs or cavernous angiomas may benefit from interventional radiology. Each location deserves specific considerations, especially if there is face, genital, or acral involvement. Surgery is the successive or primary option, depending on the extension and location [8, 13] (Fig. 49.2).

Malformations due to dilation or venous aneurysms must be treated with anticoagulant or antithrombotic therapy, with further surgical treatment. The jugular location, internal or external, is always surgical. The common femoral or external iliac poses a technical problem. Popliteal location deserves a venous reconstruction [14].

Venous compressions as those occurring in the nutcracker, May-Thurner, or Cockett syndromes deserve a special consideration. These are of complex resolution, still with interventional radiology, since they will require stent replacement in infants. Veno-venous bridges are a primary option depending on the malformation meaning [5, 15].

The generation of phleboliths, secondary to venous thrombosis, must be avoided with antithrombotic therapy. If these are symptomatic, they force a resective surgery [3].

In the Klippel-Trenaunay-Servelle syndrome, with primary or secondary hypoplasia to abnormal muscle insertions, the latter should be solved first, before blocking a marginal vein or its equivalent in other body segments. If a hemorrhage conditions the inverted therapeutic sequence, this attenuating solution shall be provided early, due to secondary overgrowth [10, 11, 16] (Figs. 49.3 and 49.4).

Complex cases include hypoplasia or agenesis of the external iliac vein with agenesis or hypoplasia of the superficial and common femoral vein. Here the marginal vein always persists, and at least one Palma operation or similar techniques should be performed.

In the Bean syndrome (blue rubber bleb nevus), if the extension forces so, it will be treated with rapamycin, but the selective intestinal hemorrhage generally forces to consider the surgical treatment. Painful lesions in the skin are also treated surgically. The multicenter gastrointestinal "nevus," diagnosed, if possible, with video capsule due to age, forces to make a surgical decision.

Primary overgrowth syndromes such as the CLOVES, Proteus, Klippel-Trenaunay-Weber, and Servelle syndromes; extensive Sotos, Weaver, Costello, and Bannayan syndromes; and congenital lipomatosis, such as Bernardino, Laurence, and Simmons syndrome, pose an important challenge. Others, such as Dercum's and Madelung's disease, are not expressed in infants [10, 11, 14, 17–19].

The growth discrepancy treatment and, in young children, the early treatment of macropodia are a priority. Podal or acral overgrowth treated late is complex. Macropodia treatment always means partial foot resections; this is possible with a good, cosmetic, and functional result. This problem in hands is complex. Macrodactyly poses a challenge, and the intention of a functional correction with metaphyseal curettage or epiphyseal arrest should always prevail. A macropodia, whether operated or not, may be hidden, for better or worse. A large and asymmetrical hand is a serious psychosocial burden. Discrepancies larger than 3 cm in the lower limbs are always surgical from 9–10 years of age.

Oncologic control is a priority (e.g., Wilms tumor in Beckwith-Wiedemann or Klippel-Trenaunay syndrome) as well as the associated possible malformations (e.g., of the urinary tract).

Lipomatous tumor resections with vascular malformation may be important challenges, since due to their extension they may be complex and risky [5].

In the case of primary lymphedema, there are 12 truncular, extratruncular, and nodal dysplasia, and they can further present hyperplasia, hypoplasia, and

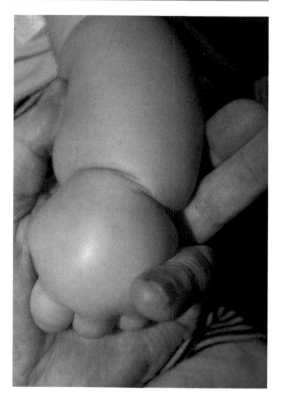

Fig. 49.5 Upper limb lymphedema in an infant

agenesis of vascular and nodal segments. There is primary lymphedema with vascular hyperplasia. Its treatment is specified in the international consensus documents (International Society of Lymphology, International Lymphoedema Framework, International Union of Phlebology), in which vascular rehabilitation is a priority. Vodder, Foldi, and Leduc techniques are used, as well as bandages and inelastic supports and taping (Fig. 49.5).

No rehabilitation can be done on what does not exist and only what was in good condition before can be rehabilitated. Rehabilitation means to go back to the initial state; therefore, in a malformed system, this could mean life rehabilitation.

Lymphatic circuits in hypertension or with interstitial hypertension (primary lymphedema, lymphangiomatosis) are pathologies with oncologic risk. This is the main reason why they should receive early treatment. The Stewart-Treves syndrome is a distant but real risk [20–23] (Fig. 49.6).

Infection, especially erysipelas, requires prevention and oral treatment protocols.

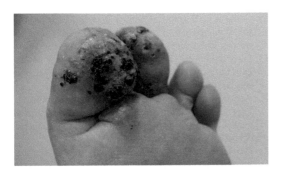

Fig. 49.6 Lymphangiomatosis, with necrobiosis, thrombosis, and hemorrhage in a foot

At present, lymphatic system dysplasia is also surgical. Lymphovenous shunt derivative techniques include Campisi (lymphatic terminal lymphovenous anastomosis or with venous bridge), Olszewski (venous lymph node anastomosis), Koshima (supermicrosurgery), or the combination of several surgical techniques. C. Becker technique is under consideration provided the blockage level is nodal. H. Brorson technique is excluded, since it is not generally possible to imagine a permanent inelastic support for the rest of somebody's life. This last alternative is valid in some syndromes with lipomatous overgrowth, which can even be a result of lymphedema. Lymphovenous bypass in areas with venous hypertension is not advisable since there is no pressure gradient, except through a Palma-like bridge (Papendieck) in the lower or upper limb [20, 21, 24, 25].

In this last respect, the standard of seeking an adequate problem-solution in every treatment should always prevail, firstly enabling survival, but within the context of seeking an appropriate psychosocial integration in the future [26, 27].

The vascular malformation treatment in infants is only possible if there is some knowledge of the pediatric clinic, surgical clinic, and angiology, further requiring a multidisciplinary team.

References

1. Mulliken JB, Gloacki J. Hemangiomas and vascular malformations in infants and children: a classification based on endothelial characteristics. Plast Reconstr Surg. 1982;59:412–20.

2. Mulliken JB, Young AE. Vascular birthmarks: hemangiomas and malformations. Philadelphia: WB Saunders; 1988.

3. Lee BB, Baumgartner I, Berlien P, Bianchini G, Burrows P, Gloviczki P, et al. Diagnosis and treatment of venous malformations consensus document of the International Union of Phlebology (IUP): updated 2013. Int Angiol. 2015;34:97–149. [Epub ahead of print]

4. Lee BB, Antignani PL, Baraldini V, Baumgartner I, Berlien P, Blei F, et al. ISVI-IUA consensus document – diagnostic guidelines on vascular anomalies: vascular malformations and hemangiomas. Int Angiol. 2015;34:333–74. [Epub ahead of print]

5. Papendieck CM. Angiodysplasias in pediatrics. Atlas color. Buenos Aires: Ed. Med Panam; 1988.

6. Papendieck CM. Lymphatic dysplasias in pediatrics. Int Angiol. 1999;18(1):5–9.

7. Papendieck CM. The big angiodysplasic syndromes in pediatrics with the participation of the lymphatic system. Prgress Lymphology. 1998;31(suppl):390–2.

8. Burrows PE. Endovascular treatment of slow-flow vascular malformations. Tech Vasc Interv Radiol. 2013;16(1):12–21.

9. Belov S, Loose DA, Weber J. Vascular Malformations. In: Periodica angiologica 16. Reinbek: Einhorn Presse Verlag; 1989. p. 29–30.

10. Klippel M, Trenaunay P. Naevus variqueux osteohypertrophique. Arch Gen Med. 1900;3:641.

11. Gloviczki P, Driscoll DJ. Klippel-Trenaunay syndrome: current management. Phlebology. 2007;22:291–8.

12. Chachaj A, Drozdz K, Chabowski H, et al. Chyloperitoneum, Chylothorax and lower extremity lymphedema in woman with sporadic lymphangioleiomyomatosis: successfully treated with sirolimus. A case report. Lymphology. 2012;45:53–7.

13. Loose D.A, Weber J. Angeborene gefaessmissbildungen. Interdiziplinaere therapie von haemangiomen und gefaessmalformationen (Angioddysplasien) Periodica Angiologica 21. Nordlanddruck GmbH Lüneburg: Hamburg; 1997.17–23.

14. Servelle M. Pathologie vasculaire. 2. Les affections veineuses. Paris: Masson; 1978.

15. Amore M, Soracco J, Gerez S, Marcovecchio L, Bengoa G, Carlevaro O, et al. Diagnostico y tratamiento endovascular del sindrome de compresion de la vena iliaca comun izquierda. Tecnicas Endovasculares. Vol XVI. N° 2. Mayo-Agosto 2013. https://issuu.com/salutaria/docs/te_2013-n__2.

16. Mattassi R, Vaghi M. Management of the marginal vein: current issues. Phlebology. 2007;22:283–6.

17. Gorham LW, Wright AN, Schulz HH, Maxon FC. Disappearing bones: a rare form of massive osteolysis. Am J Med. 1954;67:302–7.

18. Wiedemann HR. The proteus syndrome. Eur J Pediatr. 1983;149:5.

19. Alomari A, Thiex R, Mulliken JB. H. Friedberg's case report: an early description of CLOVEs Syndrome. Clin Genet. 2010;78(4):342–7.

20. International Society of Lymphology. The diagnosis and treatment of peripheral lymphedema: 2013

Consensus Document of the International Society of Lymphology. Lymphology. 2013;46:1–11.

21. Lee BB, Andrade M, Antignani PL, Boccardo F, Bunke N, Campisi C, et al. Diagnosis and treatment of primary lymphedema. Consensus document of the International Union of Phlebology (IUP) -2013. Int Angiol. 2013;32(6):541–74.

22. Hennekam RC. Syndromic lymphatic maldevelopment. Acad Med Center. Amsterdam. NLN Conf Orlando 2000. Abstr. 11–12.

23. Witte MH, Bernas MJ, Northup KA. Molecular lymphology and genetics of lymphedema-angiodysplasia syndromes. In: Foeldi M, Foeldi E, Kubik S, editors. Textbook of Lymphology. München: Elsevier; 2003. p. 471–93.

24. Campisi C, Bellini C, Campisi C, et al. Microsurgery for lymphedema. Clinical research and long-term results. Microsurgery. 2010;30(4):256–60.

25. Olszewski WL. The treatment of lymphedema of the extremities with microsurgical lymphovenous anastomosis. Int Angiol. 1988;7:312–21.

26. Acevedo L, Villanueva N, Gonzalez D, Barbosa L, Papendieck CM. Integracion psicosocial del niño con sindromes angiodisplasicos combinados. Valencia: XXXIX ESL Congess; 2013.

27. Harrison AM. Body image and self esteem. In: The development and sustaining of self esteem in childhood. New York: Inter Univ Press Inc; 1983. p. 90.

J.C. Lopez Gutierrez

General Considerations

Appropriate care of the pediatric vascular anomaly patient is multidisciplinary and requires a correct understanding of the vascular tumors or malformations encountered, as well as an in-depth knowledge of the pediatric physiology. The vascular anomalies specialist must be aware of the unique issues inherent in providing medical care for neonates, infants, and children identifying the relationship between developmental stages and age-appropriate interventions in order to avoid potential complications. As an example, average blood volume ranges, in relation to age, from 100 ml/kg in premature babies to 70 ml/kg in adolescents, while normal heart rate is 160 bpm at 1 month of life and 80 bpm at puberty.

Vascular anomalies change their appearance between the neonatal period and adolescence, and very often, children with rare vascular anomalies remain undiagnosed for years until typical symptoms and signs of the disease are noticed. In general, the younger the patient develops symptoms, the more aggressive his/her behavior of a

vascular anomaly is. There are specific vascular anomalies for each age period. Congenital hemangiomas are characteristically present at birth and never proliferate, while infantile hemangiomas are not present at birth and cannot proliferate beyond the second year of life.

Small age, size, or weight are invalid reasons to support a delay of a necessary and properly indicated treatment. Expert multidisciplinary teams in tertiary centers include skilled physicians and nurses in the modern management of premature babies needing aggressive surgical or endovascular procedures. Patients presenting with indications for surgery at an early age need a fully prepared pediatric facility with expertise in fetal medicine and surgical procedures under hypothermia and cardiopulmonary bypass, extracorporal membrane oxygenation (ECMO), large-volume blood replacement, and high-frequency ventilatory support in small children (Fig. 50.1).

Children are more sensitive to radiation received from medical imaging as they have more rapidly dividing cells exposed to the low-level radiation and a longer expected lifetime for the effects of radiation exposure. The vascular anomalies expert must consider having an accurate diagnosis with the lowest radiation dose necessary. The use of ionizing radiations should be restricted in children, and therefore ultrasonography and MRI are always indicated in children

J.C.L. Gutierrez
Vascular Anomalies Center, La Paz Children's
Hospital, University of Madrid, Paseo de la Castellana
261, 28046 Madrid, Spain
e-mail: queminfantil.hulp@salud.madrid.org

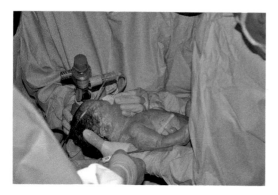

Fig. 50.1 EXIT procedure in a neonate with oral vascular malformation and upper airway involvement

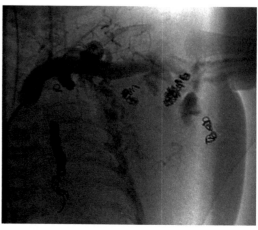

Fig. 50.2 Preoperative embolization of a thoracic arteriovenous in a 3-day-old baby with severe cardiac failure

before considering the use of procedures with high levels of radiation exposure such as CT. The radiology literature is clear and shows evidence that using adult CT protocols for pediatric patients results in estimated radiation doses to the smallest children as much as three times than given to an adult [1, 2]. Even considering that MRI is more time-consuming and expensive, machines are less available, and uncooperative patients need to be sedated; its use in the pediatric population should be promoted. Angiography must only be indicated in a small number of cases and always as a therapeutic and not diagnostic tool.

The use of contrast is also not recommended in the newborn and the diagnostic workup should consider this point. Embolization is technically possible in the very low weight patient (Fig. 50.2), but potential toxicity of sclerosing and embolizing agents and the need of small doses remain a problem when considering this therapeutic modality [3].

Recently, the use of intralesional diode laser is helping as an adjuvant treatment in the management of venous malformations by reducing the number and toxicity of endovascular procedures in the pediatric population.

The role of parents is crucial during the pre- and postoperative decision-making process (i.e., the presence of parents during anesthetic induc-

tion as a method to reduce the anxiety of children). Anesthesia in the pediatric patient remains a concern for parents and physicians, and an increased number of vascular procedures under sedation have been related to psychological disorders late in life, but currently there is not enough scientific evidence supporting a limitation of anesthetic interventions when needed [4–6].

Psychology is an important issue in the management of pediatric population with vascular anomalies, and many parents are aware of taking therapeutic decisions and delaying appropriate management. They very often prefer to transfer the responsibility of treating a non-life-threatening vascular anomaly to the patient at older age. Hospitalization in children is the origin of a significant social and emotional deprivation that can generate psychological disorders. Therefore, the emotional factor in the perioperative period may become more important than the physical condition of the child. Psychological support when needed should be recommended as a part of the multidisciplinary management.

Scarring is an active process and there is a broad agreement that small children benefit for a faster wound healing. Once the indication for surgical removal of a facial vascular anomaly has been stablished, an early approach would be recommended.

Specific Considerations

Infantile hemangiomas. Vascular anomalies specialists must be able to distinguish hemangiomas from various vascular malformations as well as appreciate their dynamic course with time. Infantile hemangioma (IH) is the most common tumor of infancy, but understanding of its etiology and pathogenesis has lagged far behind other diseases. IH are not noticeable at birth and do not proliferate in utero. About 50 % of them present a macula with a white halo at its periphery as a precursor lesion. A large vascular mass in a neonate presents at delivery does not suggest IH as final diagnosis. The proliferative phase usually begins at 10–20 days of life and is particularly rapid between during the second month of life being their final growth unpredictable. Nevertheless this clinical course is not unique and several neonatal malignant and highly vascularized tumors can show a similar growth pattern. Seven patients have been sent to our institution in the past 4 years to undergo surgical excision of nonresponders to propranolol infantile hemangiomas. Final diagnosis included congenital fibrosarcomas in two, rhabdomyosarcomas in four, and hepatic mesenchymal hamartoma in one.

Although up to 60 % of IH are small and disappear without sequelae, indications of when and how to treat them are difficult to stablish for several reasons: not all IH with similar initial size and location develop the same clinical outcome. Proliferation rate and therefore cosmetic and functional impact are frequently different. Their biological timing is unique, specific, and not comparable between two patients, so the physician in charge has to change very often indications for treatment between the third and the tenth weeks of life. Generally considered active treatment of IH is mandatory in those that endanger life (liver, airway), cause irreversible functional disorders (orbit, eyelid, central nervous system), suffer complications not responding to conventional care (i.e. progressive ulceration with significant tissue loss), persistent sore (genital and perianal IH), causing serious cosmetic disfigurement and distortion (nose, lip) and finally those in which post involutive sequelae is expected to require surgical treatment. In this regard, height, topography, surface component and edges have been proved to be effective prognostic factors. Parents can decide between therapeutic abstention, drug treatment or surgical approach depending on factors difficult to be controlled (anesthestic risk, possible pharmacological toxicity or side effects etc.).

IH are pediatric tumors responding to propranolol therapy in 99 % of the cases. Therefore, there is no indication for this treatment in any vascular tumor arising in adults. Misdiagnosis of *cavernous hemangiomas* leads to the inappropriate and non-indicated use of beta-blocker treatments in this group of age. Differential diagnosis between IH and some pediatric sarcomas proliferating in the first 4 months of life can be challenging, specifically when located in the mediastinum, orbit (intraconal), or abdomen. In those instances, a 2–3-week course of propranolol can help in differentiating them, avoiding the need of biopsy in case of significant response to beta-blocker administration.

The indication for surgical management of IH is basically the result of a wrongly delayed treatment with beta-blockers or unresponsiveness to this therapy, currently estimated at 1 % of the cases. If IH continues to proliferate during the first months of life, surgical treatment is advisable in the following situations: visual, airway, or gastrointestinal obstruction, recurrent bleeding, painful and persistent ulceration, and progressive facial deformity [7].

Congenital hemangiomas proliferate in utero and never proliferate after birth. While non-involuting congenital hemangiomas (NICH) can be present beyond adolescence, rapidly involuting congenital hemangiomas (RICH) are not noticeable in the second decade of life unless its involution is not complete (PICH, partially involuting congenital hemangiomas). "Wait-and-see" policy is recommended in the first year of age unless severe thrombocytopenia and/or cardiac failure due to their large size is present. Abnormal skin contour with fat atrophy and the presence of relevant enlarging veins in the subcutaneous tissue are the typical signs of a fully involuted

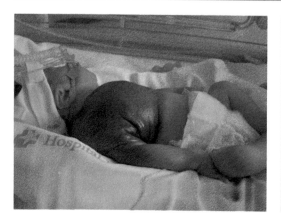

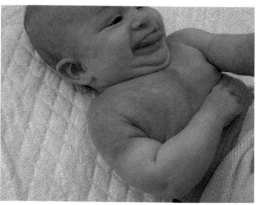

Fig. 50.3 Newborn with a thoracic kaposiform hemangio-endothelioma developing Kasabach-Merritt phenomenon

Fig. 50.4 Successful response to pharmacological treatment

RICH. Current management of this sequelae includes vein sclerosis, vein ablation with diode laser, and lipofilling, in order to improve their cosmetic outcome. Surgical resection is indicated for cosmetically unacceptable residual tumors [8].

Kaposiform hemangioendothelioma and tufted angioma can be diagnosed from neonatal period to elderly, but they behave more aggressively early in life, with a higher tendency for Kasabach-Merritt phenomenon development, as size in children is usually bigger [9]. In fact current treatment options are pharmacological in the pediatric population (vincristine at 0.05 mg/kg/week IV associated with oral aspirin and ticlopidine at 10 mg/kg/day and, more recently (Figs. 50.3 and 50.4), sirolimus at 0.8 mg/m²/dose twice a day), while surgical resection of smaller tumors remains the more frequently performed treatment in adults [10, 11]. Although the number of treated patients with mTOR inhibitors is still limited, response has been uniformly good in the reported cases as well as in our two cases experience with excellent tolerability and an easier oral administration.

In any case and before taking the decision of treating or not, it is important to consider that the natural history of those tumors is represented by a slow tendency to sclerosis and fibrosis being the main goal in their treatment, to control, when present, severe thrombocytopenia. Once the platelet count is normal, there is no risk for the patient even though the tumor does not show signs of regression.

Angiosarcomas, Epithelioid, Composite, and Retiform Hemangioendotheliomas are exceedingly rare in children. Histologically, they can be difficult to differentiate, but, most of all, their behavior is not similar, being much more aggressive in adults than children. Mortality is uncommon in the first decade of life so the pediatric patient with diagnosis of epithelioid hemangioendothelioma deserves a specific approach [12].

Arteriovenous malformations are very often unable to be cured, and therefore the main objective in their management is to control its progression, keeping the patient under a good quality of life. Blood or urine markers giving information about aggressive behavior of an AVM are not available. Considering that an AVM can be dormant for decades, there is no indication for treatment in the neonatal period unless cardiac failure is present. AVMs in Schöbinger I stage should be conservatively managed during early childhood, and preventive surgical excision is only indicated in small lesions at affordable locations. AVMs in Schöbinger II stage need an appropriate evaluation and indication of surgical treatment considering reconstructive needs. Ulceration, bleeding episodes, and cardiac failure are extremely rare in the pediatric age [13].

Lymphatic malformations are the vascular malformations needing treatment most frequently at very early age (Fig. 50.5). Only patients with a minor LM are considered candidates for a wait-and-see protocol till their adulthood [14]. Prenatal treatment is sometimes indicated, and different

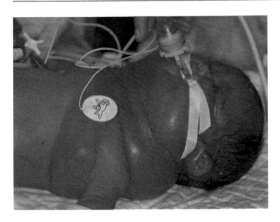

Fig. 50.5 Massive cervicothoracic lymphatic malformation

fetal procedures have been reported in order to avoid airway compromise during pregnancy. In fact the EXIT procedure is frequently indicated at delivery in order to prevent perinatal hypoxemic episodes. The neonate with airway involvement in the context of an oral or cervical LM needs a careful examination by an expert team. Immediate bronchoscopy has to be performed in order to confirm tracheal mucosa infiltration. In this eventuality a tracheostomy has to be considered as appropriate treatment will take years. If the upper airway shows signs of compression and not infiltration, total or subtotal surgical excision remains the best option in order to achieve a prompt extubation. Recently, we have developed a new strategy in this group of patients. In case of difficulty for extubation in the first week of life, we administrate rapamycin at 1 mg/kg/day for 2–3 more weeks. Reduction in the volume and size of the lymphatic mass very often helps in the process of extubating the patient, and therefore the surgical or sclerosing procedure can be delayed 6–12 months. Surgical resection of large LM in neonates is the origin of frequent neural damage as facial nerve branches are difficult to identify, monitor, and preserve.

Therapeutic strategy in infants and children depends on LM size, type (micro-/macrocystic), and location. As most of LM develop enlargement, lymphangitis, and bleeding episodes in addition to significant body contour deformity, delay in their treatment is not indicated. When to perform surgical excision or sclerosis remains an unsolved debate by radiologists and surgeons. Bleomycin and doxycycline are less toxic than ethanol derivatives and therefore more frequently used in the pediatric population.

Venous malformations are slowly progressive vascular anomalies resulting in most cases from TIE-2 mutation. Vein dilatation, blood flow speed reduction, coagulopathy, and pain are developing proportionally to the extent of malformation and therefore are not commonly found in the newborn and infant, so the treatment is usually delayed for several years until pain or severe deformity arises [15]. A large unique venous malformation present at birth is the hallmark of blue rubber bleb nevus syndrome. If anemia or multiple cutaneous VM appear, an upper and lower GI tract endoscopy has to be performed in order to confirm the extent of digestive tract involvement. One more unique presentation of VM in neonates is the sinus pericranii represented by a communication between midline intra- and extracranial venous flow from maxillary to occipital areas. Despite being present at birth, SP is uniformly asymptomatic and treatment usually delayed.

Combined vascular anomalies are commonly seen in newborns and infants in the form of capillary lymphatic venous malformations and frequently associated with segmental overgrowth. The newborn with a vascular anomaly and overgrowth deserves special attention as appropriate differential diagnosis is crucial in order to stablish accurate prognosis. Parents from affected children show significant stress until information regarding vascular anomaly clinical course is available. A multidisciplinary workup must include a specialist in genetics and neonatal dysmorphology. Management of CLOVES, Klippel-Trenaunay, Parkes-Weber, Proteus, PTEN hamartoma tumor, megalencephaly-capillary malformation, or CLAPO syndromes and diffuse capillary malformation with overgrowth differs significantly, and a correct identification of the vascular anomaly in the first month of life will facilitate the initiation of a diagnostic and therapeutic protocol. The presence of a PIK3CA mutation investigation in blood and affected tissue has to be investigated in this group of patients [16].

References

1. Karmazyn B, Ai H, Liang Y. Effect of body size on dose reduction with longitudinal tube current modulation in pediatric patients. Am J Roentgenol. 2015; 204(4):861–4.
2. Schüz J, Espina C. Villain P European Code against Cancer 4th edition: 12 ways to reduce your cancer risk. Cancer Epidemiol. 2015;9(15):127–37.
3. Cohen MD. Safe use of imaging contrast agents in children. J Am Coll Radiol. 2009;6(8):576–81.
4. Aker J, Block RI, Biddle C. Anesthesia and the developing brain. AANA J. 2015;83(2):139–47.
5. Bailey KM, Bird SJ, McGrath PJ, Chorney JE. Preparing parents to be present for their child's anesthesia induction: a randomized controlled trial. Anesth Analg. 2015;121:1001–10.
6. Fortier MA, Kain ZN. Treating perioperative anxiety and pain in children: a tailored and innovative approach. Paediatr Anaesth. 2015;25(1):27–35.
7. Léauté-Labrèze C, Hoeger P, Mazereeuw-Hautier J, et al. A randomized, controlled trial of oral propranolol in infantile hemangioma. N Engl J Med. 2015; 372(8):735–46.
8. Hoeger PH, Colmenero I. Vascular tumours in infants. Part I: benign vascular tumours other than infantile haemangioma. Br J Dermatol. 2014;171(3):466–73.
9. Croteau SE, Liang MG, Kozakewich HP, Alomari AI, Fishman SJ, Mulliken JB, Trenor CC 3rdrd.

Kaposiform hemangioendothelioma: atypical features and risks of Kasabach-Merritt phenomenon in 107 referrals. J Pediatr 2013;162(1):142–7.
10. Fernandez-Pineda I, Lopez-Gutierrez JC, Chocarro G. Long-term outcome of vincristine-aspirin-ticlopidine (VAT) therapy for vascular tumors associated with Kasabach-Merritt phenomenon. Pediatr Blood Cancer. 2013;60(9):1478–81.
11. Uno T, Ito S, Nakazawa A. Successful treatment of kaposiform hemangioendothelioma with everolimus. Pediatr Blood Cancer. Pediatr Blood Cancer. 2015;62(3):536–8.
12. Flucke U, Vogels RJ, de Saint Aubain Somerhausen N, et al. Epithelioid Hemangioendothelioma: clinicopathologic, immunhistochemical, and molecular genetic analysis of 39 cases. Diagn Pathol. 2014;9:131.
13. Lee BB, Baumgartner I, Berlien HP. Consensus document of the International Union of Angiology (IUA)-2013. Current concept on the management of arterio-venous management. Int Angiol. 2013;32(1): 9–36.
14. Bagrodia N, Defnet AM, Kandel JJ. Management of lymphatic malformations in children. Curr Opin Pediatr. 2015;27(3):356–63.
15. Dasgupta R, Patel M. Venous malformations. Semin Pediatr Surg. 2014;23(4):198–202.
16. Kulungowski AM, Fishman SJ. Management of combined vascular malformations. Clin Plast Surg. 2011; 38(1):107–20.

Epilogue

The process of completing this handbook has been an enjoyable experience collaborating with so many renowned experts in the field of congenital vascular malformation (CVM). Memories of obscure, difficult medical terms with no clear treatment guidelines dot my memories of CVM, circa my bygone medical school days. Uncertainties associated with this disease left a trail of frustrated clinicians as well as disappointed patients in its wake.

From the inception of this handbook to the conclusion, it was clear that there are still varied concepts of CVM among the field's experts. We invited many chapter authors from five continents (Asia, Australia, Europe, North America, and South America in alphabetical order) and attempted to cover all aspects of CVM including pathogenesis, definition, classification, diagnosis and management.

Though some minor differences and overlapping content are present, we felt it to be more important to respect and accept each author's original input. My deepest heartfelt gratitude is owed to all of the authors. Thank you.

All of this would not have been possible without the strong support of Dr. BB Lee, who lead us the entire process from the invitation of authors to editorial reviewing. He has been dedicated to the enrichment of knowledge of CVM throughout his career and spared no resources in bringing this book to fruition.

I wish this book will be a good guide to those who yearn for clarity in the field of CVM, and serve as a springboard for further advances in this field of medical science.

Young-wook Kim, MD, FACS
Professor, Vascular Surgery
Samsung Medical Center
Sungkyunkwan University School of Medicine
Seoul, South Korea
April, 2016

© Springer-Verlag Berlin Heidelberg 2017
Y.-W. Kim et al. (eds.), *Congenital Vascular Malformations*, DOI 10.1007/978-3-662-46709-1

Index

A

Abdominal superficial location, 272
Abnormal origin of right subclavicular artery, 10
Absence of suprarenal inferior vena cava, 12
Absolute alcohol, 100, 101
Activin receptor-like kinase 1 (ALK1), 18
AKT signaling, 17
Anatomical surgery, 297–298
Anatomic variations, 36
Anesthesia, 370
Aneurysmal dilatation, 155
Angiodysplasia syndrome, 364
Angiogenesis, 8
Angiographic classification, 55–60
Angiography, 109, 111, 151–152, 370
Angioma racemosum, 134–135
Angiosarcomas, 162, 372
Angiostat, 199
Anomalous development
    of aortic arch, 10
    of lymphatic system, 12–13
    of superior and inferior vena cava, 12
Antiangiogenic therapy, 343–346
Anti-cancer, 325
Anticoagulant, 364
Antifungal, 325
Antithrombotic therapy, 364
Aplasia, 155
    of deep veins, 291
    and hypoplasia, 295
Arterial malformations, 134–135
Arterial system, 7–10
    development of, 7–10
Arteriographic classification, 63–68, 276
Arteriovenous fistulae (AVF), 43
Arteriovenous malformations (AVMs), 55–58, 74, 105,
        201, 233–239, 259–260, 343–344, 372
    coils, 234
    embolic agents, 233–234
    ethanol, 234–237
    extratruncular, 76, 275
    indications for treatment, 233
    NBCA, 234
    nidus, 224
    Onyx, 234
    particle embolic agents, 233–234
    sclerosing agent, 234–237
    stent graft, 237–238
    treatment, 233–239
    truncular, 74
Aspirin, 372
Ataxia-telangiectasia (Louis-Bar syndrome), 131
Avastin/bevacizumab, 325
AV CVMs, 365
Avitene, 198

B

Back scattering, 315
Bare fiber contact vaporization, 318–319
Bean syndrome, 84, 366
Bevacizumab, 19
Biochronogram, 364
Biological approaches, 343–346
Bleeding, 229
Bleomycin, 253, 363, 364
Blue rubber bleb nevus syndrome
        (BRBNS), 84, 326
B mode, 155
Bogota Congenital Malformations Surveillance
        Program (BCMSP), 31
Bone involvement, 162

C

Capillary-lymphatic malformations, 132–133
Capillary malformations (CMs), 35, 74, 136
Capillary/microvascular form, 52
Capillary vascular malformations, 129
CAPRT time resolved imaging, 151
Caput medusae, 3
Cardiovascular and pulmonary, 262–263
Catheter venogram, 93
Cavernous angiomas, 364
    cavernoso cara, 365
Cavernous/capillary hemangioma, 43
Cerebrovascular events, 263–264
Charles' operation, 298
Children, 369
Cho-Do peripheral vascular classification, 63

© Springer-Verlag Berlin Heidelberg 2017
Y.-W. Kim et al. (eds.), *Congenital Vascular Malformations*, DOI 10.1007/978-3-662-46709-1

Cho, S.K., 56
Chronological diagrams, 7
Chylo-cutanea fistula, 358
Cirsoid aneurysm, 3
Coarctation of the aorta (CoA), 10
Cockett syndrome, 365
Coils, 199
CO_2 laser, 316
Color Doppler imaging (CDI), 107
Combined and complex malformations, 242
Combined approach, 285, 286
Combined embolization and sclerotherapy, 352
Combined treatment, 276
Combined vascular anomalies, 373
Complex decongestive therapy (CDT), 307–312
Complications, 229, 257
Compression after sclerotherapy, 251
Compression garments, 309
Compression therapy, 99, 310
Computed tomography (CT), 99, 141
Computed tomography angiography (CTA), 75, 108
Congenital hemangiomas, 369, 371
Congenital lipomatous overgrowth, vascular
      malformation, epidermal nevus, scoliosis
      (CLOVES), 27, 364
Congenital vascular bone syndrome (CVBS), 335–341
   clinical features, 336–337
   diagnosis, 337–339
   management, 339–341
   pathophysiology, 335–336
   prevalence, 335
   risk factors, 337
Congenital vascular malformations (CVMs), 31, 35, 41,
      73, 257–265
   drugs in, 325–326
   epidemiology, 31, 363–364
   incidence, 31
   neonatal and infant, 363–367
Conservative measures, 248
Conservative treatment, 323
Contrast agent, 185–186
Contrast-enhanced CT, 142
Contrast enhancement computed tomography (CT), 161
Contrast venography, 99
Cranial nerve palsy, 226
Cutis Marmorata Telangiectatica Congenita
      (Van Lohuizen Syndrome), 130–131

D
Deep vein thrombosis (DVT),264
Detachable balloons, 200
Differential diagnosis, 155
Diffuse, intramuscular infiltrating malformations, 271
Direct puncture, 227
Direct surgical excision, 298–299
Distal embolism, 265
Doppler examination, 156
Double aortic arch, 10
Double inferior vena cava, 12

Double superior vena cava, 12
Doxycycline, 19, 252, 325, 373
Duplex ultrasonography, 75, 93, 141
Duplex ultrasound, 98, 155, 244
Dynamic contrast enhanced MRI (dceMRI),
      115, 143, 148–150
Dysplasia, 367

E
Embolic agents, 202–208
Embolization, 19, 226, 351
Embolotherapy, 198, 224, 352
Embryogenesis, 41
Embryological development, 7
Embryological stage, 32
Embryologic basis, 241
Encephalon, 364
Endoglin (ENG), 18
Endoscopic laser resection, 249
Endosurgical skills, 197
Endovascular approach, 225
Endovascular coils, 100
Endovascular laser ablation (EVLA), 248–249
Endovascular therapy, 100
Endovascular treatment, 197–208, 223–230
   complications of, 257–265
Epiphysiodesis, 339
Estrogen and progesterone, 326
Ethanol, 227, 254
Ethyl alcohol, 200
EUROCAT, 31
Evolution potential, 332
Exercises, 308
EXIT procedure, 371
Extratruncular, 42, 51, 53, 291
Extra-truncular lymphatic malformations (LMs),
      242, 243
Extratruncular malformations, 129

F
Facial PWS, 135
Fibroadipose vascular anomaly (FAVA), 86
Flap interposition, 300
Flow characteristics, 141, 142
Flow motion, 180–181
Fluoroscopy/CDI techniques, 227
Functional impairment, 310
Functional surgery, 300

G
Gadobenate dimeglumine, 185
Gastrointestinal bleeding, 320
Gelfoam, 198
Generalized essential telangiectasia
      (angioma serpiginosum), 131–132
Genetic mutations, 23
Genetic studies, 246

Genital chylous cutanea fistulas, 357
Genital lymphedema, 309
Genomic mutations, 23, 27
Glomangioma, 134
Glomuvenous malformations, 84
Glues, 198
Gorham-Stout-Haferkamp syndromes, 364
Greater omentum lymphangiomatosis, 364

H

Hemangiopericytoma, 162
Haemoglobinuria, 264–265
Hamburg classification, 42, 51, 74, 91, 331
Hamburg consensus classification, 284
Head and neck, 223–230
    lymphedema, 309
Hemangioblast, 47
Hemangioendothelioma, 50
Hemangiomas, 43, 73, 78–79, 363
Hemodynamic features, 155
Hemolymphatic malformation (HLM), 41, 97
    multidisciplinary team approach, 99
Hemostatic agent, 228
Hereditary hemorrhagic telangiectasia (HHT), 18
Hereditary lymphedema type I, 122
Hereditary lymphedema type II, 122
High-flow arteriovenous malformation (AVM),
    162, 258
High flow congenital vascular malformations, 275
High-flow vascular malformations (HFVMs), 141, 151
Homans' operation, 298–299
Hormonal changes, 35–36
Houdart classification, 64
Houdart's CNS classification, 64
Hygroscopicus, 325
Hyperkeratotic capillary malformation, 133
Hypertrophy, 364
Hypoplasia, 155
    of deep veins, 292

I

Iatrogenic provoking factors, 36–37
Indocyanine green (ICG) lymphography, 173–177
    classification, 176–177
    dynamic, 173–174
    fluorescent, 174
    LE pattern, 177
    lymphatic image, 177
    lymphatic surgery, 174
    NE pattern, 177
    pattern, 175
Infantile hemangiomas, 371
Inguinal incision, 358
Inguinal lymph nodes, 190
Inhibition, 325
Intense pulsed light (IPL), 315
Intermittent pneumatic compression pump (IPC),
    309–310

International Society for the Study of Vascular
    Anomalies (ISSVA), 113, 223
    classification, 23, 42–43, 47–50, 77, 91, 284
International Union of Phlebology (IUP), 114
Interpretation, 186–191
Interventional procedures, 257
Intraarticular malformations, 272
Intraconal, 371
Intralesional lignocaine, 251
Intraluminal techniques, 317
Intramicrolymphatic flow, 180
Intraosseous A-V shunt, 156
Intraosseous VM, 273
Ionizing radiations, 369
Isobutyl 2-cyanoacrylate (IBCA), 199
ISSVA Classification of Vascular Anomalies, 2014, 48

J

Jahnke syndrome, 136

K

Kaposiform hemangioendothelioma (KHE),
    80, 81, 326, 372
Kasabach-Merritt phenomenon, 80, 372
Kasabach-Merritt syndrome, 364
Klippel-Trenaunay patients, 162
Klippel-Trenaunay-Servelle syndrome, 365
Klippel-Trenaunay syndrome (KTS), 48, 75,
    93, 97, 242, 364
    endovenous thermal ablation, 101–102
KTP, 315

L

Laser coagulation, 319
Lasers, 249
Lateral marginal vein, 291–296
Left superior vena cava (SVC), 12
Lifestyle modification, 323
Limb length discrepancy (LLD), 291, 335–341
    development of, 335
    two-cm threshold of, 337
Limited intramuscular VM, 270–271
Liposuction, 250, 299
Localized complications, 260–262
Localized intravascular coagulopathy (LIC), 319, 324
Location on the hand, 272
Lower extremity scanogram, 337
Lower limbs, 272–273
Low-flow CVM, 269
Low-flow malformations, 147
Low molecular weight heparin (LMWH), 324, 364
Lymphangiectasia, 244
Lymphangioleiomyomatosis, 364
Lymphangioma, 113–119
    extratruncular, 113–119
Lymphangiomatosis, 127–128
Lymphatic circulation, 181

Lymphatic drainage patterns, 188–190
Lymphatic-lymphatic bypass, 300
Lymphatic malformations (LMs), 74, 113, 161,
        241–254, 260, 372
    classification, 113–114
    clinical presentation, 114–115
    combined, 115
    diagnosis, 115
    extratruncular, 74
    high flow, 114
    low flow, 114
    macrocystic, 115, 161–162
    macrocystic lesions, 242, 248, 250
    microcystic, 115, 162
    microcystic lesions, 242, 249–250
    mixed lesions, 242
    mucosal lesions, 249–250
    pathophysiology, 114
    sclerotherapy, 116, 248, 250–254
    surgery, 249
    surgical debulking, 250
    surgical resection, 249
    thrombosed lesions, 245
    treatment, 115–119, 246–250
    truncular, 114, 241, 242
    truncular forms, 75
Lymphaticovenular anastomosis, 300
Lymphatic scintigraphy, 158
Lymphatic system
    development of, 12
    malformations, 122
Lymphedema, 134, 181
    Chylous reflux, 125
    confirmation, 190–191
    congenital, 121
    inherited, 122
    surgical treatment for, 275–281
    in syndromes, 124–125
Lymphedema-distichiasis syndrome, 13
Lymphogenesis, 113
Lymphoscintigraphy, 165, 168
Lymphovenous bypass, 300

M
Macrodactyly, 366
Macropodia, 366
Maffucci syndrome, 365
Magnetic resonance (MR), 228
Magnetic resonance angiography (MRA), 147–152
Magnetic resonance imaging (MRI), 75, 86, 93, 99,
        108–109, 147–152, 246, 369
Mammalian target of rapamycin (MTOR), 344
Marginal vein (MV), 292, 295
Masson's tumor, 18
May-Thurner syndrome, 365
Medical treatment, 248, 323
Meticulous care of skin and nail, 308
Microcatheter systems, 199
Microcystic ("solid") lymphatic malformation, 317–318

Microlymphographs, 180
Microlymphography, 179, 181
Microscopic lymphangiography, 179–183
Milles syndrome, 136
Milroy-Meige syndrome, 13
Modified Hamburg classification, 114
Morphologic characteristics, 190
Mosaicism and clinical genetics, 24
MR lymphangiography (MRL), 122–123, 185–191
Mulliken, J.B., 47
Multidetector CT venography, 162
Multidirectional blood flow, 141
Multidisciplinary team approach, 331–333
Multilayered short-stretch bandaging, 309
Multiple diagnostic modalities, 147
Mutations, 23

N
Naevus Unna, 130
N-butyl cyanoacrylate (NBCA), 234
Nd:YAG laser, 315
Near infrared, 315
Nerve injury, 262
Neurocutaneous and dysplasia syndromes/phakomatois,
        136–137
Neuropletic sedation, 227
Nidus, 55, 66, 162, 276
Non contact method, 318
Non-involuting congenital hemangioma (NICH), 50
Nonparasitic secondary lymphedema, 364
Nonresponders, propranolol infantile hemangiomas, 371
Nutcracker syndrome, 365

O
Octreotide, 326
OK-432 (Picibanil), 100, 254, 364
Onyx, 100, 200
Orthostatism, 156
Overgrowth, 35, 335

P
Pain and swelling, 260–261
Parkes Weber syndrome (PWS), 26, 75, 242
Partially involuting congenital hemangiomas (PICH), 79
Patent ductus arteriosus (PDA), 10
Pediatric vascular anomaly, 369
Pelvic arteriovenous malformation (AVM)
    angiographic anatomy, 351
    demographic and clinical features of patients, 350
    diagnosis, 349–350
    symptoms, 349
    treatment, 351–352
Perivascular tumescent anaesthesia, 251
Persistent marginal vein (MV), 92
Phakomatosis, 129
Phlebographic classification, 58
Phlebography, 58

Phleboliths, 93, 142, 158, 365
Phosphatase and tensin homolog (PTEN), 344
Picibanil, 319, 364
Plain films, 141
Plain radiography, 141
Pleurodesis, 359
Polidocanol (POL), 100, 212, 252–253
Polyvinyl alcohol foam, 199
Popcorn effect, 318
Port-wine skin lesion (capillary malformation), 92
Port-wine stain (PWS), 129–130, 316
Praecox, 121
Pregnancy, 36
Preoperative embolization, 226, 370
Preoperative embolotherapy, 285, 286
Primary lymphedema, 121, 173, 182
    and chylous reflux, 358
    with chylous reflux by transnodal pathway, 358
    classification, 121–124
    clinical manifestations, 121
    family history, 121
    truncular, 121–128
Primary/secondary lymphedema, 364, 366
Progression, 326
Prophylactic Antibiotics for the Treatment of Cellulitis
        at Home (PATCH), 324
Propranolol, 363
Protective embolization, 226
Protein-losing enteropathy, 127
Proteus syndrome, 27, 316
Provoking factor, 35
Provoking maneuver, 142
Psychological support, 323
Psychology, 370
PTEN, 19
Puig classification, 60
Pulse duration, 315

Q
Qualitatively and morphological observation, 188–191
Quantitative analysis, 186

R
Radiofrequency ablation (RFA), 249
Radiolabeled erythrocytes (99mTc-RBC), 95
Radionuclide scintigraphy, 165
    diagnosis, 168
    SPECT, 165–167
    TLPS, 165, 167
    WBBPS, 165–167
Rapamycin, 325
Rapidly involuting congenital hemangiomas (RICH), 50, 79
RASA1, 18
Rathke's diagram, 7
Rendu-Osler-Weber syndrome (hereditary hemorrhagic
        telangiectasia), 135–136
Rhabdomyosarcoma, 162
Riley-Smith syndrome, 137

S
Scattering, 315
Schobinger classification, 275
Sciatic vein, 295
Sclerosant, 251
Sclerosing/embolic agents, 258, 259
Sclerotherapy, 18, 86, 100
Selective catheter arteriography, 200
Selective catheterization, 200
Self-management phase, 309
7th nerve neuropraxi, 229
Short-tau inversion recovery (STIR) images, 149
Sildenafil, 325, 363, 364
Single cystic lymphangioma, 132
Sinus pericranii, 373
Sirenomelia, 3
Sirolimus, 325
Sistrunk's operation, 299
Skin necrosis, 261
Slow flow-high flow, 155
SMAD4, 18
Small age, 369
Sodium tetradecyl sulphate (STS), 252
Soft tissue phlebectasias, 134
Soft tissue sarcoma, 162
Somatic mutations, 26, 27
Sotradecol, 200
Spetzler and Martin grading system, 55
Spider nevus (nevus araneus), 132
Sturge-Weber syndrome, 27, 136
Subcardinal veins, 10
Subischial leg length, 339
Superficial and deep capillary malformation, 129–137
Superficial dilated dysplastic veins, 269–270
Superficial VM of limbs, 272
Supracardinal veins, 10
Swan-Ganz and arterial line monitoring, 227

T
Tarda, 121
Telangiectasias, 132
Thalidomide, 19, 325
Thompson's operation, 299
Thoracic duct, 356
Thorax location, 272
TIE2, 17–18
Time resolved echo-shared angiographic
        techniques (TREAT), 149
Time resolved imaging of contrast kinetics (TRICKS), 148
Timolol, 363
TLPS. See Transarterial lung perfusion scintigraphy
        (TLPS)
Tracheostomy, 227
Transarterial lung perfusion scintigraphy (TLPS),
        111, 141, 143, 165, 167
Transcutaneous ice cube-cooled Nd:YAG
        laser technique, 319
Treatment, 292
Truncal, 48

Truncular, 42, 51, 291
Truncular venous malformations (VMs), 91, 364
Tufted angioma, 372
T1-weighted and hyperintense on T2-weighted, 148
T2-weighted spin-echo sequences, 142, 147
Types of surgical treatment, 298
Tyrosine kinase receptor TIE2, 17, 83

U
Ultrasonography, 86, 155–158
Undergrowth, 335
Upper limb lymphedema, 366

V
Vascularized lymph node transfers (VLNT), 300–301
Vascular malformations (VMs), 48, 51, 77–78
    extratruncular, 97, 98
    truncular, 97, 98
Vascular tumor(s), 48, 51, 77–78
Vasculogenesis, 8, 32, 129, 241
Vasomotion, 180–181
Venous aneurysms, 270
Venous hypertension, 66, 364
Venous malformations (VMs), 17, 58–60, 74, 83,
        134, 211, 260, 373
    ethanol, 212
    extratruncal, 211–219

extratruncular, 74, 75
in head, 271
localized outside muscles, 271
on neck, 271–272
outcome, 219
percutaneous embolization, 211–219
polidocanol, 212
sclerotherapy, 211–219
STS, 212
truncal, 219, 220
truncular, 74, 75
Venous system, 7, 10–12
    development of, 7, 10–12
Venous truncular defects, 269

W
Waldmann disease, 360, 364
Whole body blood pool scintigraphy (WBBPS),
        92, 143, 165–167
Wyburn-Mason syndrome/Bonnet-Decaume-Blanc
        syndrome, 135

Y
Yakes AVM classification system, 63–68, 202–208
    embolic agents, 65–66
    therapeutic implications, 65